SLOW VIRUS INFECTIONS OF THE CENTRAL NERVOUS SYSTEM

SLOW VIRUS INFECTIONS OF THE CENTRAL NERVOUS SYSTEM

Investigational Approaches to
Etiology and Pathogenesis of These Diseases

Edited by
VOLKER ter MEULEN / MICHAEL KATZ

WITH 97 ILLUSTRATIONS

Springer-Verlag
New York   Heidelberg   Berlin

Proceedings: Workshop on Slow Virus Infections:
University of Würzburg: March 24–26, 1975

Volker ter Meulen, M.D.   Michael Katz, M.D.
Institut fuer Virologie   College of Physicians and Surgeons
8700 Wuerzburg   Columbia University
Verbascher Landstr. 7   630 West 168th Street
West Germany   New York, N. Y. 10032

Library of Congress Cataloging in Publication Data

Workshop on Slow Virus Infections, University of Würzburg, 1975.
    Slow virus infections of the central nervous system.

Includes bibliographical references and index.
1. Virus diseases, Slow—Congresses. 2. Nervous
system—Diseases—Congresses. I. ter Meulen, Volker,
1928-   II. Katz Michael. III. Title
RC114.6.W67 1975   616.8'04'194   77-1570
ISBN 0-387-90188-4

9 8 7 6 5 4 3 2 1

ISBN 0-387-90188-4 Springer-Verlag New York

ISBN 3-540-90188-4 Springer-Verlag Berlin Heidelberg

Preface

This book is a result of a Workshop held at the Institute of Virology of the University of Würzburg, Germany in March of 1975. The Workshop was organized to bring together investigators of slow virus infections and other scientists, who have not engaged in such research, but who were leaders in the field of biologic investigations. The conveners hoped that these latter would be more objective critics, who would express their views freely and who would offer recommendations for new directions and new approaches to the investigations of slow virus infections. These expectations were fulfilled as the organization of the Workshop permitted much free time for discussion as well as time for directed critiques. This volume represents an extensive summary of the proceedings and the discussions that followed. We believe it will be of interest to all investigators of slow virus infections and to the students of host-parasite relationships.

Volker ter Meulen
Michael Katz

Contents

Contents

PART III / MULTIPLE SCLEROSIS

List of Contributors

Ellsworth C. Alvord, Jr.
Department of Pathology
School of Medicine
University of Washington
Seattle, Washington 98105

Luiz H. Barbosa
National Institute of Neurological and
Communicative Diseases and Stroke
Bethesda, Maryland 20014

H. Becht
Justus Liebig–University Giessen
6300—Giessen
Frankfurter Str. 107
West Germany

Hans J. Bertrams*
Institute for Medical Virology and
Immunology
University of Essen,
Gesamthohochschule
Essen, West Germany

A. D. Bloom
Departments of Pediatrics and Genetics
and Human Development
College of Physicians and Surgeons
Columbia University, New York 10032

Purnell W. Choppin
The Rockefeller University
New York, New York 10021

Kurt Danner
Institute of Medical Microbiology
Infectious and Epidemic Diseases
Veterinary Faculty
University of Munich
West Germany

Alan G. Dickinson
A. R. C. Animal Breeding Organisation
Edinburgh EH9 3JQ, United Kingdom

Monique Dubois-Dalcq
Unit of Electron Microscopy
Infectious Diseases Branch, IRP
National Institute of Neurological and
Communicative Disorders and Stroke
National Institutes of Health
Bethesda, Maryland 20014

Hugh Fraser
Moredun Research Institute
Edinburgh EH17 7JH, United Kingdom

D. Carleton Gajdusek
Laboratory of Central Nervous System
Studies
National Institute of Neurological and
Communicative Disorders and Stroke
National Institutes of Health
Bethesda, Maryland 20014

Clarence J. Gibbs, Jr.
Laboratory of Central Nervous System
Studies
National Institute of Neurological and
Communicative Disorders and Stroke
National Institutes of Health
Bethesda, Maryland 20014

John E. Greenlee
Department of Neurology
The Johns Hopkins University
School of Medicine
Baltimore, Maryland

Donald H. Harter†
Departments of Neurology and
Microbiology
College of Physicians and Surgeons
Columbia University
New York, New York 10032

* Present address: Department for Laboratory Medicine, Elisabeth Hospital, Essen, West Germany.

† Present address: Department of Neurology, The Medical School, Northwestern University, Chicago, Illinois 60611.

Casper Jersild
Tissue Typing Laboratory
Blood Bank and Blood Grouping
Department
University Hospital (Rigshospitalet)
DK-2100 Copenhagen, Denmark

Richard T. Johnson
Department of Neurology
The Johns Hopkins University
School of Medicine
Baltimore, Maryland 21205

Michael Katz
Departments of Public Health and
Pediatrics
College of Physicians and Surgeons
Columbia University
New York, New York 10032

Adalbert Koestner
Department of Veterinary Pathobiology
The Ohio State University
Columbus, Ohio 43210

Hilary Koprowski
The Multiple Sclerosis Research Center
Wistar Institute
University of Pennsylvania
Philadelphia, Pennsylvania 19104

Ernst K. Kuwert
Institute for Medical Virology and
Immunology
University of Essen,
Gesamthochschule
Essen, West Germany

Edwin H. Lennette
State of California
Department of Health
2151 Berkeley Way
Berkeley, California 94704

Hans Ludwig
Professor of Virology
Justus Liebig–University Giessen
6300—Giessen
Frankfurter Str. 107
West Germany

Brian MacMahon
Department of Epidemiology
School of Public Health
Harvard University
Boston, Massachusetts 02115

Volker ter Meulen
Institute of Virology and Immunobiology
University of Würzburg
Versbacher Landstrasse 7
8700 Würzburg, West Germany

Cedric A. Mims
Department of Microbiology
Guys Hospital Medical School
London Bridge
London SE 1, England

Opendra Narayan
Department of Neurology
The Johns Hopkins University
School of Medicine
Baltimore, Maryland 21205

Erling Norrby
Department of Virology
Karolinska Institutet
Stockholm, Sweden

Gudmundun Petursson
Tilraunastod Haskolans 1 Meinafraedi
Keldur Vid Reykjavik, Iceland

David Porter
Department of Pathology
School of Medicine
University of California
Los Angeles, California 90024

Ludvik Prevec
Department of Biology
McMaster University
Hamilton, Ontario, Canada

Donald D. Reid
Department of Epidemiology
London School of Hygiene and
Tropical Medicine
London, WCIE 7HT, England

Andreas Scheid
The Rockefeller University
New York, New York 10021

Steven Krakowka
Department of Veterinary Pathobiology
The Ohio State University
Columbus, Ohio 43210

Duard L. Walker
Department of Microbiology
Medical School
The University of Wisconsin
Madison, Wisconsin 53706

Eberhard Wecker
Institute fur Virologie und
Immunbiologie Der Universitat Würzburg
Versbacher Landstrasse 7
8700 Würzburg, West Germany

Leslie P. Weiner
Department of Neurology
The Johns Hopkins University
School of Medicine
Baltimore, Maryland 21205

Julius S. Younger
Department of Microbiology
School of Medicine
University of Pittsburgh
Pittsburgh, Pennsylvania 15261

OTHER PARTICIPANTS

Althaus, H. H., *Göttingen, Germany*
Appel, M., *Ithaca, USA*
Askonas, B. A., *London, UK*
Bachmann, P., *München, Germany*
Bauer, H., *Göttingen, Germany*
Becht, H., *Giessen, Germany*
Behrens, F., *Marburg/Lahn, Germany*
Blechschmidt, H., *Göttingen, Germany*
Bodo, G., *Wien, Austria*
Bornkamp, G., *Erlangen, Germany*
Brody, J. A., *Hiroshima, Japan*
Darai, G., *Heidelberg, Germany*
Dörfler, W., *Köln, Germany*
Drzeniek, R., *Hamburg, Germany*
Eggers, H. J., *Köln, Germany*
Enders-Ruckle, G., *Stuttgart, Germany*
Fischer, F., *Bonn, Germany*
Frick, E., *München, Germany*
Friss, R. R., *Giessen*
Fuccillo, D., *Bethesda, USA*
Haas, R., *Freiburg, Germany*
Hall, W., *Würzburg, Germany*
zur Hausen, H., *Erlangen, Germany*
Hewlett, G., *Wuppertal, Germany*
Hofschneider, P. H., *München, Germany*
Homma, M., *Yamagata City, Japan*
Horak, I., *Würzburg, Germany*
Jacob, H., *Marburg/Lahn, Germany*
Jungwirth, C., *Würzburg, Germany*
Kabat, E., *New York, USA*
Käckell, Y. M., *Göttingen, Germany*
Kaplan, M., *Geneve, Switzerland*
Kersting, G., *Bonn, Germany*
Kibler, R., *Würzburg, Germany*

Klenk, H., *Giessen, Germany*
Koschel, K., *Würzburg, Germany*
Kreth, H. W., *Göttingen, Germany*
Kratsch, V., *Würzburg, Germany*
Kurland, L. T., *Rochester, Minn., USA*
Lehmann-Grube, F., *Hamburg, Germany*
Loh, W., *Würzburg, Germany*
Löhler, J., *Hamburg, Germany*
Martin, S. J., *Belfast, UK*
Meyermann, R., *Göttingen, Germany*
Mannweiler, K., *Hamburg, Germany*
Mussgay, M., *Tübingen, Germany*
Naujoks, R., *Würzburg, Germany*
Petersen, P., *Freiburg, Germany*
Roggendorf, M., *Bonn, Germany*
Rott, R., *Giessen, Germany*
Schäfer, W., *Tübingen, Germany*
Schaltenbrand, G., *Würzburg, Germany*
Schimpl, A., *Würzburg, Germany*
Schneweis, K. E., *Bonn, Germany*
Schneider, J., *La Jolla, Cal., USA*
Schneider, L. G., *Tübingen, Germany*
Schulte-Holthausen, H., *Erlangen, Germany*
Scriba, M., *Wien, Austria*
Sluga, E., *Wien, Austria*
Straub, O. C., *Tübingen, Germany*
Ströder, J., *Würzburg, Germany*
Thomssen, R., *Göttingen, Germany*
Wechsler, W., *Köln, Germany*
Weiss, E., *Giessen, Germany*
Wiegers, W., *Hamburg, Germany*
Winnacker, E.-L., *Köln, Germany*
Yung, L. L., *Würzburg, Germany*
Zander, H., *München, Germany*

PART I
UNCONVENTIONAL AGENTS

CHAPTER 1

Scrapie: Pathogenesis in Inbred Mice: An Assessment of Host Control and Response Involving Many Strains of Agent

A. G. DICKINSON / H. FRASER

INTRODUCTION

Scrapie is a fatal progressive degenerative disorder of the central nervous system that occurs as a natural infection in sheep and goats. It is transmissible experimentally to various species, including mice, but the disease has not been produced in all species that have been tested, such as, rabbits and guinea pigs. There are many strains of the agent that causes scrapie, and their molecular structure is probably outside the range for conventional viruses. Consequently, they display very high resistance to inactivation by a wide range of physical and chemical treatments. Although scrapie agents remain infectious after treatment with very large doses of 254 nm UV irradiation, this finding does not necessarily exclude nucleic acids as the informational molecule in scrapie, as many have assumed. It is possible that nucleic acids can be protected chemically, or repaired, in ways not yet known. Because of these uncertainties many workers have preferred to use the operational term "agent" rather than "virus."

The many unusual properties have prompted various hypotheses about the nature of these agents, though none of them can now accommodate all the findings. An unfortunate corollary has been the uncritical acceptance of various unlikely "findings" that would quickly be recognized as experimental errors, if conventional microorganisms were involved. The only agreed remnant of these hypotheses is that most of the infectivity, detectable by present methods in brain homogenates from mice with advanced disease, accompanies cell membranes, and it is assumed that this association is present in the living animal. It is unknown whether this applies to most of the agent earlier in incubation or in tissues other than brain. Neither the form of this association with membranes nor its significance, if any, for agent replication or protection is known.

Infectivity assays in whole animals are the only available tests for the presence of the agent: There are no immunologic, electron microscopic, or tissue culture findings on which to base *in vitro* tests. Many attempts have

3

been made to grow tissues (usually brain) from affected animals in which the agent could be shown to be replicating, but there has only been satisfactory evidence of success in one case (2).

AGENT REPLICATION

Agent Replication during Incubation in Mice

The importance of the lymphoreticular system (LRS) in the early pathogenesis of scrapie first became apparent from a time-sequence study involving 13 organs (14). The same general pattern appears to be followed by various agent strains, at least in the most widely used mouse strains, but the different host/agent combinations vary widely in the absolute time intervals involved.

The sequence of events follows. The earliest rise in titer occurs in organs of the LRS, such as the spleen, after either intracerebral (i.c.) or extraneural injection. Agent titer rises at a later stage in other tissues, such as the lungs, the intestines, and the uterus, but only later, if the extraneural injection in the spinal cord and brain led to death after a relatively short clinical course. It is unknown how the agent is transported from the site of injection to the LRS and, with peripheral injections, eventually from the LRS to the brain. No convincing "viremic" phase has been detected, with the exception of the brief one occurring immediately after i.c. or intravenous injection. Presently, it is reasonable to assume that rise of titer in an organ indicates that replication is occurring there. In the case of an i.c. injection, the extraneural events seem to be irrelevant to the course of the disease because the agent that remains in the brain starts to replicate there much sooner than it would have after extraneural injection, though still not as soon as it does in the spleen. It is possible that the agent that has received some types of treatment (e.g., heating) (7, 13) may not do so, but with ordinary inocula, there are several reasons for concluding that the agent replicates in the brain after an i.c. injection: Incubation is shortest after i.c. injection, even when sterile i.c. injection-trauma accompany intraperitoneal (i.p.) injection of the agent; splenectomy (or genetic asplenia) has no effect after an i.c. injection but increases incubation after an i.p. injection (8, 18); the effective titer of an inoculum is higher by the i.c. than the i.p. route (Fig. 1.1); neonatal and young mice are easier to infect by the i.c. than the i.p. route (27); the *supression* of susceptibility with large doses of steroids does not apply to i.c. injections.

Replication in the spleen can occur fairly quickly. It is possible that there is a short delay of a day or so before replication commences in the spleen in the quicker host/agent combinations (e.g., ME7 agent in C57BL mice, with 160-day incubation period after an i.c. injection of 10^5 LD_{50} units). But this then proceeds with a doubling time of about 2 days, and the process is complete 4 to 5 weeks later. Afterward, there is a titer plateau phase for the remaining 17 weeks before death. The amount of agent dur-

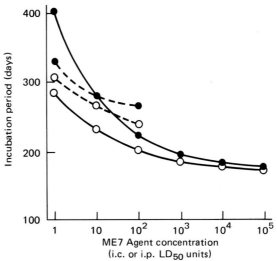

Figure 1.1.
Dose response curves for ME7-infected brain homogenate from BALB/c mice, titrated i.c. (solid line) or i.p. (broken line) in BALB/c mice (closed circles) or BRVR mice (open circles). Log_{10} LD_{50} estimated titers per 2 milligrams of brain: i.c. in BALB/c, 6.5; i.c. in BRVR, 6.6; i.p. in BALB/c, 4.0; i.p. in BRVR, 4.1.

ing this plateau is only about 1 i.c. LD_{50} unit/50 spleen cells, but in the brain the concentration of agent eventually reaches about one infective unit per cell. It is unknown whether the infectivity is evenly distributed between cells or highly concentrated in a few of them.

Various procedures can interfere with these events, but they all relate to the earliest phase of the process. It seems possible to reduce the effective susceptibility of mice to infection either physiologically, pharmacologically, or genetically, and these appear to act by preventing infection from taking place or by delaying the start of replication. Once replication has commenced, it appears to proceed inexorably. It must be emphasized that there is no evidence that scrapie is ever present as a latent infection of a type that can be activated by random events within the host or the environment.

Effects on Agent Replication

With all the mouse-passaged agents that have been tested, there is a *precise* inverse relationship between dose and incubation period, but the absolute dose/time details depend on the particular mouse strain/agent strain combination and the route of injection (Figs. 1.1 and 1.2).

The limitation imposed by only having one method of assay is not always appreciated: We have no means of knowing how much agent is functionally present in a tissue—functional, that is, for replication of more agent, or "stored" but able to produce damage—we can only estimate an operational titer and *assume* that it bears a direct relationship to the functional concentration. Another independent method of assay could give some perspective on the validity of this assumption, and an indication of the uncertainty of the present position is given by the fact that assays by i.p. injection give estimates 10 to 500-fold lower than by the i.c. route and that assay in different strains of mice using the same route can differ to a similar extent (5, 11).

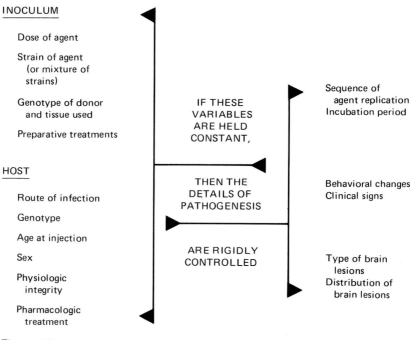

Figure 1.2.
Principal sources of variation in the pathogenesis of scrapie.

The Maturation of Susceptibility

The effect of age at injection on an incubation period in mice differs according to the route of injection. With i.c. injections there is a slight decrease in incubation with increasing age from birth to, at least, halfway through the lifespan (e.g., with ME7 in C57BL a decrease of about 1 day/20 days of age). Also with i.c. injections there is no indication that susceptibility varies with age, but this is not so with i.p. injections, when the younger mice are *less* susceptible.

The maturation of susceptibility appears to follow the same time course as the maturation of immune responses, which become well developed in the second postnatal week. Given the extreme stability of scrapie agents, it is surprising that all or most of the infectivity in the inoculum does not persist in the young mouse for the few days before the animal becomes susceptible. Very large doses of the agent do appear to persist and can produce an unexpectedly short incubation. The infectivity in intermediate and lower doses, however, appears to be quickly removed, even though it is unknown whether this is done by excretion or, more probably, by some degradation processes. It is easy to see that these could be "swamped" by very large doses of the agent. It seems reasonable to expect that these processes also occur in the older mice and that the maturation of susceptibility does not mean that they cease, but that they are involved in the development of readily accessible cellular sites where the agent can be protected from degradation and can, as a result, replicate.

Treatment of mice with prednisone acetate tends to restore the neonatal

6

state of insusceptibility (28), but as age increases, larger or repeated doses of prednisone are needed for this effect. It is unlikely that this effect is the result of T-cell suppression because adult thymectomy (plus irradiation) does not affect incubation after i.p. injection (24). However, the general feature of scrapie presented so far makes some other types of cells in the LRS an attractive possibility for agent replication. Treatment of mice with arachis oil has an effect similar to, but less dramatic than, those of prednisone (29). It remains to be determined whether the oil acts because of its unsaturated fatty acids or because it contains traces of potent anti-inflammatory substances.

Agent Strain Variation and Strain-Typing Techniques

A common strategic mistake has been to use only those combinations of agent strain, mouse strain, and route of injection that give the shortest incubation period as a basis for generalizations about "scrapie in the mouse." There is great variation in the timing of events during incubation between different strains of the agent and also between mice differing in their alleles of the gene *sinc* (abbreviation for *s*crapie *inc*ubation), which controls the incubation period.

It is unfortunate that most work with scrapie has stemmed from sources (SSBP/1 sheep or "drowsy" goats) that contain several agent strains and that the majority of natural cases of scrapie in sheep appear to be infected with more than one strain (6). In retrospect, it can be seen that claims about modification of "the agent" by passage in different species can be explained by recognizing that the starting material was a mixture of strains that become more homogeneous on passage, due to the new hosts restricting replication of some of them.

As a consequence, it is no longer possible to interpret gross agent changes due to passage history in terms that imply modification of the structure of the infective units, unless it can be established that the starting material was a homogeneous agent strain. Cloning of agents, by serial passage in inbred mice from end-point dilution cases is the only practicable starting point for critical studies. Even with such cloned agents, the possibility of "mutation" (or whatever the scrapie equivalent is) has to be taken into account, because roughly 2^{20} replications occur between injection and death and there is no information on the frequency of replication errors.

We have developed various agent-typing techniques during the last decade, and they have recently been employed to probe some of the molecular events in agent replication and its control by the host. Although recent results have shown that strains of agents can differ in thermal stability—22C being much more labile than 22A (13)—all the basic techniques for identifying agents stem from the differences in pathogenesis. These are of two types, which are largely independent of each other: tests that use the absolute and relative differences in the speed of incubation in a standard array of inbred and F_1 mice (4, 5, 12) and tests that use quantitative and qualitative aspects of the brain lesions (15–17, 19).

Histopathology: Quantitative and Qualitative Aspects

The brain lesions can include vacuolation of gray and white matter, astrocytic hypertrophy, and amyloid deposits, but there is no inflammatory reaction. There is extensive variation in the nature of the lesions present and in their intensity and regional distribution. However, if the variables shown in Fig. 1.2 are held constant, then the "lesion profiles" are extremely repeatable, as are the incubation periods. The constancy of gray and white matter lesion profiles can be used to identify different strains of agents (e.g., Fig. 1.3), and it is fortunate that the dose of the agent has virtually no effect on the profiles, which enhances their usefulness.

The bilateral symmetry of scrapie vacuolation had become a long-standing dogma, but it has now been found that some strains of agent tend to have asymmetrical lesions, and surprisingly, these are the agents that produce the highest frequencies of amyloid plaques (15, 17). When the reason for this association is known, it is likely to have a fundamental significance for the understanding of this type of disease, especially if the suspicion is confirmed that amyloid plaques are evidence of a disorganized immune response. The range of plaque morphology now known in scrapie includes those similar to senile plaques in humans (1, 32). There is some evidence that plaque formation can be an earlier morphological lesion than vacuolar degeneration. Vacuolation starts to appear during the second half of incubation at a stage determined by the variables shown in Fig. 1.2, which also control the extent to which vacuolation lags behind agent replication in the brain.

Compared with i.c. injections, i.p. injections generally produce less vacuolation, and it can be somewhat differently distributed. However, it must be stressed that although some combinations (e.g., ME7 agent i.c. in A2G or VM mice) develop extremely spongy lesions, others have very little vacuolation. Therefore the term "spongiform" is quite misleading for these

Figure 1.3.
Gray matter lesion profiles in VM mice for three different scrapie agents that have been passaged from 3 to 8 times i.c. in VM mice (solid lines, i.c. profiles; broken line; i.p. profile). Positions in brain: 1, medulla; 2, cerebellum; 3, midbrain tectum; 4, hypothalamus; 5, thalamus; 6, hippocampus; 7, para-terminal body; 8 and 9, posterior and anterior midline cerebral cortex.

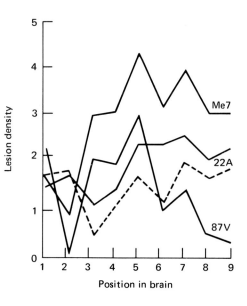

diseases, a conclusion emphasized by some types of sheep scrapie and transmissible mink encephalopathy that lack these diagnostic lesions (15, 23). Although the more vacuolated areas appear to have the higher agent titers (3, 20), there is no close correlation, because those mouse strain/ agent strain/route combinations that have hardly any vacuolation have brain titers within the same tenfold range as combinations with over a thousand times as much vacuolation.

It is doubtful, therefore, whether the visible lesions are the direct cause of death. Undetermined biochemical lesions produce behavioral changes from an early stage of incubation (22, 25, 31), and these lesions are the more likely cause of death. Even if the histologic lesions are a secondary issue, the precision and variety of the profiles pose perplexing questions about the specificity of the "targeting" processes within the brain, which they must reflect.

Genetic Control of Agent Replication

The incubation period is used as the basis for a set of agent-typing characteristics that are largely independent of the histologic ones. An absolute incubation period depends on many factors (Fig. 1.2), especially dose, agent strain, and mouse genotype, but the *relative* incubation period of the same dose in different genotypes is specific for each agent. With high doses, most agents have longer incubation periods in males than females, but with some agents (e.g., ME7) incubation tends to be equal in both sexes.

The gene *sinc* controls agent replication at a basic level, and this is seen as the difference in incubation periods (12). Although more evidence is needed, it appears that a major role of *sinc* is the control of the stage at which agent replication commences in each tissue. There are two subgroups of scrapie agents (22A group and ME7 group), which differ fundamentally in their control by the two alleles, $sinc^{s7}$ and $sinc^{p7}$. The ME7-group agents have shorter incubation in inbred mice carrying $sinc^{s7}$ (e.g., C57BL, C3H, BALB/c, A2G, RIII, BRVR, BSVS) than in ones carrying $sinc^{p7}$ (e.g., VM); conversely, 22A-group agents have prolonged incubation in the $sinc^{s7}$ mouse strains and shorter incubation in the $sinc^{p7}$ mice. In addition to this reversal of gene action in the homozygotes according to the agent group, individual agents in the s7p7 heterozygote differ markedly in the effect of the allelic interaction on the incubation period. Some agents show no dominance, whereas others are subject to various degrees of dominance of either of the alleles. Some agents (e.g., 22A) even show overdominance of the s7 allele so that the incubation period is longer in the F_1 mice than in either parental strain.

Incubation periods in VM and C57BL mice and their F_1 cross are shown in Fig. 1.4 for large i.c. doses of various agents. The lifespan of inbred mice averages 2 to 2.5 years, and it can be seen that incubation in some cases takes more than half the lifespan, even for high i.c. doses. With low doses of some of the agents given i.p., the length of incubation would

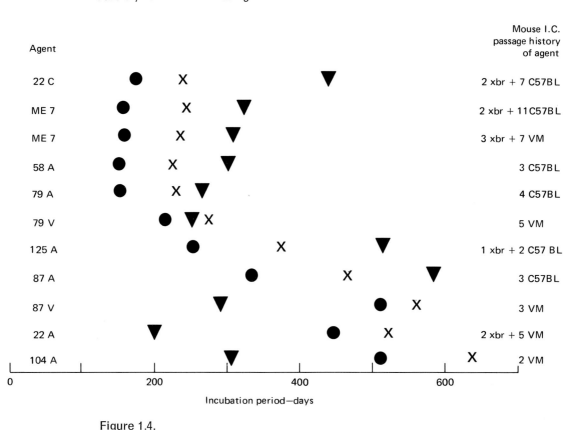

Figure 1.4.
Incubation periods of different scrapie agents in C57BL mice (●), VM mice (▼), and their F₁ cross (X) after i.c. injection with 5% mouse brain homogenates whose passage history is shown on the right-hand side of the figure.

be greater than the natural lifespan, which is paradoxical. This conclusion is based on the fact that the agent is replicating in the spleen close to the end of the lifespan but that there are no brain lesions or clinical signs. When higher doses of the same agent are used, replication starts earlier in the spleen and clinical signs and lesions can develop in the old animals (11). An example of this is the 22A agent injected i.p. in C57BL mice. However, it is puzzling that no agent replication can be detected in the C57BL spleen for at least 1 year after i.p. injection with doses below about 1,000 VM i.c. LD$_{50}$ units of 22A. It is not known where infectivity might be detected during this long interval, and the spleen may not, in this combination, be the first location for replication. If the sequence of events in these C57BL's is the usual one, this long-drawn-out tempo may be useful in determining the sequence of early cellular events. It would, of course, be quite incorrect to describe the many months' absence of infectivity from these spleens as an "eclipse phase," because we do not know whether infectivity is present in some other organ during this interval. Until a great deal more is known about scrapie and other related diseases—kuru, Creutzfeldt–Jakob disease, and TME—it is unwarranted to use such virologic categories as "eclipse phase," "maturation phase," agent "redirecting host-cell metabolism," or agent "assembly" (in the absence of virion assembly).

The aforementioned finding concerning genetic overdominance involving the gene *sinc* with some agents (e.g., 22A, 104A) has important implications for an understanding of the molecular events on which agent replication depends. Overdominance indicates that the two alleles present in the diploid genome do not act independently of each other. By analogy with the molecular events associated with allelic complementation in microorganisms (33), it has been proposed that the gene product of *sinc* is a multimeric structure. In the heterozygote then both alleles contribute subunits to form a heteromeric multimer. This may be structurally analogous to an enzyme and acts as the replication site for scrapie agents: Its still unknown function in the normal mouse could be crucial for a wider understanding of these diseases (12). If there is free association of monomers, then the observation of overdominance can only be explained if the total effective number of replication sites is relatively small.

The Scrapie Replication Site Hypothesis

The great diversity of scrapie incubation periods and modes of gene action of *sinc* can be explained in terms of the multimeric replication site model. The accessory condition for the free association version of the model, namely the limited number of sites, also helps to explain a variety of other features of the disease. These include (a) the observed plateau phase of agent titer (e.g., in the spleen) where site saturation and slow agent turnover produce a plateau; (b) the absence of the spleen, which would reduce the number of sites, if a considerable proportion were in the spleen, giving longer incubation of the extraneurally injected agent, which is the effect observed; (c) the expectation that different agents would compete if the site number were small and different agents used the same sites, and this is the effect found (9); and (d) the fact that the removal of the spleen, if the spleen contains an important proportion of the extraneural sites, should only affect the incubation period when the amount of agent i.p. injected is large but that the prolongation should not occur at high dilution when the number of infective units is less than the remaining number of sites (preliminary results support this possibility).

The conditions for agent strain competition experiments follow. Mice are given an injection of an operationally slow agent (e.g., a 22A-group agent in *sinc*[s7] mice), and after an interval of weeks or months, a second injection of an operationally quick agent is given (e.g., an ME7-group agent in these *sinc*[s7] mice). The exact result depends on the particular agents and recipients used, the routes of injection, the doses of the agent, and the interval between injections. The details can be arranged so that the second agent kills the mice, and competition is detected as an increased incubation period of this lethal agent. Analysis of the lesion profiles can establish which agent killed the mice or even whether both contributed. The time intervals between injections required for competition are much greater than any known to be necessary for conventional immune or inter-feron responses. More recently, combinations have been found in which the infectivity of the second agent is completely lost: Low i.p. doses were used, and 22A was followed 100 to 300 days later by 22C in $sinc^{s7}$ mice (10). If the site-blocking explanation is correct, then it must be remarkably efficient and obviously raises the question of whether the normal product of the *sinc* specified site can also exert a scrapie-blocking effect. Even if this explanation is wrong, the results add to others (e.g., age and steroid effects) to confirm the presence of some processes that can degrade scrapie in-fectivity.

Additional experiments have established that blocking can occur in VM mice using the agents ME7 and 22A, both of which had been passaged several times in VM mice. This rules out the possibility that donor tissue differences in the inocula are responsible for the effect. No blocking occurs by the i.p. route if the dose of the first (i.e., blocking) agent is just below the i.p. infective dose but still contains infectivity for the i.c. assays. Even though blocking depends on operational infectivity, recent evidence sug-gests that the effect begins before the blocking agent has started to repli-cate (3).

It is obviously important to devise experiments that have a potential for disproving the hypothesis, and a vigorous search is needed for alterna-tive models that can explain as wide a range of the facts as economically as does the scrapie replication site hypothesis.

WHY IS SCRAPIE THIS TYPE OF DISEASE?

Can a coherent explanation concerning the *slow, degenerative,* and *en-cephalopathic* characteristics of scrapie-like diseases now be evolved?

The evidence is growing that scrapie agents use some infrequent cell-types in the LRS, such as Trojan horses, where they can replicate and perhaps be transported to the CNS. The use of LRS cells without provoking inflammatory and immune responses requires that either (a) the doses of functionally exposed agent are at tolerogenic rather than immunogenic levels, (b) these agents are able to disarm specific inflammatory and other LRS responses, or (c) the agent's structure may be essentially similar to the postulated informational molecules used for normal communication between LRS cells (21, 26, 30). Knowledge of the normal function of *sinc* should help to decide among these possibilities.

Understanding why these are degenerative diseases is simplest if the agents do not modify cell function by providing new information that redirects the cell's metabolism. If the agent has a structure and code that simply permits it to be replicated by the normal course of events in the cell, and if the amount of replication is under strict control, then damage will merely reflect the extent to which the agent hinders cell function by its presence. Such marginal damage may be lost in the normal course of cell replacement and only appear as histologic change in those tissues where cells are permanent or have low turnover rates, a description that fits the

CNS. Diseases produced by this type of agent would, therefore, tend to be degenerative encephalopathies.

Some of these conjectures also account for the slowness of these diseases, but the crux of the matter relates to the ability of the host to limit agent replication—positively rather than by default—within cells and tissues. The gene *sinc* appears to provide such control, and its fuller investigation is essential.

REFERENCES

1. Bruce, M.E., and Fraser, H. (1975). Amyloid plaques in the brains of mice infected with scrapie: Morphological variation and straining properties. *Neuropathol. Appl. Neurobiol. 1*, 189–202.
2. Clarke, M. C., and Haig, D. A. (1970). Evidence for the multiplication of scrapie agent in cell culture. *Nature 225*, 100–101.
3. Dickinson, A. G. Unpublished data. 1974.
4. Dickinson, A. G. Classification of scrapie agents based on histological and incubation period criteria in mice. *Proceedings VI International Congress of Neuropathology*, pp. 841–842. Masson, Paris. 1970.
5. Dickinson, A. G. (1975). Host-pathogen interactions in scrapie. *Genetics 79* (Suppl.), 387–395.
6. Dickinson, A. G. (1976). Scrapie in sheep and goats. In *Slow Virus Diseases of Animals and Man* (R. H. Kimberlin, ed.), pp. 209–241. Elsevier, Amsterdam.
7. Dickinson, A. G., and Fraser, H. (1969). Modification of the pathogenesis of scrapie in mice by treatment of the agent. *Nature 222*, 892–893.
8. Dickinson, A. G., and Fraser, H. (1972). Scrapie: Effect of Dh gene on incubation period of extraneurally injected agent. *Heredity 29*, 91–93.
9. Dickinson, A. G., Fraser, H., Meikle, V. M. H., and Outram, G. W. (1972). Competition between different scrapie agents in mice. *Nature [New Biol.] 237*, 244–245.
10. Dickinson, A. G., Fraser, H., McConnell, I., Outram, G. W., Sales, D. I., and Taylor, D. M. (1975). Extraneural competition between different scrapie agents leading to loss of infectivity. *Nature 253*, 556.
11. Dickinson, A. G., Fraser, H., and Outram, G. W. (1975). Scrapie incubation time can exceed natural lifespan. *Nature 256*, 732–733.
12. Dickinson, A. G., and Meikle, V. M. H. (1971). Host-genotype and agent effects in scrapie incubation: Change in allelic interaction with different strains of agent. *Mol. Gen. Genet. 112*, 73–79.
13. Dickinson, A. G., and Taylor, D. M. Unpublished data. 1974.
14. Eklund, C. M., Kennedy, R. C., and Hadlow, W. J. (1967). Pathogenesis of scrapie virus infections in the mouse. *J. Infect. Dis. 117*, 15–22.
15. Fraser, H. (1976). The pathology of natural and experimental scrapie. In *Slow Virus Diseases of Animals and Man* (R. H. Kimberlin, ed.), pp. 267–305. Elsevier, Amsterdam.
16. Fraser, H., and Bruce, M. E. (1973). Argyrophilic plaques in mice inoculated with scrapie from particular sources. *Lancet i*, 617.
17. Fraser, H., Bruce, M. E., and Dickinson, A. G. (1975). Quantitative pathology for understanding the nature and pathogenesis of scrapie, using different strains of agent. *Proceedings VII International Congress of Neuropathology*, in press.
18. Fraser, H., and Dickinson, A. G. (1970). Pathogenesis of scrapie in the mouse: The role of the spleen. *Nature 226*, 462–463.
19. Fraser, H., and Dickinson, A. G. (1973). Scrapie in mice: Agent-strain differences in the distribution and intensity of grey matter vacuolation. *J. Comp. Pathol. 83*, 29–40.

20. Hadlow, W. J. Personal communication.
21. Gottlieb, A. A., and Straus, D. S. (1969). Physical studies on the light density ribonucleoprotein complex of macrophage cells. *J. Biol. Chem. 244*, 3324–3329.
22. Heitzman, R. J., and Corp, C. R. (1968). Behaviour in emergence and open-field tests of normal and scrapie mice. *Res. Vet. Sci. 9*, 600–601.
23. Marsh, R. F. (1976). Subacute spongiform encephalopathies. In *Slow Virus Diseases of Animals and Man* (R. H. Kimberlin, ed.), pp. 359–380. Elsevier, Amsterdam.
24. McFarlin, D. E., Raff, M. C., Simpson, E., and Nehlsen, S. H. (1971). Scrapie in immunologically deficient mice. *Nature 233*, 336.
25. Outram, G. W. (1972). Changes in drinking and feeding habits of mice with experimental scrapie. *J. Comp. Pathol. 82*, 415–427.
26. Outram, G. W. (1976). The pathogenesis of scrapie in mice. In *Slow Virus Diseases of Animals and Man* (R. H. Kimberlin, ed.), pp. 325–357. Elsevier, Amsterdam.
27. Outram, G. W., Dickinson, A. G., and Fraser, H. (1973). Developmental maturation of susceptibility to scrapie in mice. *Nature 241*, 536–537.
28. Outram, G. W., Dickinson, A. G., and Fraser, H. (1974). Reduced susceptibility to scrapie in mice after steroid administration. *Nature 249*, 855–856.
29. Outram, G. W., Dickinson, A. G., and Fraser, H. (1975). Slow encephalopathies, inflammatory responses, and arachis oil. *Lancet i*, 198–200.
30. Reanney, D. C. (1975). The regulatory role of viral RNA in eukaryotes. *J. of Theor. Biol. 49*, 461–492.
31. Savage, R. D., and Field, E. J. (1965). Brain damage and emotional behaviour: The effects of scrapie on the emotional responses of mice. *J. Anim. Behav. 13*, 443–446.
32. Wisniewski, H. M., Bruce, M. E., and Fraser, H. (1975). Infectious etiology of neuritic (senile) plaques in mice. *Science*, 190, 1108–1110.
33. Zimmermann, F. K., and Gundelach, E. (1969). Intragenic complementation, hybrid enzyme formation and dominance in diploid cells of Saccharomyces cerevisiae. *Mol. Gen. Genet. 103*, 348–362.

CHAPTER 2
Kuru, Creutzfeldt–Jakob Disease, and Transmissible Presenile Dementias

D. CARLETON GAJDUSEK / CLARENCE J. GIBBS, JR.

INTRODUCTION

We have long used scrapie virus as our model, in the hope of elucidating the molecular structure and growth characteristics of at least one of these unconventional viruses. We tend to be more conservative than most other groups in our interpretation of the data and call these agents "viruses" in most of our publications. We argue that they are viruses, as viruses were originally defined, and then we play the semantic trick of calling them the "unconventional group of viruses." As our hypotheses on the minimal number of codons the virus ribonucleic acid (RNA) or deoxyribonucleic acid (DNA) should have in order to code for a virus transcriptase or virus structural proteins collapse, and as other conventionally assumed behavior of the virus on ultraviolet (UV) inactivation or hot formaldehyde treatment of RNAse and DNAse treatment is found not to occur, we are pushed further and further into a difficult position with the scrapie virus which was so beautifully pointed out by Dickinson.

We selected scrapie as the animal virus model in our study of kuru, after Hadlow pointed out the neuropathologic similarities between scrapie and kuru. Kuru is a chronic neurologic disease restricted to cannibal, stone age Melanesian peoples in the highlands of Papua, New Guinea. Our goal was the elucidation of the cause of kuru. Our initial attempts to demonstrate that the kuru epidemic was due to an infectious or postinfectious phenomenon had failed. A search for virus etiology by conventional techniques had been unsuccessful. Our attempts to demonstrate that it might possibly be of genetic origin were equally a failure. We had observed hundreds of cases and had records of over 1,000 cases in genealogies; this series was adequate to demonstrate that Mendelian ratios of frequency of kuru in maternal and paternal sides of the family were wrong for our genetic hypothesis of an autosomal trait dominant in the female. Although all cases were familial with a history of the disease in close relatives and no contact cases to be found, it was unreasonable to believe that an epidemic with such a high gene frequency could have developed in the absence of any recognized genetic advantage to heterozygotes, which were lost to the breeding pool before the end of their reproductive period. Thus, we continued to wonder whether an infectious process might be involved in kuru, perhaps as a late sequel to an earlier acute infection, as appeared to be the case in von Economo's encephalitis after World War I in Europe with its postencephalitic parkinsonism.

This trail from scrapie experiments led to our transmitting kuru, after long incubation periods, first to the chimpanzee, later to a half dozen species of New World monkeys, and, more recently, to a half dozen species of Old World monkeys. Such transmission occurred when we used bacteria-free filtrates of brain from kuru patients inoculated intracerebrally or only peripherally into nonhuman primates.

SIMILARITIES BETWEEN KURU AND CREUTZFELDT–JAKOB DISEASE

We finally asked the question: Why is this strange epidemic of kuru restricted to a small group of people, highly related to one another genetically, in the highlands of New Guinea? Is there the same or similar disease in other populations? In the CJD-type of presenile dementia, we found the worldwide occurrence of a kurulike transmissible disease. When Igor Klatzo originally described the neuropathology in kuru (1959), he pointed out that were he studying the brain of only one or two adults he would have called the neuropathologic picture Creutzfeldt–Jakob disease (CJD). However, since CJD was never reported as an epidemic disease affecting hundreds of children and adults, but was a very rare, sporadic presenile dementia, he did not consider the CJD diagnosis and only referred to the neuropathologic similarities between this disease and kuru.

This early analogy between kuru and the CJD-type of presenile dementia is of interest, since it was made without awareness of two other pathologic analogies that have subsequently been demonstrated, namely: (a) the presence of areas of status spongiosus in gray matter in most cases of both diseases; and (b) the presence of kurulike amyloid plaques in 12% of CJD patients, similar to the amyloid-containing plaques found in 60% of kuru patients. Only later work on both these diseases revealed these other neuropathologic similarities. For example, on passage of kuru to the chimpanzee or monkey, the neuronal vacuolation and occasional restricted areas of status spongiosus that characterize kuru in man became a dominant feature of the experimental disease. Thus we were forced to ask where in human neuropathology such an extensive status spongiosus of gray matter was encountered. Once again our neuropathologist colleagues studying human diseases pointed out that this was seen almost exclusively in CJD. Similarly, veterinary neuropathologists had shown that natural sheep scrapie is characterized by vacuolation of neurons, but this does not progress to a true spongiform degeneration of gray matter. However, on transmission of scrapie from sheep to other sheep or to goat, hamster, or mouse, the spongiform degeneration becomes a dominant feature of the experimentally induced disease. Yet, even with these similarities on the neuropathologic level, it was difficult to interpret these findings as virus-induced lesions.

16

TABLE 2.1 / Naturally Occurring Slow Virus Infections Caused by Unconventional Viruses (Subacute Spongiform Virus Encephalopathies)

Of Man	Of Animals
Kuru	Scrapie
Transmissible virus dementia	In sheep
Creutzfeldt–Jakob disease	In goats
Sporadic	Mink encephalopathy
Familial	
Familial Alzheimer's disease	

However, we have now proved this to be the case. In this presentation we will review some of our previous work and present newer data on the subacute spongiform virus encephalopathies.

Degenerative slow virus diseases include some caused by unconventional viruses with extremely unusual properties (Table 2.1) and others caused by conventional viruses, such as measles (Table 2.2). Most so-called subacute and chronic progressive degenerative diseases of the central nervous system (CNS) have been classified as disorders of unknown etiology. Although some are genetically determined, many cases of the same disorders are sporadic and do not have a history of the disease in a close relative. It is curious that apparently heredofamilial forms of some progressive degenerative disorders are as transmissible as their sporadic counterparts. We must consider the possibility of pathogenesis regulated by a genetically determined susceptibility, or a turning on, or derepression, of a usually masked or latent potentially slow virus.

TABLE 2.2 / Slow Infections Caused by Conventional Viruses

Infection	Virus
Subacute sclerosing panencephalitis (SSPE)	Measles—defective
Subacute panencephalitis as a late sequela following congenital rubella	Rubella—defective
Subacute postmeasles leukoencephalitis	Measles—defective
Multiple sclerosis	? defective myxovirus or paramyxovirus
Progressive multifocal leukoencephalopathy (PML)	Papovavirus (JC and SV-40 strain)
Cytomegalovirus brain infection	Cytomegalovirus
Progressive congenital rubella	Rubella
Subacute encephalitis	Herpes simplex
	Adenovirus type 32
Epilepsia partialis continua in USSR (Kozhevnikov's epilepsy)	Tick-borne encephalitis virus (RSSE)
Focal epilepsy with chronic encephalitis	?
Crohn's disease	? RNA virus
Ulcerative colitis	?
Homologus serum jaundice	Hepatitis B
Infectious hepatitis	Hepatitis A
	Hepatitis B
	Hepatitis C

KURU IN NEW GUINEA PROMPTS THE STUDY OF SLOW VIRUS INFECTIONS OF THE CENTRAL NERVOUS SYSTEM OF MAN

This study was an outgrowth of our attempts to solve the riddle of an epidemic of a fatal subacute degenerative neurologic disease, kuru, in New Guinea highland natives, which had attained enormous proportions in an isolated primitive population still using stone tools and practicing endo-cannibalism (23, 24, 49). This exotic model was chosen for such intensive study because of the obvious implications its solution would have for other CNS degenerative diseases, which it resembled in basic pathologic lesions, and even in degenerative processes active in all aging brains (1, 2, 32). Thus kuru became the first chronic human disease proved to be a slow virus infection (20, 21). Soon thereafter, the presenile dementias of the CJD-type were proved equivalents of kuru, of worldwide nonexotic distribution (3, 28). Both the sporadic and familial forms were shown to be transmissible (12, 42, 46).

Subsequently, others demonstrated that subacute sclerosing panencephalitis (SSPE) (7, 30, 41, 43) and progressive multifocal leukoencephalopathy (PML) (39, 48, 50) were also slow virus diseases. Some data now accumulating suggest that multiple sclerosis (MS) and Parkinson's disease may also be slow virus infections.

In our laboratory, MS, Parkinson's disease, Alzheimer's disease, Pick's disease, Huntington's chorea, amyotrophic lateral sclerosis, chronic encephalitis, focal epilepsy, progressive supranuclear palsy, and degenerative reactions to schizophrenia are among the other diseases under investigation (15, 18, 21). Our attempts at transmitting any of them to animals have been unsuccessful.

SLOW VIRUS INFECTIONS IN MAN

Kuru

Kuru, a descriptive name in the Fore language, is characterized by cerebellar ataxia and a tremor that progresses to complete motor incapacity and death in about 1 year. It is confined to a number of adjacent valleys in the mountainous interior of New Guinea and has occurred in 160 villages with a total population of just over 35,000 (Fig. 2.1). Eighty percent of kuru cases occur among the people with a prevalence of about 1%. Originally, it was found to affect all ages beyond infancy and was common in children of both sexes and in adult females, but it was rare in adult males. The marked excess of deaths of adult females over males has led to a male to female ratio of over 3:1 in some villages, and of 2:1 for the whole south Fore group (16, 23, 24).

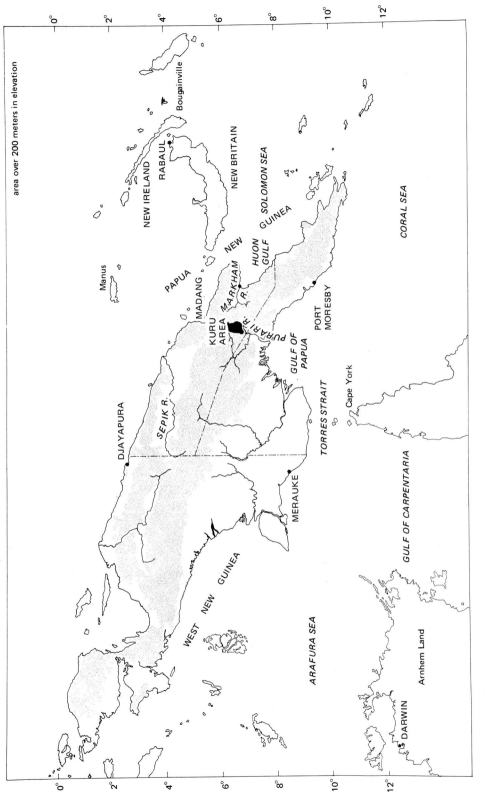

Figure 2.1.
The irregular black area within the rectangle in the highlands on the eastern side of the islands is the region in New Guinea from which all kuru patients have come. Over 35,000 people living in 160 villages (census units) here have experienced kuru. All kuru-affected hamlets lie between 1000- and 2500-m elevation.

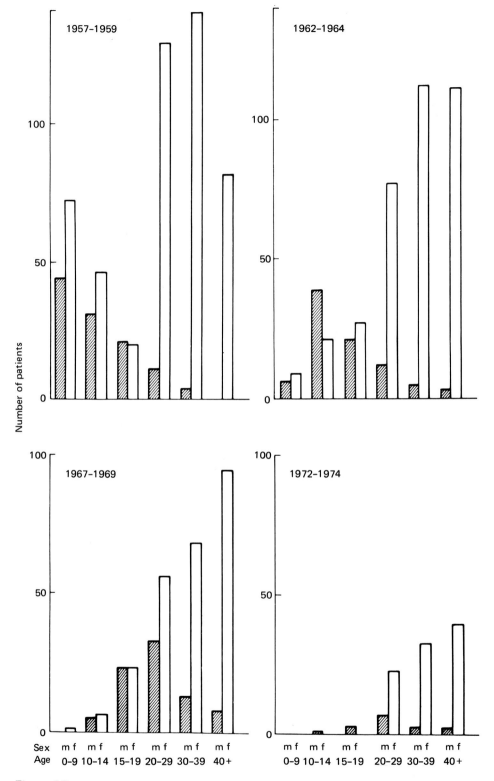

Figure 2.2.
Incidence of kuru in male and female patients by year since its discovery in 1957 through 1974. m-male; f-female. Age is given in years.

Incidence

Incidence of kuru has gradually decreased during the past 15 years (Fig. 2.2). It is no longer seen in preadolescent children or adolescents (Fig. 2.2). Perhaps this change is the result of the cessation of ritual cannibalism as a rite of mourning and respect for the dead kinsmen, since the transmission probably occurred through conjunctival, nasal, and skin contamination during the rite (Figs. 2.2, 3, 4, and 2.5a, b, c) (16).

Origin and Transmission of Kuru

Unanswered crucial questions posed by all of these unconventional agents are related to their biologic origin and mode of survival in nature. The diseases they evoke are natural not artificial ones, produced by researchers tampering with cellular macromolecular structures. We do not know the mode of their dissemination or the mechanism of their long term persistence.

In the case of Fore kuru, the contamination of close kinsmen within a mourning family group by the opening of the skull of dead victims in a rite of cannibalism, during which all adult females and children of the

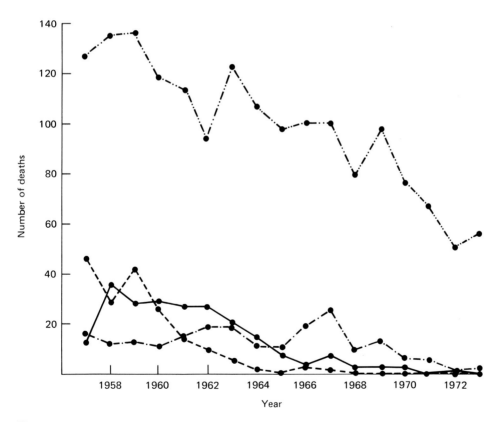

Figure 2.3.
Kuru deaths by year. 20 years and older (line broken by 2 dots); 15–19 years (line broken by 1 dot); 10–14 years (solid line); 4–9 years (broken line).

21

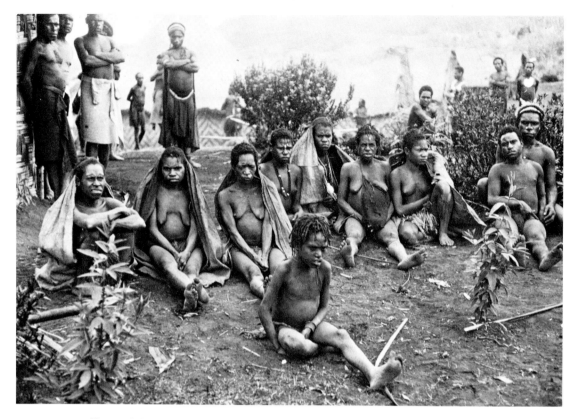

Figure 2.4.
Nine victims of kuru assembled one afternoon in 1957 from several villages in the Purosa valley (total population about 400) in the South Fore region. The victims include six adult females, one adolescent female, one adolescent male, and a prepubertal male. All died of their disease within 1 year after this picture was taken.

kuru victim's family were thoroughly contaminated with the virus, seems to provide a full explanation of the unique epidemiologic findings in kuru and their change over the past two decades (14–16). However, this does not provide a satisfactory explanation for the origin of kuru. Was it the unlikely event of a sporadic case of worldwide CJD that produced a unique epidemic in the unusual cultural setting of New Guinea? We now have the report of a spontaneous case of CJD in a native Chimbu New Guinean from the central highlands; his clinical diagnosis was proved by light and electron microscopic examination of a brain biopsy specimen (Gajdusek, unpublished data). Serial passage of brain in man in successive cannibalistic rituals might have resulted in a change in the clinical picture of the disease, with modification of the virulence of the original agent.

If such spontaneous CJD is not related to the origin of kuru, another possibility might be that the serial brain passage, which occurred in this ritual inoculation of brain from successive victims in multiple sequential passages into their kinsmen, may have yielded a new neurotropic strain of virus from some well-known virus. Finally, in view of what occurs in the defective replication of measles virus in patients with SSPE, we must wonder whether a ubiquitous or, at least, a well-known virus may not be modified into a defective, incomplete, or highly integrated or repressed agent *in vivo* in the course of its long masked state in the individual host. Such a new breed of virus may no longer be easily recognizable antigenically or structurally, because of failure of full synthesis of viral subunits or of their assembly into a known virion. Thus, we may ask whether kuru contains some of the subunits of a known agent, modified by its unusual passage history (14, 15, 18).

Isolation of the Virus

Original isolation was accomplished in chimpanzees (Figs. 2.6a, b, and 2.7) (18, 20), but ultimately transmission to other species was accomplished. For example, several species of New and Old World monkeys were successfully infected. The incubation periods in these animals were much longer than in chimpanzees. (Tables 2.3 and 2.4) (19, 27). We have now transmitted kuru to mink, the first nonprimate host that proved to be susceptible (Table 2.5).

The virus has been regularly isolated from the brain tissue of kuru patients. It attains titer of $\geqq 10^8$ infectious doses/g. In peripheral tissue, namely, liver and spleen, it has been found only rarely at the time of death and in much lower titers. Urine, blood leukocytes, cerebrospinal fluid, and placenta and embryo membranes of patients with kuru have not yielded the virus.

Transmissible Virus Dementia (Creutzfeldt–Jakob Disease)

Creutzfeldt–Jakob disease is a rare, unusually sporadic, presenile dementia found worldwide; it has a familial dominant autosomal pattern of inheritance in about 10% of the cases (Fig. 2.8). The typical clinical picture includes myoclonus, paroxysmal bursts on the electroencephalogram, and evidence of widespread cerebral dysfunction. The disease is regularly transmissible to chimpanzees (3, 28), New and Old World monkeys (Tables 2.3 and 2.4), and the domestic cat (Table 2.6) (19, 27). Pathologic findings for these animals are indistinguishable at the cellular level from those in the natural human disease or in experimental kuru (3, 33) (Fig. 2.9). Transmission of CJD from human brain to guinea pig (36) and from human brain to mice (5) has been reported.

A wide range of clinical syndromes involving dementia in middle and late life actually have been shown to be CJD. These include cases of brain tumors (glioblastoma, meningioma); brain abscess; Alzheimer's disease; senile dementia, or stroke; and Köhlmeier–Degos disease (23, 38, 46). It is important, therefore, to define the whole spectrum of subacute and chronic neurologic illnesses caused by or associated with CJD. One pathologic characteristic of these diseases is the amyloid plaque. Some 14% of CJD

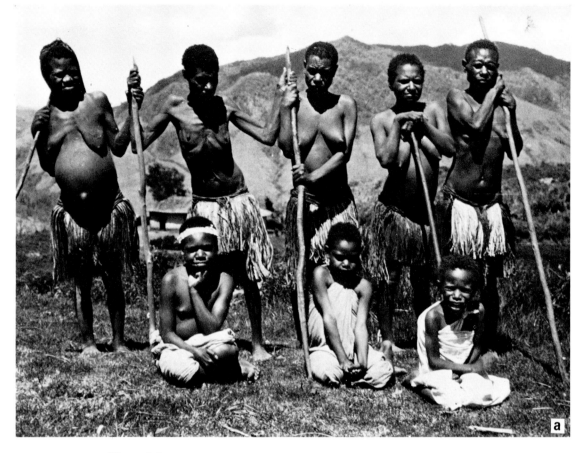

Figure 2.5.
New Guinea kuru patients in 1957 at the Kuru Research Hospital. All died within
1 year. Shown are many preadolescent victims of kuru, an age group in which kuru
has not occurred in recent years.
a. Eight kuru patients in the first, or ambulatory, stage of the disease. Five adult
females are holding sticks to maintain their balance. Three adolescent girls who are
still able to walk without the aid of a stick, but with severe ataxia, sit in front.
b. Eight preadolescent children, four boys and four girls, with kuru, The girl at the
far right in her father's lap is the same child as that on the left in Fig. 2.5**a,** now
2 months later and in the second, or sedentary, stage of kuru.
c. Five children with kuru: two boys in the center, a girl on each side; the adolescent boy supporting the girl on the left is a kuru victim himself, but in an earlier
stage of the disease. All are just passing from the first, or ambulatory, to the second,
or sedentary, stage of the disease, and can no longer stand without support.

cases show such plaques; they are also found in kuru and Alzheimer's
disease. In addition, CJD and the other diseases have status spongiosus
and astrogliosis (37, 38, 46). Therefore, we have started to refer to these
transmissible disorders as transmissible virus dementia (TVD).

Incidence

Since our first transmission of CJD, we have obtained brain biopsy or early
postmortem brain tissue in more than 130 cases of pathologically confirmed

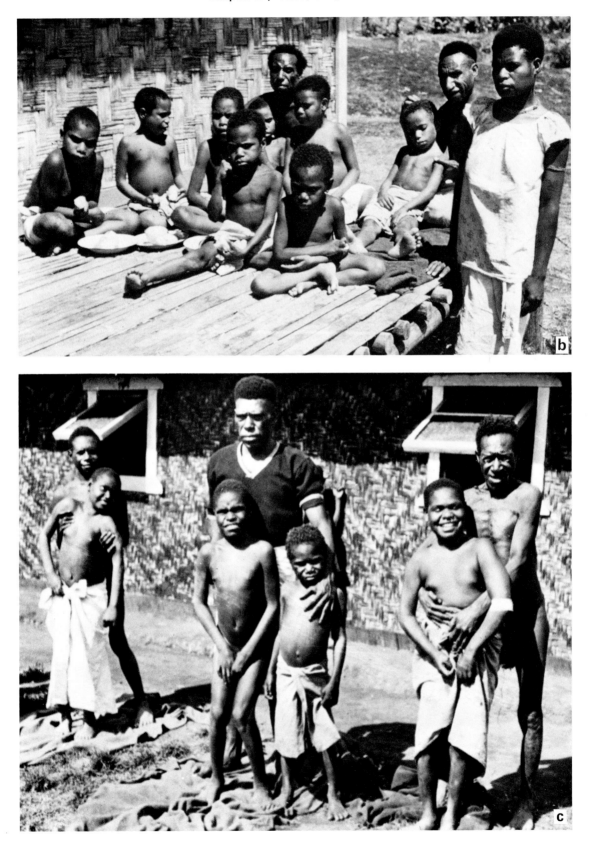

Figure 2.6.
a. Chimpanzee with early experimental kuru eating from the floor without use of prehension. This "vacuum cleaner" feeding was a frequent sign in early disease in the chimpanzee when tremor and ataxia were already apparent.
b. Range of movement in forelimbs in walking: left, normal chimpanzee; right, chimpanzee in the second stage of experimental kuru. Quantitative assessment was made by studying individual frames of Research Cinema Film [from Gajdusek and Gibbs (19)].

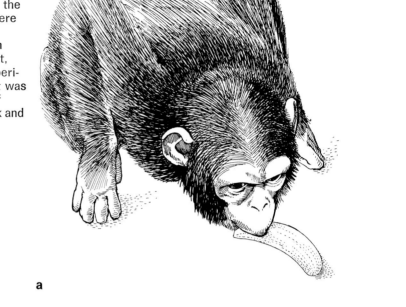

a

b

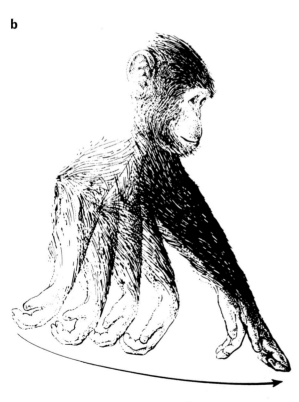

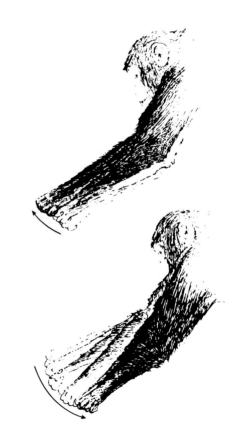

TABLE 2.3 / Species of Laboratory Primates Susceptible to the Subacute Spongiform Virus Encephalopathies[a]

OF MAN

Kuru	*Apes*	chimpanzee, gibbon
	New World monkeys	capuchin, marmoset, spider, squirrel, woolly
	Old World monkeys	cynomolgus macaque, mangabey, rhesus, pig-tailed macaque
Creutzfeldt–Jakob disease	*Apes*	chimpanzee
	New World monkeys	capuchin, marmoset, spider, squirrel, woolly
	Old World monkeys	African green, baboon, bushbaby, cynomolgus macaque, mangabey, patas, pig-tailed macaque, rhesus, stump-tailed macaque, talapoin

OF ANIMALS

Scrapie	*New World monkeys*	capuchin, spider, squirrel
	Old World monkeys	cynomolgus macaque, rhesus
Transmissible mink encephalopathy	*New World monkeys*	squirrel
	Old World monkeys	rhesus, stump-tailed macaque

[a] As of July 1, 1975.

TABLE 2.4 / Species of Laboratory Primates Susceptible to Subacute Spongiform Encephalopathies[a]

	Incubation Periods in Months[b]			
	Kuru	CJD	Scrapie	TME
APES				
Chimpanzee (*Pan troglodytes*)	10–82	11–71	(111)	(61)
Gibbon (*Hylobates lar*)	+(10)	NT	NT	NT
NEW WORLD MONKEYS				
Capuchin (*Cebus albifrons*)	10–15	29–34	NT	NT
Capuchin (*Cebus apella*)	11–60	11–44.5	32–35.5	NT
Spider (*Ateles geoffroyi*)	10–63	23–50	38	NT
Squirrel (*Saimiri sciureus*)	9.5–44	11–47	14–35	8–13
Marmoset (*Saguinus* sp.)	31–38	43	NT	NT
Woolly (*Lagothrix lagothricha*)	33	21	NT	NT
OLD WORLD MONKEYS				
African green (*Cercopithecus aethiops*)	(98)	33–48	(109)	NT
Baboon (*Papia anubis*)	(99)	47.5	NT	NT
Bushbaby (*Galago senegalensis*)	(89)	16	NT	NT
Cynomolgus macaque (*Macaca fascicularis*)	16	52.5–60	27–65	NT
Patas (*Erythrocebes patas patas*)	(107)	47	NT	NT
Pig-tailed macaque (*Macaca nemestrina*)	70	+(2)	NT	NT
Rhesus (*Macaca mulatta*)	15–103	43–68	30–37	17–33
Sooty mangabey (*Cercocebus atys*)	+(2)	+(2)–43	NT	NT
Stump-tailed macaque (*Macaca arctoides*)	(105)	60	NT	13
Talapoin (*Cercopithecus talapoin*)	(1+)	64.5	NT	NT

[a] As of July 1, 1975.
[b] NT = no transmission

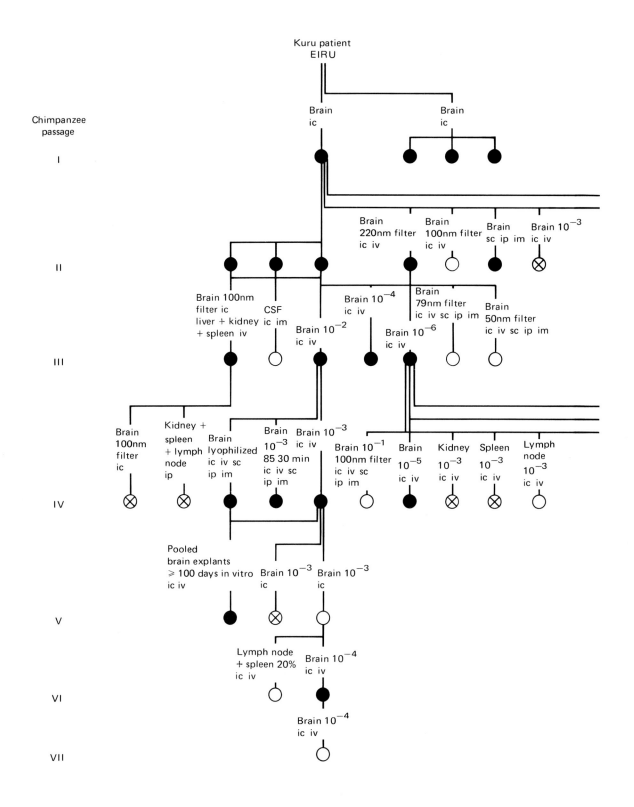

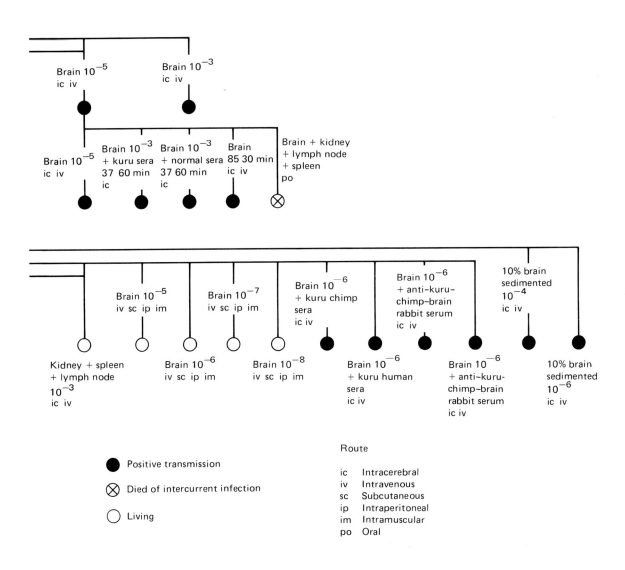

Figure 2.7.
Kuru transmission experiments in chimpanzees.

**TABLE 2.5 / Nonprimate Hosts for Experimental
Subacute Spongiform Encephalopathies**[a]

OF MAN
Kuru	Mink
Creutzfeldt–Jakob disease	Cat, ? guinea pig (New Haven) (35), ? mouse (Bristol) (5)

OF ANIMALS
Scrapie	Gerbil, goat, hamster, mink, mouse, rat, sheep, vole
Transmissible mink encephalopathy	Ferret, goat, hamster, mink, racoon, sheep, skunk

[a] As of July 1, 1975.

CJD. The clinical, laboratory, and virus investigation of these cases have been summarized in a recent report (46) that extends our earlier report of 35 cases (42). We have been aware of occasional clustering of cases in small population centers, admittedly lacking in natural boundaries, and the unexplained absence of any cases over periods of many years in some large population centers where they were found earlier. Matthews has recently made a similar observation in two clusters in England (37). This geographic and temporal clustering does not apply, however, to the majority of cases and cannot be explained for 10% of the cases that are familial. There are

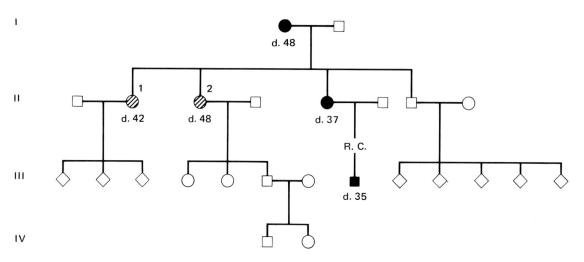

Figure 2.8.
A family with five cases of CJD over three generations. Autosomal dominant inheritance is suggested. The disease was transmitted from the patient R.C. to a chimpanzee. It has been similarly transmitted to chimpanzees or new world monkeys from an additional six patients with transmissible virus dementia of a familial type. Ten percent of CJD patients have a history of similar disease in kinsmen (46). Creutzfeldt–Jakob disease was a rare, almost unknown disease; now cases of transmissible virus dementia are regularly found wherever they are looked for. Better ascertainment of cases, the study of familial aggregations and an unusually high prevalence in Libyan Jews, and the possibility of occupational hazard and transmission through corneal transplant provide promising epidemiologic leads to the understanding of the natural history of the disease, and hence to its prevention. Solid box or circle, CJD confirmed pathologically; hatched box or circle, probable CJD; arrow, transmitted to chimpanzee from brain tissue inoculated intracerebrally.

TABLE 2.6 / Incubation Period and Duration of Experimental Disease in Cats on Primary Inoculation with CJD and/or Serial Passage in Cats[a]

Inoculum	Incubation (months)	Duration (months)
Human brain	30	2
Cat brain	19–24	4–5.5

[a] As of July 1, 1975.

two reports of conjugal disease with husband and wife dying of CJD within a few years of each other. (25, 37).

The prevalence of CJD has varied markedly throughout the United States and Europe; the diagnosis tends to be more frequent in many neurologic clinics since attention has been drawn to the syndrome by its transmission to primates (3, 28). For many large population centers of the United States, Europe, Australia, and Asia, we have found a prevalence approaching one per million with an annual incidence and a mortality of about the same magnitude, since the average duration of the disease is 8 to 12 months. Matthews (37) found an annual incidence of 1.3 per million in one of his clusters, which was over 10 times the annual incidence for the past decade for England and Wales (0.09 per million). Recently, Kahana et al. (31) reported annual incidence of CJD ranging from 0.4 to 1.9 per million in various ethnic groups in Israel. They noted, however, a 30-fold higher incidence of CJD in Jews of Libyan origin.

Transmission

Man-to-man transmission of CJD has been reported in a recipient of a corneal graft that was taken from a donor who in retrospect had pathologically confirmed CJD (11). The disease occurred 18 months after the transplant, an incubation period just average for chimpanzees inoculated with human CJD brain tissue (27, 46). Finally, the recognition of TVD in a neurosurgeon (22, 27) has raised the question of possible occupational infection, particularly in those exposed to infected human brain tissue during surgery, or at postmortem examination (45, 47). The unexpectedly high incidence of previous craniotomy in CJD patients, noted first by Nevin et al. (38) and, more recently, by Matthews (37) and ourselves (46), raises the possibility of brain surgery either affording a mode of entry for the agent or of precipitating the disease in patients already carrying a latent infection.

Two of the patients with TVD were neither diagnosed clinically nor neuropathologically as having CJD, but rather as having Alzheimer's disease (46). In both of these cases the disease was familial; in one (Fig. 2.10), there were six close family members with the disease in two generations. In the second, both the patient's father and sister died of presenile dementia. The disease transmitted to primates from both cases was typical subacute

31

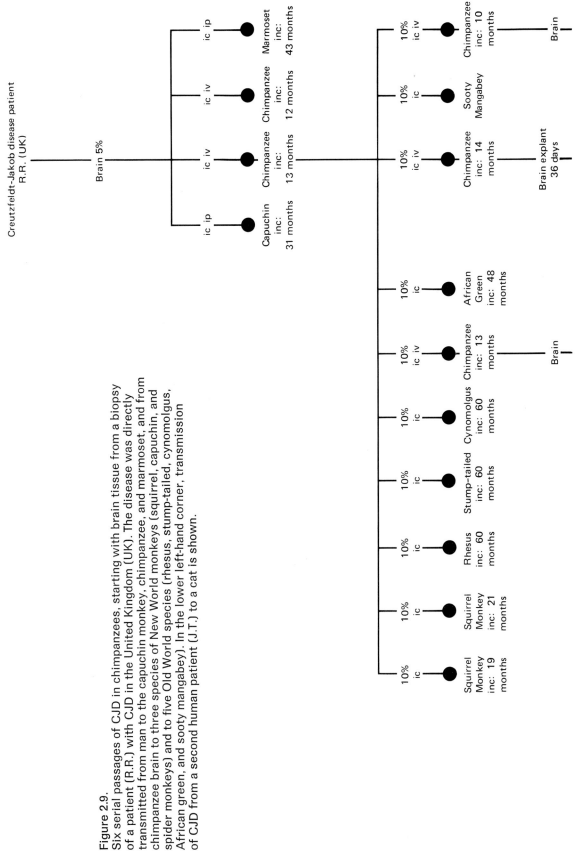

Figure 2.9.
Six serial passages of CJD in chimpanzees, starting with brain tissue from a biopsy of a patient (R.R.) with CJD in the United Kingdom (UK). The disease was directly transmitted from man to the capuchin monkey, chimpanzee, and marmoset, and from chimpanzee brain to three species of New World monkeys (squirrel, capuchin, and spider monkeys) and to five Old World species (rhesus, stump-tailed, cynomolgus, African green, and sooty mangabey). In the lower left-hand corner, transmission of CJD from a second human patient (J.T.) to a cat is shown.

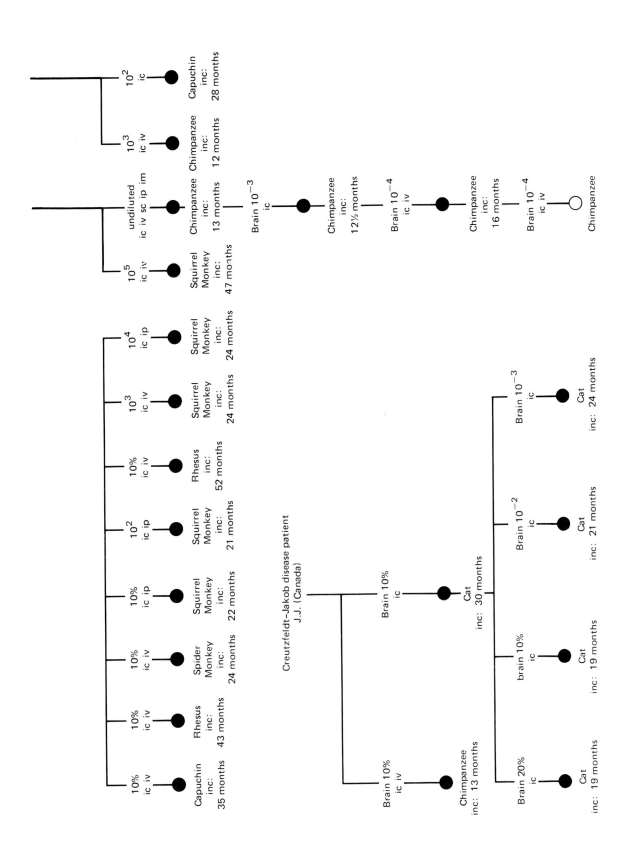

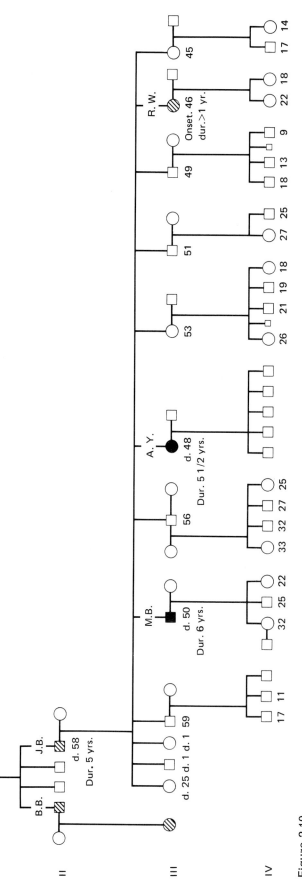

Family of A. Y.

Figure 2.10.
A family with six cases of Alzheimer's disease in two generations. Two of the cases were proved by pathologic examination. From the patient A.Y., a subacute spongiform encephalopathy was transmitted to a squirrel monkey on primary inoculation and successfully passed from this animal into two squirrel monkeys. Brain tissue from a second patient with familial Alzheimer's disease (in both father and sister) also caused subacute spongiform encephalopathy in an inoculated squirrel monkey. Box with diagonal rules, clinical evidence of Alzheimer's disease; solid box, clinical and pathologic evidence of Alzheimer's disease.

spongiform virus encephalopathy without the pathologic features of Alzheimer's disease. Over 30 additional specimens of brain tissue from Alzheimer's disease patients have been inoculated into TVD susceptible primates without producing disease. Thus we cannot claim to have transmitted the classic sporadic Alzheimer's disease to primates, but we are confronted with the fact that inoculation of brain tissues from the familial form of Alzheimer's disease has led to transmission of CJD.

SLOW VIRUS INFECTIONS IN ANIMALS

Scrapie

The clinical picture and histopathologic findings of scrapie closely resemble those of kuru; this permitted Hadlow (29) to suggest that both diseases might have similar etiologies. In 1936, Cuillé and Chelle (6) transmitted scrapie to the sheep; its filterable nature and other viruslike properties were demonstrated two to three decades ago (21). Since scrapie is the only one of the subacute spongiform virus encephalopathies that has been serially transmitted in mice, much more virologic information is available about this agent than about the viruses causing the human diseases.

Transmission

Scrapie may spread from naturally infected sheep to uninfected sheep and goats, although such lateral transmission has not been observed from experimentally infected sheep or goats. Both sheep and goats, as well as mice, have been experimentally infected orally. It appears to pass from ewes to lambs, even without suckling; the contact of the lamb with the infected ewe at birth appears to be sufficient, since the placenta itself is infectious (40). Transplacental versus oral, nasal, eye, or cutaneous infection in the perinatal period are unresolved possibilities. Older sheep are infected only after long contact with diseased animals; however, susceptible sheep have developed the disease in pastures previously occupied by scrapied sheep.

Both field studies and experimental work have suggested genetic control of the occurrence of the disease in sheep. In mice, there is evidence of genetic control of the length of the incubation period and of the anatomic distribution of the lesions that is also dependent on the strain of scrapie agent used. Scrapie has been transmitted in our laboratory to five species of monkeys (Tables 2.3 and 2.4) (19, 26, 27). Such transmission has occurred using infected brain from naturally infected sheep and experimentally infected goats and mice (Fig. 2.11). The disease produced is clinically and pathologically indistinguishable from experimental CJD in these species.

Unconventional Properties

The scrapie virus has been partially purified using fluorocarbon precipitation of proteins and density gradient banding, using the zonal rotor (Fig.

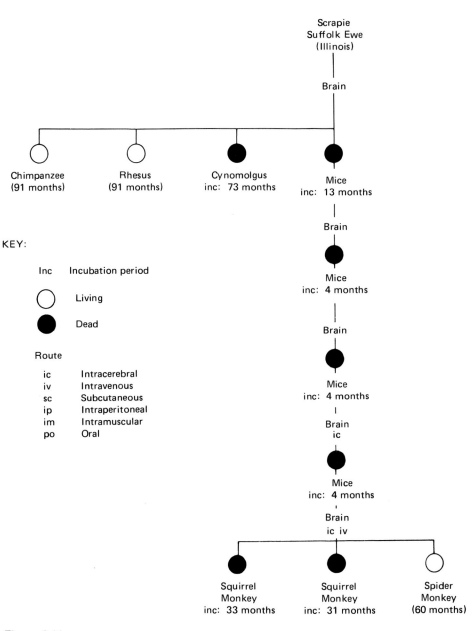

Figure 2.11.
Transmission of scrapie from the brain of a scrapie-infected Suffolk ewe in Illinois to a cynomolgus monkey and a mouse, and from the fourth mouse passage of this strain of scrapie virus to two squirrel monkeys.

2.12) (44). Other semipurified preparations have been made using ultra-filtration and repeated complete sedimentation and washing of the scrapie virus using ultrasonication for resuspension of the virus-containing pellets. As shown in Figs. 2.13a and b, the sucrose–saline density gradient banding of scrapie virus in mouse brains produced wide peaks of scrapie infectivity at densities of 1.14 to 1.23. A second smaller peak of high infectivity at densities of 1.26 to 1.28 disappeared on filtration of the crude suspension through 200 nm porous membranes (see Fig. 2.13b). On electron microscopic examination, fractions of high infectivity (10^7–10^8 LD_{50}/ml) revealed only smooth vesicular membranes with mitochondrial and ribosomal debris and no structures resembling recognizable virions. The UV absorptions at 260 and 280 nm (A_{260}; A_{280}) and the ratios of A_{260}/A_{280} for each of the fractions plotted against density are illustrated in Figs. 2.14a and b. Lysosomal hydrolases (N-acetyl-β-D-glucosaminidase, β-galactosidase, acid phosphatase) and mitochondrial marker enzyme (INT-succinate reductase) showed most of their activity in fractions of lower density than the region of high scrapie infectivity (Fig. 2.15) (44).

We have confirmed the previously noted resistance of scrapie virus to UV inactivation at 254 nm and UV inactivation action spectrum with a sixfold increased sensitivity at 237 nm over that at 254 or 280 nm (35). This may not be taken as proof that no genetic information exists in the scrapie virus as DNA or RNA molecules, since work with viroids indicates a similar resistance to UV inactivation in crude, infected plant-sap preparation. There is also a great effect of small RNA size on UV sensitivity, as has been shown by the high resistance with the purified, very small RNA (about 80,000 daltons) of tobacco ring spot satellite virus (8, 9). Partial purification by fluorocarbon treatment only slightly increases UV sensitivity at 254 nm (35) (Figs. 2.16a and b).

Fluorocarbon purified scrapie was not inactivated by RNAse I or III or by DNAse I. Autoclaving (121°C/20 psi/45 min) completely inactivates scrapie virus in crude suspensions of mouse brain.

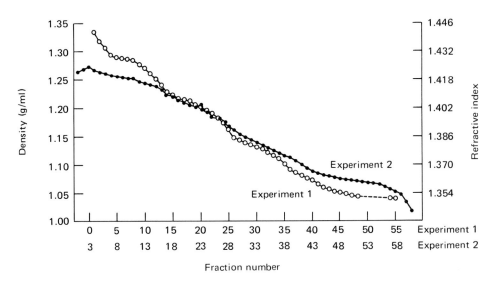

Figure 2.12.
Sucrose density profiles of scrapie-infected mouse brain of two zonal gradient experiments. The scale of *Experiment 2* has been shifted three fractions to the left, in order to obtain overlap of the curves. Refractive indices of the fractions have been converted to absolute densities.

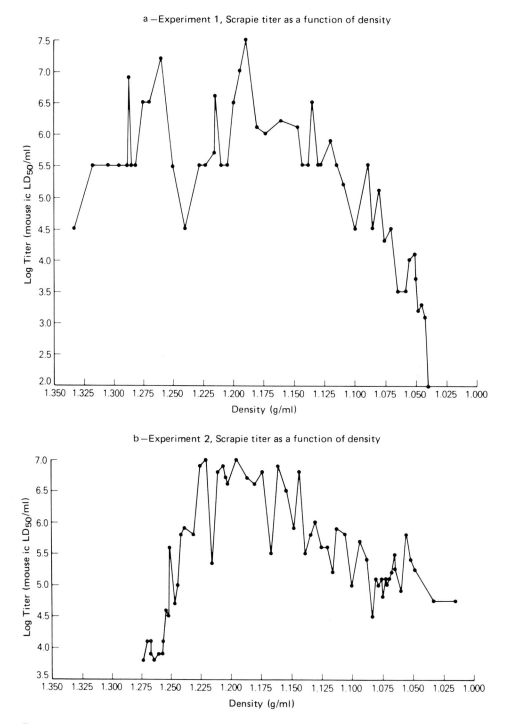

Figures 2.13**a** and **b**.
Infectivity titers of individual zonal fractions of scrapie-infected mouse brain,
expressed as mouse i.c. LD_{50}/ml, plotted against density for each of two experiments. Titers were computed by the method of Reed and Muench. The total recovery
of scrapie in (**a**) *Experiment 1* was 1.1% of the 1.7×10^{11} infective units added to
the gradient; in (**b**) *Experiment 2* it was 20% of the 9.5×10^{9} input infectivity. The
calculated standard error for infectivity titrations is ±0.24 with a final titration
error estimated to be ±0.50 log LD_{50}/ml.

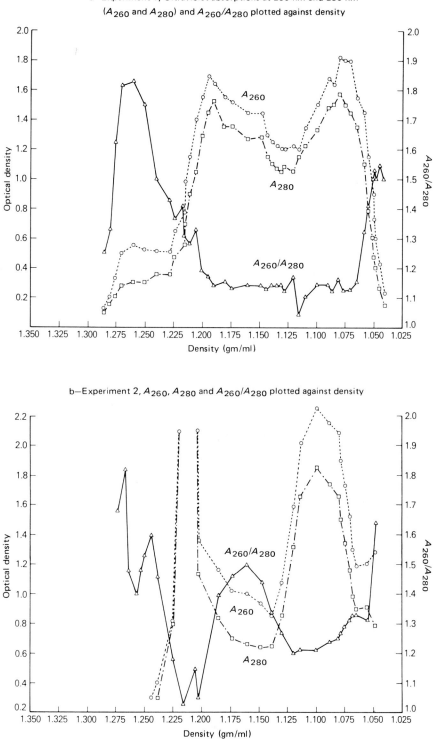

a—Experiment 1, Ultraviolet absorptions at 260 nm and 280 nm (A_{260} and A_{280}) and A_{260}/A_{280} plotted against density

b—Experiment 2, A_{260}, A_{280} and A_{260}/A_{280} plotted against density

Figures 2.14a and **b.**
Optical densities of zonal gradient fractions of scrapie-infected mouse brains plotted relative to their average density to facilitate comparison of two separate experiments.

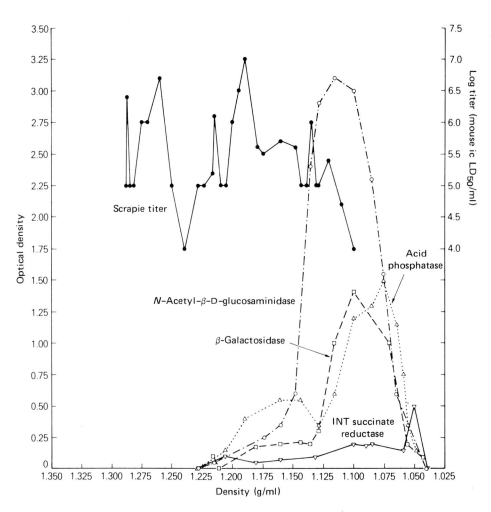

Figure 2.15.
Activity of three lysozomal enzymes and one mitochondrial enzyme plotted against density. Superimposed is a curve showing the scrapie infectivity titers of various fractions of given densities. The major part of all enzyme activity is at lower densities than the infectivity peaks.

Freeze Fracture Electron Microscopic Studies

Freeze fracture studies of membranes in the scrapie-affected mouse cerebellar cells have been initiated in the hope of better defining the membrane subunit structure we assume is the infectious agent of scrapie (10). Preliminary studies reveal no unique structures obviously related to virus particles inside the membranes, even those forming the walls of vacuoles. However, the innermost limiting membranes of vacuole in neurons and astrocytes show large areas devoid of usual 8 to 13 nm intramembranous particles. The astrocyte membranes around the vacuoles show abnormally high numbers of "assemblies," which are specific structures for astrocytes. The latter membrane changes might be an aspect of the astrocytic hypertrophy known to occur in scrapie. Preliminary studies already reveal the

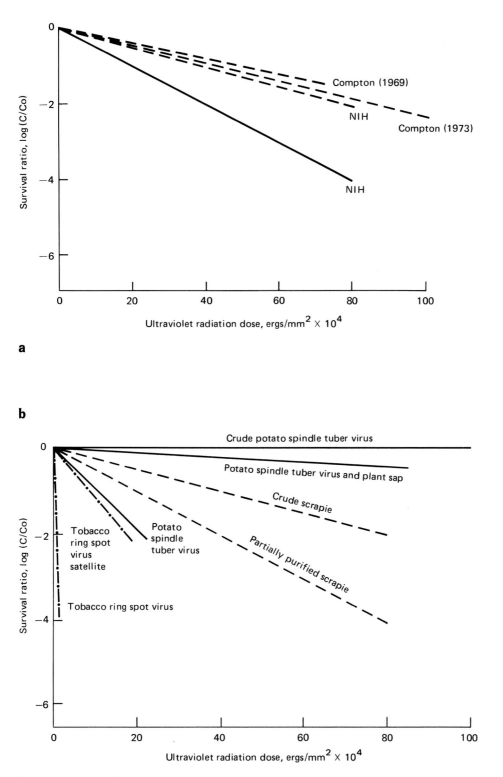

Figures 2.16a and **b.**
Inactivation of scrapie virus by UV irradiation **(a)** Dashed line, crude scrapie; solid line, partially purified scrapie. Comparison with potato spindle tuber viroid (PSTV) **(b)**.

same type of changes in CJD-affected cells. Too little is known about the appearance of various pathologic states in freeze fractured neural membranes to say whether any of these changes are specific to scrapie and CJD.

Transmissible Mink Encephalopathy

Transmissible mink encephalopathy (TME) is very similar to scrapie in clinical picture and pathologic lesions. On ranches where it developed, the carcasses of scrapie-infected sheep had been fed to the mink; presumably the disease is scrapie. The disease is indistinguishable from that induced in mink by inoculation of sheep or mouse scrapie. Like scrapie, TME has been transmitted orally, but transplacental or perinatal transmission from the mother has not been demonstrated. Physicochemical study of the virus has thus far revealed no differences between it and the scrapie virus.

The disease has been transmitted to the squirrel monkey, rhesus monkey, and stump-tailed monkey (Tables 2.3 and 2.4) (Fig. 2.17) and to many nonprimate hosts, including the sheep, goat, and ferret, but it does not transmit to mice (Table 2.5). In monkeys, the illness is indistinguishable from experimental CJD in these species.

SUBACUTE SPONGIFORM VIRUS ENCEPHALOPATHIES

Caused by Unconventional Viruses

Kuru and TVD belong to a group of slow virus infections that we have described as subacute spongiform virus encephalopathies, because of their similar cytopathic lesions (Table 2.1). The basic neurocytologic lesion in kuru, CJD, scrapie, and TME is a progressive vacuolation in the dendritic and axonal processes of neurons and, to a lesser extent, in astrocytes and oligodendrocytes; an extensive astroglial hypertrophy and proliferation; and finally, spongiform change or status spongiosus of gray matter (1, 2, 32, 33, 34). These atypical infections differ from other slow infections of the human brain in that they do not evoke an inflammatory response in the brain; they usually show no pleocytosis or any rise in protein in the cerebrospinal fluid throughout the course of infection; and they show no evidence of an immune response.

These unconventional viruses have unusual resistance to UV radiation and ionizing radiation (35); ultrasonication; heat; proteases and nucleases; and formaldehyde, β-propionolactone, ethylenediamine, and sodium deoxycholate. They are moderately sensitive to most membrane disrupting agents such as phenol (90%), chloroform, ether, urea (6 M), periodate (0.01 M), 2-chloroethanol, alcoholic iodine, acetone, and chloroform–butanol. They are not associated with a recognizable virion on electron microscopic study of infected cells *in vivo* or *in vitro*, neither are they concentrated in virus preparations by density gradient banding in the zonal rotor (44). This has led to the speculation (44) that they represent infectious agents lacking a nucleic acid, perhaps even a self-replicating membrane fragment. A major

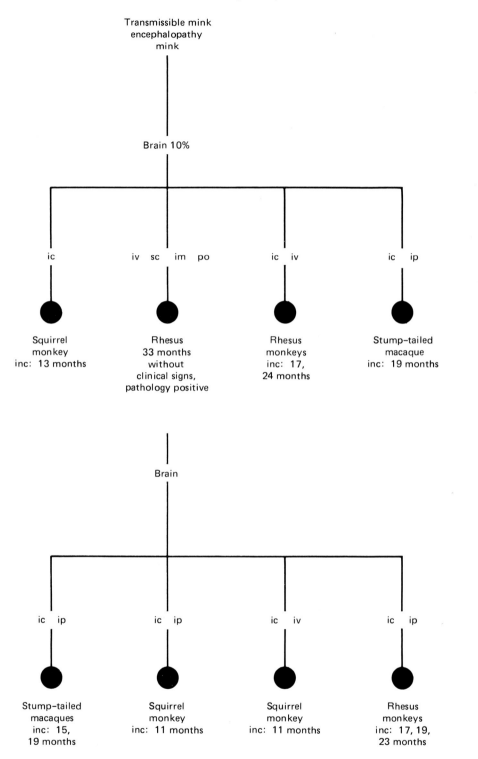

Figure 2.17.
Transmission of transmissible mink encephalopathy (TME) from mink to New and Old World monkeys. [Adapted from R. F. Marsh and R. J. Eckroade, personal communications.]

effort in this laboratory has been directed toward the molecular biologic elucidation of the nature and structure of this group of atypical viruses.

Conjectural Natural History: Hypothetical Origin of Creutzfeldt–Jakob Disease, Kuru, and Transmissible Mink Encephalopathy from Natural Sheep Scrapie

Scrapie has now been found to cause a disease clinically and neuropathologically indistinguishable from experimental CJD in three species of New World monkeys and two species of Old World monkeys (Table 2.3). This disease occurs after either intracerebral or peripheral inoculation. Natural sheep scrapie, as well as experimental goat and mouse scrapie, strains of virus have caused disease in the monkeys. One of the strains of scrapie virus (Compton strain), as a result of such passage through primates, develops an altered host range, for it no longer produces disease in inoculated mice. This is not true of the other strains of the virus that have been serially transmissible from monkeys to mice. However, a similar situation prevails when scrapie is produced in ferrets or mink; the mink or ferret brain virus is no longer pathogenic for mice.

Two years after inoculation in the squirrel monkey, CJD or kuru viruses may produce an acute central nervous disease and death in a few days, or simply sudden death without disease. In the spider monkey after incubation periods of 2 years or more, the same strains of kuru and CJD viruses produce chronic clinical disease closely mimicking the human disease. The time sequence of disease progression also mimics that in man, ranging from several months to more than a year. A single strain of kuru or CJD virus may cause severe status spongiosus lesions in many brain areas, particularly the cerebral cortex in chimpanzees and spider monkeys with minimal or no involvement of the brain stem or spinal cord, whereas this same virus strain may cause extensive stem and cord lesions in the squirrel monkey.

From the previous findings, it is clear that neither incubation periods nor host range nor the distribution or severity of neuropathologic lesions can be interpreted as having any significance toward unravelling the possible relationships of the four viruses causing the subacute spongiform virus encephalopathies.

We have presented in Fig. 2.18 a schematic conjectural natural history of the subacute spongiform virus encephalopathies in which the hypothetical origin of CJD, kuru, and TME from natural scrapie in sheep is proposed with possible routes of transmission indicated. In the absence of evidence of antigenicity or identified infectious nucleic acid in the agents, neither serologic specificity nor nucleic acid homology can be used to answer the compelling question of the relationship among the viruses of kuru, TVD, scrapie, and TME.

It is possible that the viruses of all four of the subacute spongiform virus encephalopathies are different strains of a single virus that has been modified in different hosts. The passage of sheep scrapie into other sheep and goats by feeding them material contaminated with placenta and em-

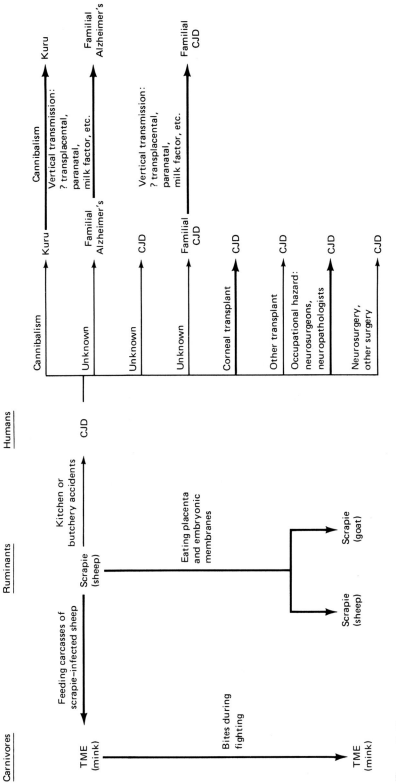

Figure 2.18.
Hypothetical origin of CJD, kuru, and TME from natural sheep scrapie. Established or highly probable routes of infection are indicated in bold face.

bryonic membrane (40) is an established method, as is transmitting scrapie into mink feeding on carcasses of scrapied sheep. In view of the experimental transmission of scrapie to monkeys, there is serious cause for wonder whether kitchen and butchery accidents involving the contamination of skin and eyes are a possible source of CJD in man. We believe that contamination during the cannibalistic ritual was the sole source of transmission of kuru from man to man, and have conjectured that a spontaneous case of CJD may have given rise to the chain of kuru transmissions (16). The mode of transmission, which at first sight would appear to be vertical in the cases of familial CJD or Alzheimer's disease, remains unknown (4, 12, 37, 46). Whether infection is transovarian, occurs *in utero* or during parturition, or can be obtained from a milk factor or some other neonatal infection also remains unknown, although from epidemiologic study of kuru (i.e., failure to see kuru in children born to kuru-affected mothers since the cessation of cannibalism), we have no evidence for such transmission (16).

PROSPECT

The elucidation of the etiology and epidemiology of a rare, exotic disease restricted to a small population has brought us to worldwide considerations that have importance for all of medicine and microbiology. For neurology, specifically, we have considerable new insights into the whole range of presenile dementias and, in particular, to the large problems of Alzheimer's disease and the senile dementias. The implications of vertical transmission of slow virus infections, host genetic control of disease expression for all genetic diseases, and the relationship of these slow virus infectious processes to those that may lead to neoplastic transformation are obvious.

However, the major problems among the degenerative diseases—MS, amyotrophic lateral sclerosis, and Parkinson's disease—remain unsolved, although there are tantalizing laboratory and epidemiologic data pointing to the possible role of viruslike agents in these diseases. Perhaps the masked and defective slow infections with conventional viruses such as are seen in PML and SSPE may give us the best leads for studying these diseases.

The foci of high incidence of amyotrophic lateral sclerosis with associated high incidence of parkinsonism–dementia complex among the Chamorro people on Guam and the Japanese of the Kii Peninsula remain continuing challenges. Our discovery (13) and reevaluation (17) of the very small but very intense focus of such motor neuron disease with associated high incidence of parkinsonism, parkinsonism–dementia, and other peculiar bradykinetic and myoclonic dementia syndromes among the Auyu and Jaqai people in a remote population of West New Guinea strongly suggests that some common etiologic factor may underlie the occurrence of all these very different syndromes. These relationships may be valid since they occur only in this one small population and not in the much larger, surrounding populations.

For a now-disappearing disease in a small primitive population to have brought us thus far is ample reason for pursuing intensively the challenges offered by the still inexplicable high incidence and peculiar profusion of different neurologic syndromes, pathologically distinct yet apparently somehow related to each other, which have been discovered in the several small population enclaves (13, 17).

REFERENCES

1. Beck, E., Bak, I. J., Christ, J. F., Gajdusek, D. C., Gibbs, C. J. Jr., and Hassler, R. (1975). Experimental kuru in the spider monkey. Histopathological and ultrastructural studies of the brain during early stages of incubation. *Brain* 98, 595–612.
2. Beck, E., Daniel, P. M., and Gajdusek, D. C. (1966). A comparison between the neuropathological changes in kuru and in scrapie, a system degeneration. In *Proceedings of the Fifth International Congress of Neuropathology* (F. Luthy and A. Bischoff, eds.), pp. 213–218. Excerpta Medica International Congress Series No. 100, Amsterdam.
3. Beck, E., Daniel, P. M., Matthews, W. B., Stevens, D. L., Alpers, M. P., Asher, D. M., Gajdusek, D. C., and Gibbs, C. J., Jr. (1969). Creutzfeldt–Jakob disease: The neuropathology of a transmission experiment. *Brain* 92, 699–716.
4. Bobowick, A., Brody, J. A., Matthews, M. R., Roos, R., and Gajdusek, D. C. (1973). Creutzfeldt–Jakob disease: A case control study. *Am. J. Epidemiol.* 98, 381–394.
5. Brownell, B., Campbell, M. J., and Greenham, L. W. (1975). The experimental transmission of Creutzfeldt–Jakob disease. Fifty-first Annual Meeting, American Association of Neuropathologists, May 30–June 1, New York, Program Abstract #32, pp. 46.
6. Cuillé, J., and Chelle, P.-L. (1936). Pathologie animale—La maladie dite tremblante du mouton est-elle inoculable? *C. R. Acad. Sci. [D] (Paris)* 203, 1552–1554.
7. Dawson, J. R., Jr. (1933). Cellular inclusions in cerebral lesions of lethargic encephalitis. *Am. J. Pathol.* 9, 7–16.
8. Diener, T. O. (1973). Similarities between the scrapie agent and the agent of potato spindle tuber disease. *Ann. Clin. Res.* 5, 268–278.
9. Diener, T. O. (1974). Viroids: The smallest known agents of infectious disease. *Ann. Rev. Microbiol.* 28, 23–39.
10. DuBois-Dalcq, M., Reese, T. S., Gibbs, C. J., Jr., and Gajdusek, D. C. (1975). Freeze fracture study of structural changes in the neural membrane of mice affected with scrapie. Abstracts, International Virology 5, Third International Congress for Virology, Madrid, Spain, September 10–17, Vol. 2, p. 48.
11. Duffy, P., Wolf, J., Collins, G., DeVoe, A. G., Streeten, B., and Cowen, D. (1974). Possible person-to-person transmission of Creutzfeldt–Jakob disease. *New Engl. J. Med.* 299, 692–693.
12. Ferber, R. A., Wiesenfeld, S. L., Roos, R. P., Bobowick, A. R., Gibbs, C. J., Jr., and Gajdusek, D. C. (1974). Familial Creutzfeldt–Jakob disease: Transmission of the familial disease to primates. In *Proceedings of the Tenth International Congress of Neurology* (A. Subirana and J. M. Burrows, eds.), pp. 358–380. Excerpta Medica International Congress Series No. 319, Amsterdam.
13. Gajdusek, D. C. (1963). Motor-neuron disease in natives of New Guinea. *New Engl. J. Med.* 268, 474–476.
14. Gajdusek, D. C. (1972). Spongiform virus encephalopathies. In *Host Virus Reactions with Special Reference to Persistent Agents* (G. Dick, ed.). *J. Clin. Pathol.* 25 Supplement, 78–83.
15. Gajdusek, D. C. (1973). Kuru and Creutzfeldt–Jakob disease. Experimental models of non-inflammatory degenerative slow virus diseases of the central nervous system. *Ann. Clin. Res.* 5, 254–261.

16. Gajdusek, D. C. (1973). Kuru in the New Guinea Highlands. In *Tropical Neurology* (J. D. Spillane, ed.), Chapter 29, pp. 376–383. Oxford Univ. Press, New York.

17. Gajdusek, D. C. (1975). Focus of high incidence of motor neuron disease associated with high incidence of parkinsonism and dementia syndromes in a small population of Auyu West New Guineans, unpublished data.

18. Gajdusek, D. C., and Gibbs, C. J., Jr. (1972). Subacute and chronic diseases caused by atypical infections with unconventional viruses in aberrant hosts. In *Perspectives in Virology: Persistent Virus Infections* (M. Pollard, ed.), Vol. 8, pp. 279–311. Academic Press, New York.

19. Gajdusek, D. C., and Gibbs, C. J., Jr. (1975). Familial and sporadic chronic neurological degenerative disorders transmitted from man to primates. In *Primate Models of Neurological Disorders* (B. S. Meldrum and C. D. Marsden, eds.). *Adv. Neurol. 10*, 291–317. Raven Press, New York.

20. Gajdusek, D. C., Gibbs, C. J., Jr., and Alpers, M. (1966). Experimental transmission of a kuru-like syndrome to chimpanzees. *Nature 209*, 794–796.

21. Gajdusek, D. C., Gibbs, C. J., Jr., and Alpers, M., eds. (1965). *Slow, Latent and Temperate Virus Infections*, NINDB Monograph No. 2, National Institutes of Health, PHS Publication No. 1378. U.S. Government Printing Office, Washington, D.C.

22. Gajdusek, D. C., Gibbs, C. J., Jr., Earle, K., Dammin, C. J., Schoene, W., and Tyler, H. R. (1974). Transmission of subacute spongiform encephalopathy to the chimpanzee and squirrel monkey from a patient with papulosis atrophicans maligna of Köhlmeier-Degos. In *Proceedings of the Tenth International Congress of Neurology* Barcelona, September 9–14. (A. Subirana and J. M. Burrows, eds.), pp. 390–392. Excerpta Medica International Congress Series No. 319, Amsterdam.

23. Gajdusek, D. C., and Zigas, V. (1957). Degenerative disease of the central nervous system in New Guinea. The endemic occurrence of "kuru" in the native population. *New Engl. J. Med. 257*, 974–978.

24. Gajdusek, D. C., and Zigas, V. (1959). Kuru: Clinical, pathological and epidemiological study of an acute progressive degenerative disease of the central nervous system among natives of the Eastern Highlands of New Guinea. *Am. J. Med. 26*, 442–469.

25. Garzuly, F., Jellinger, K., and Pilz, P. (1971). Subakute Spongiose Encephalopathie (Jakob-Creutzfeldt-Syndrom). Klinische-morphologische Analyse von 9 Fällen. *Arch. Psychiatr. Nervenkr. 214*, 207–227.

26. Gibbs, C. J., Jr., and Gajdusek, D. C. (1972). Transmission of scrapie to the cynomolgus monkey (*Macaca fascicularis*). *Nature 236*, 73–74.

27. Gibbs, C. J., Jr., and Gajdusek, D. C. (1975). Studies on the viruses of subacute spongiform encephalopathies using primates, their only available indicator. First Inter-American Conference on Conservation and Utilization of American Non-Human Primates in Biomedical Research, June 2–4, Lima, Peru. Scientific Publication No. 317, pp. 83–109, Pan American Health Organization, Pan American Sanitary Bureau, Regional Office of the World Health Organization, Washington, D.C.

28. Gibbs, C. J., Jr., Gajdusek, D. C., Asher, D. M., Alpers, M. P., Beck, E., Daniel, P. M., and Matthews, W. B. (1968). Creutzfeldt–Jakob disease (subacute spongiform encephalopathy): Transmission to the chimpanzee. *Science 161*, 388–389.

29. Hadlow, W. J. (1959). Scrapie and kuru. *Lancet ii*, 289–290.

30. Horta-Barbosa, L., Fuccillo, D. A., London, W. T., Jabbour, J. T., Zeman, W., and Sever, J. L. (1969). Isolation of measles virus from brain cell cultures of two patients with subacute sclerosing panencephalitis. *Proc. Soc. Exp. Biol. Med. 132*, 272–277.

31. Kahana, E., Alter, M., Braham, J., and Sofer, D. (1974). Creutzfeldt–Jakob disease: Focus among Libyan Jews in Israel. *Science 183*, 90–91.

32. Klatzo, I., Gajdusek, D. C., and Zigas, V. (1959). Pathology of kuru. *Lab. Invest. 8*, 799–847.

33. Lampert, P. W., Gajdusek, D. C., and Gibbs, C. J., Jr. (1972). Subacute spongiform virus encephalopathies. Scrapie, kuru and Creutzfeldt–Jakob disease. *Am. J. Pathol. 68*, 626–646.
34. Lampert, P., Hooks, J., Gibbs, C. J., Jr., and Gajdusek, D. C. (1971). Altered plasma membranes in experimental scrapie. *Acta Neuropathol. (Berl.) 19*, 81–93.
35. Latarjet, R., Gajdusek, D. C., and Gibbs, C. J., Jr. (1975). The UV action spectrum on scrapie virus. In preparation.
36. Manuelidis, E. E. (1976). Transmission of Creutzfeldt–Jakob disease from man to the guinea pig. *Proc. Nat. Acad. Sci. 73*, No. 1, pp. 223–227.
37. Matthews, W. B. (1975). Epidemiology of Creutzfeldt–Jakob disease in England and Wales. *J. Neurol. Neurosurg. Psychiatry 38*, 210–213.
38. Nevin, S., McMenemy, W. H., Behrman, S., and Jones, D. P. (1960). Subacute spongiform encephalopathy—A subacute form of encephalopathy attributable to vascular dysfunction (spongiform cerebral atrophy). *Brain 83*, 519–564.
39. Padgett, B. L., ZuRhein, G. M., Walker, D. L., Eckroade, R. J., and Dessel, B. H. (1971). Cultivation of papova-like virus from human brain with progressive multifocal leukoencephalopathy. *Lancet i* (7712), 1257–1260.
40. Pattison, I. H., Hoare, M. N., Jebbett, J. N., and Watson, W. A. (1972). Spread of scrapie from sheep and goats by oral dosing with fetal membranes from scrapie affected sheep. *Vet. Rec. 90*, 465–468.
41. Payne, F. E., Baublis, J. V., and Itabashi, H. H. (1969). Isolation of measles virus from a patient with subacute sclerosing panencephalitis. *New Engl. J. Med. 281*, 585–589.
42. Roos, R., Gajdusek, D. C., and Gibbs, C. J., Jr. (1973). The clinical characteristics of transmissible Creutzfeldt–Jakob disease. *Brain 96*, 1–20.
43. Sever, J. L., and Zeman, W., eds. (1968). Conference on Measles Virus and Subacute Sclerosing Panencephalitis. *Neurology 18*, 192.
44. Siakotos, A. N., Bucana, C., Gajdusek, D. C., Gibbs, C. J., Jr., and Traub, R. D. (1975). Partial purification of the scrapie agent from mouse brain by pressure disruption and zonal centrifugation in a sucrose–sodium chloride gradient. *Virology 70*, 230–237.
45. Traub, R. D., Gajdusek, D. C., and Gibbs, C. J., Jr. (1974). Precautions in conducting biopsies and autopsies on patients with presenile dementia. *J. Neurosurg. 41*, 394–395.
46. Traub, R., Gajdusek, D. C., and Gibbs, C. J., Jr. (1975). Transmissible virus dementias. The relation of transmissible spongiform encephalopathy to Creutzfeldt–Jakob disease. In *Aging, Dementia and Cerebral Function* (M. Kinsbourne and L. Smith, eds.). Spectrum Publishing, Inc., Flushing, N.Y.
47. Traub, R. D., Gajdusek, D. C., and Gibbs, C. J., Jr. (1975). Precautions in autopsies on Creutzfeldt–Jakob disease. *Am. J. Clin. Pathol. 64*, 2 (August), 287.
48. Weiner, L. P., Herndon, R. M., Narayan, O., Johnson, R. T., Shah, K., Rubinstein, L. J., Preziosi, T. J., and Conley, F. K. (1972). Isolation of virus related to SV-40 from patients with progressive multifocal leukoencephalopathy. *New Engl. J. Med. 286*, 385–390.
49. Zigas, V., and Gajdusek, D. C. (1957). Kuru: Clinical study of a new syndrome resembling paralysis agitans in natives of the Eastern Highlands of Australian New Guinea. *Med. J. Austr. 2*, 745–754.
50. ZuRhein, G. M., and Chou, S. (1968). Papova virus in progressive multifocal leukoencephalopathy. In *Infections of the Nervous System, Proceedings* (H. M. Zimmerman, ed.), Association for Nervous and Mental Diseases, Vol. 44, pp. 254–280. Williams and Wilkins, Baltimore.

Discussion/Chapters 1-2

Dr. Dickinson pointed out that his classification of the various scrapie agents was more agent-oriented than animal-oriented. Therefore, in his presentation, it was one strain of scrapie that produced more plaques than some other strain, rather than one genotype of mice that tended to have more plaques than some other genotype. The host component, he added, obviously could not be ignored, but the agent component was by far more important. This does not necessarily apply to other species, and might be the explanation for the difference between behavior of scrapie in mice and kuru in man.

In regards to amyloid, Dr. Kabat pointed out that it can be of two types: One type is composed of light chains of immunoglobulins and the other has a different composition. He thought that sequence analyses of the amyloid from these characteristic plaques might indicate whether it resulted from an immune response on the part of the host. Such an analysis might be relatively simple and quite fast, since the first half dozen amino acids on the end terminus would reveal whether the composition was an immunoglobulin light chain or something else.

Dr. Gajdusek agreed and added that in human diseases, such as Creutzfeldt-Jakob and Altzheimer's presenile dementia, the plaques could be readily obtained. This would be especially easy, because—as stated by Dr. Kabat—this analysis could be carried out on formalinized brain material.

At this point, Dr. Porter directed the discussion toward the consideration of size of scrapie. If one used the data obtained through radiation target size measurements, the size of this agent appeared to be between 100,000 and 150,000 daltons. Therefore scrapie and the related agents might be viroids. Dr. Porter claimed, however, that some of the experiments in his laboratory would tend to indicate that scrapie is not a viroid. He proposed that the agent in all probability is a conventional virus, but that it is being protected either by binding to the host cell membrane or by an active repair mechanism of the nucleic acid that gives erroneously small radiation inactivation target sizes.

At this point the discussion turned to the transmissibility of kuru and Creutzfeldt-Jakob disease (CJD), and Dr. Kurland suggested that missionaries—like neurosurgeons in Dr. Gajdusek's concept—were at an added risk for the development of this type of a disease. He cited a case of a 48-year-old minister who visited the highlands of New Guinea during a round-the-world trip and had come in contact with the Fore people. On the day of his arrival in the highlands, he became ill with an upper respiratory infection, but otherwise had remained well throughout the trip. Ten months later, he developed dysphagia, progressive weakness with rigidity, ataxia, myoclonus, dementia, and finally died after an illness of 4 months. On the basis of the clinical course and histopathology, the man's disease was diagnosed as CJD. The brain was homogenized and inoculated into squirrel monkeys. Eighteen months after the inoculation, one monkey began showing symptoms of a central nervous system disease, which histologically resembled a spongiform encephalopathy. The question remains whether this was kuru or CJD. Dr. Gajdusek concluded that it was CJD, because in his laboratory inoculation of this man's brain material into chimpanzees resulted in spongiform encephalopathy in 11 months, an incubation period that was much shorter than that for laboratory-transmitted kuru, but quite consistent with the incubation period of laboratory-transmitted CJD.

The discussion concluded with some comments about a resistance of these infectious agents to treatment with lipid solvents and proteolytic enzymes. This was in response to a question by Dr. Wecker whether a gentle extraction of lipids from the membrane fractions of the infectious material rendered the material non-infectious. Although this type of extraction had not been carried out, Dr. Gajdusek stated, all the lipid solvents such as chloroform, ether, 6 *M* urea, ethanol, and so on, do reduce the infectivity of scrapie, but do not inactivate it 100%. The extreme resistance of scrapie to these solvents and to nucleases, proteases, and formalde-hyde, as well as their extreme resistance to trichloroacetic acid, ethylene diamine, and β-proprionelactone is an established fact. Even treatment with hot formaldehyde of moderately purified material containing membranes has not sterilized it.

Comment/Chapters 1-2
C. A. Mims

All future basic research on scrapie must be with scrapie in the mouse, if only because this is such a simple, cheap, and comparatively short way of doing this work. My reaction to the preceeding papers was amazement at how precise and respectable research is becoming in this area, thanks especially to the efforts of people such as Dickinson and Gajdusek. Compared with scrapie research 20 years ago or so, coming upon Gajdusek and Gibbs' research is like coming upon the periodic table or the double helix after studying some medieval text on alchemy. The whole subject is alive and moving; the problems are being dissected and understood.

The agents causing these diseases may be regarded as conventional agents in the sense that they spread and multiply in the infected host during an incubation period. They are unconventional in a number of characteristics, but it is very important not to attribute a special mystique to them. Fundamentally, they multiply very slowly, at least as judged by the production of infectious units in the animal. For example, a scrapie growth curve calculated for an infected mouse brain indicates a doubling time of something from 4 to 7 days depending on the experiment. This is a very slow rate of replication. Two things follow from this very slow rate of replication. First, if there is even a trace of a host response, whether immune, interferon, or phagocytic, it would have a major inhibitory effect during this slow replication. Yet there is not the slightest flicker of such a response. The phagocytic response, which is a principal antimicrobial defense mechanism, has not been studied in these diseases, not even in scrapie in the mouse. What happens to scrapie in the phagocytes, in the polymorphonuclear cells, or in the macrophages? More careful studies of this sort should be carried out because phagocytosis may hold the key to the persistence of these agents in the body and might be of central importance in understanding the pathogenesis of these diseases. Second, once multiplication has begun, it continues inexorably. However, if there were any thermal inactivation of the sort seen in most other virus infections, scrapie would be destroyed faster than it was produced. Of course it is possible that it spreads without producing stable offspring in the infected host. Freshly formed scrapie would not have to be stable for more than 1 or 2 hours if it entered a new set of cells within that time. Thus thermal stability is of no consequence within a host, but it is much more important when it comes to transmission to a new host. How this spread to the new host takes place under natural circumstances remains a complete mystery.

Partly because of its thermal stability, scrapie can stay in the body for long periods. Many years ago, the group in Wisconsin showed that if the agent of transmissible mink encephalopathy is injected intraperitoneally into chickens or cattle, it is still detectable in the spleen 1 to 1.5 years later. We may presume that it does not replicate in either host, but if it persists in the spleen, we can ask in which cells it persists. Perhaps it will persist in macrophages or in lymphoid cells.

The whole story of scrapie research reveals an almost total neglect of the extraneural events in the pathogenesis of the disease. We are very much in danger of reaching the situation in which poliovirus research found itself 30 years ago after concentrating on highly neurotropic brain passaged strains of the virus. This led to an obsession with the behavior of poliovirus in the nervous system and a failure to appreciate the extraneural events that are responsible for the spread of the virus through the body. Scrapie research is getting into this sort of danger, and we need to make far more thorough studies of its extraneural pathogenesis.

We must ask intelligent questions. Immunologists can take cells apart, separate them, and make numerous subtle studies of their functional behavior. We must, therefore, get down to study of the spleen in scrapie and not be content with the mere identification and titration of the agent in this organ. Let us take the spleen out, take it apart, and identify the cells in which scrapie resides. Eklund showed many years ago that there is a very high titer of scrapie in the salivary glands of the mouse. Salivary glands provide a way out to the exterior, and thus could be involved in the spread of scrapie. No study of the salivary glands has been done except for titrations.

Gajdusek commented on the totally negative evidence for the spread of kuru either through placental transfer or breast milk. The ancestral virus might well have behaved differently, and one wonders whether neurologic passage has changed its properties, so that now we should not expect it to spread naturally from individual to individual. It is clear that we must look for the extraneural equivalent of kuru, as well as for the extraneural equivalent of Creutzfeldt–Jakob disease (CJD). The fact that CJD occurs in five continents in the world must mean that there is some common undercurrent of extraneural infection occurring in people all over the world, giving no pathology, evoking no antibody response, and only rarely giving rise to the neurologic disease.

Gajdusek and Gibbs' study presents several guidelines for the future. We must study extraneural scrapie and study the agent in phagocytic cells. We must look for an extraneural agent from this group, which is present as a common infection in man. An understanding of the replication and pathogenesis of these agents will come from studies of scrapie in the mouse.

CHAPTER 3
Sheep Progressive Pneumonia Viruses

DONALD H. HARTER

INTRODUCTION

Sheep throughout the world are susceptible to a viral progressive interstitial pneumonia. Recently, agents responsible for this disorder have been the object of much scientific scrutiny. On the one hand, they behave as conventional viruses; on the other, they produce disease after very long incubation periods. Moreover, they have many properties similar to those of RNA tumor viruses.

CLINICAL AND PATHOLOGIC FEATURES

Sheep progressive pneumonia was first described by Marsh in Montana flocks in 1923 (39). Similar afflictions have now been found in sheep flocks from many different countries. Most thoroughly studied have been maedi in Iceland (52, 75) and zwoegerziekte in Holland (10). The entity has also been reported in sheep from South Africa, France, Kenya, Scotland, India, and Germany. Sheep progressive pneumonia has been of serious economic consequence. In The Netherlands, the annual mortality reached 15% on individual farms (47). In Iceland, sacrifice of almost 200,000 sheep was necessary to control the disease (52).

Symptoms of sheep progressive pneumonia develop gradually with a 1- to 4-year incubation period. Affected sheep often lag behind the flock and breathe heavily, particularly when they are moving up a slope. There is little cough and no marked fever. As the disease progresses, the animal becomes emaciated; death occurs as the result of asphyxia.

At the time that maedi occurred in Iceland, a neurologic disease called visna was also observed (53, 54, 75). Signs of visna first appear after an incubation period of 1 month to 6 years and include unsteadiness of gait and abnormal head posture. Weakness of the hind legs occurs later and progresses to total limb paralysis. Fever is absent. The disease is invariably fatal. Before neurologic signs become manifest, virus can be recovered from spinal fluid, and there is persistent elevation of the spinal fluid cell count and protein content (17, 53, 54). Antibodies appear in serum during the asymptomatic phase of the disease (16, 17, 63, 75).

At death, virus can be recovered from brain, spleen, lung, kidney, salivary gland, and mediastinal lymph nodes (17). Gross pathologic changes include hyperplastic mediastinal lymph nodes and maedi-like pulmonary lesions (17).

Major histologic changes are limited to the nervous system (46, 54, 56). They consist of glial and pericapillary infiltration by lymphocytes, histiocytes, and plasma cells; glial fibrosis; and foci of demyelination. White matter lesions are seen at all levels of the nervous system; they are sub-ependymal or subpial in location and irregularly disseminated, and have no relationship to blood vessels.

At autopsy, the lungs do not collapse when the chest is opened, because they are consolidated. The only findings outside the lungs are enlarged bronchial and mediastinal lymph nodes. Histologic features are a chronic interstitial inflammation with dense cellular infiltration, hyperplasia of the smooth muscle in alveolar septa, and epithelial proliferation in small bronchi and bronchioles (14, 47). Frank neoplasms have not been reported.

VIRUS ISOLATION

Transmission of progressive pneumonia by intrapulmonary or intravenous inoculation of sheep with suspensions of lung and mediastinal lymph nodes from naturally affected Montana sheep was accomplished by Creech and Gochenour in 1936 (9, 11). Similar transmission of maedi, zwoegerziekte, and visna has been accomplished by inoculating healthy sheep with lung or brain suspensions from diseased sheep (10, 48, 53, 55).

Visna virus was the first member of the sheep progressive pneumonia virus group to be isolated in tissue culture (57). Isolates were initially obtained by inoculating infected brain homogenate into cell cultures obtained from ependyma and white matter of normal sheep brain. Visna virus was also recovered in explant cultures derived from the choroid plexus of sheep afflicted with visna. Virus was then passaged in tissue cultures prepared from explanted or trypsin-dispersed choroid plexus from normal sheep. Tissue culture-passaged visna virus has been found to cause characteristic visna disease after inoculation into unaffected animals (57).

Maedi virus was recovered from the lungs of Icelandic sheep using similar sheep choroid plexus (SCP) cell cultures (51). Maedi disease was produced in healthy sheep by injection of viral strains isolated in tissue culture (18). Lesions in the central nervous system indistinguishable from visna were also observed.

Most subsequent studies of visna and maedi viruses have employed SCP cultures, but cells derived from other sheep organs, including kidney, lung, liver, and testicles, have also been used. The Montana isolate, progressive pneumonia virus (PPV), and the Dutch zwoegerziekte agent replicate in similar sheep cell cultures (10, 29).

After inoculation of sheep cell cultures at multiplicities from 4 to 10 $TCID_{50}$/cell, progeny virus is first detected after a 16- to 20-hour latent period. An exponential increase in infective virus takes place over the next 15 to 36 hours (24, 66, 71). Virus development is accompanied by cytopathic changes culminating in destruction of practically the entire monolayer. The changes include the formation of elongated fibroblastic cells with refractile cytoplasm and large multinucleated cells with stellate process (Fig. 3.1).

When susceptible cells are inoculated with visna virus or PPV at high multiplicity (ca. 30 $TCID_{50}$/cell), cell fusion begins within 30 to 60 minutes; it progresses to involve the entire monolayer in 5 to 6 hours resulting in total destruction of the monolayer (15, 24, 37). Visna virus also promotes fusion of cells derived from a number of different animal species, including rodents, grazing mammals, and nonhuman primates (1, 3, 24).

VIRUS ULTRASTRUCTURE

Electron microscopy of visna virus-infected cells reveals two types of extracellular particles (8, 65) (Fig. 3.2). One is 65 to 100 nm in diameter and contains a 20- to 30-nm electron-dense core often surrounded by a membrane. It appears to represent the infective virus particle (Fig. 3.3). The

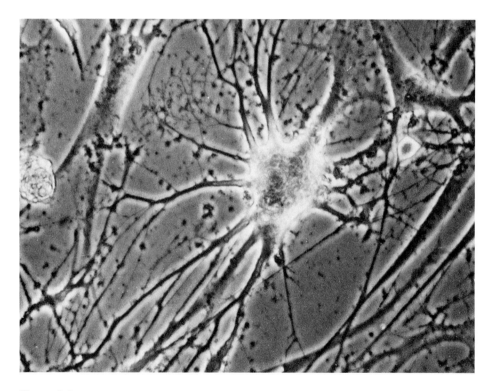

Figure 3.1.
Phase contrast photomicrograph of polykaryocytes with elongated cellular processes present in SCP culture 96 hours after visna virus inoculation. ×240 (courtesy of Dr. Joe E. Coward)

Figure 3.2.
Budding forms and extracellular particles in SCP culture 120 hours after
inoculation with visna virus. Smaller
particles containing electron dense
cores appear to represent mature
virions. ×50,000 (courtesy of Dr. Joe
E. Coward)

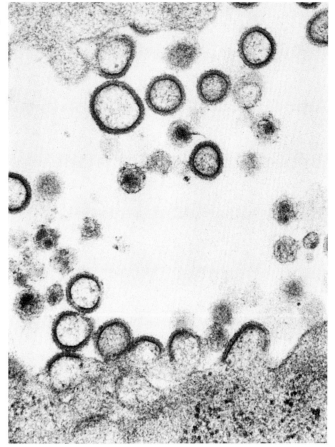

other is larger (100–140 nm), lacks a central dense region, and contains
material that is similar in appearance to the cell cytoplasm. It probably
originates from crescent-shaped budding structures at the cell membrane.
The budding forms, particles with electron-dense cores, and coreless particles are all antigenically related to visna virus as shown by indirect
immunoferritin staining (11).

In addition, visna- and PPV-infected sheep testicular cells and fetal
sheep lung cells contain intracytoplasmic multilayered spherical structures
(7, 38, 61) (Fig. 3.4). These concentric or spiral layers are 13 to 14 nm
thick and consist of a dense membranous component and a finely granular
zone of lesser density.

Negatively stained visna virus particles appear as pleomorphic spherical
structures varying in diameter from 900 to 1200 A (45, 60, 73). Projections
50 to 100 A long, surround the outer membrane of the virus.

Visna virions disrupted under controlled conditions and examined by
negative staining have a spherical nucleoid 800 A in diameter within the
viral envelope. The nucleoid contains filamentous structures 25 A in diameter coiled into a nucleocapsid helix of 70 to 80 A diameter (45).

COMPARISONS

Antigenic Relationships

Antibodies to visna virus have been demonstrated by neutralization, complement fixation, precipitation and immunofluorescence in serums from sheep with natural or experimentally induced visna or maedi (16, 57, 63, 72). Antibodies detected by immunofluorescence are formed in sheep shortly after infection but before neutralizing antibodies are detectable. Visna virus antibodies have also been identified by the use of a passive hemagglutination test with tanned sheep erythrocytes (28). The relationship between the appearance of antibodies and the slow evolution of the disease is not yet clear (75). Neutralizing antibodies are present chiefly in the IgG_1 class; low activity can be associated with IgM, but no significant activity is noted in the IgG_2 class (40).

Partial cross reaction has been found between visna and maedi viruses in neutralization tests (74). Some sheep afflicted with zwoegerziekte or Montana sheep disease develop neutralizing antibodies to visna virus (69). Cell cultures infected with PPV show immunofluorescence staining when exposed to visna virus antiserum (61). The currently available information appears to indicate that the viruses of the progressive pneumonia complex are immunologically related.

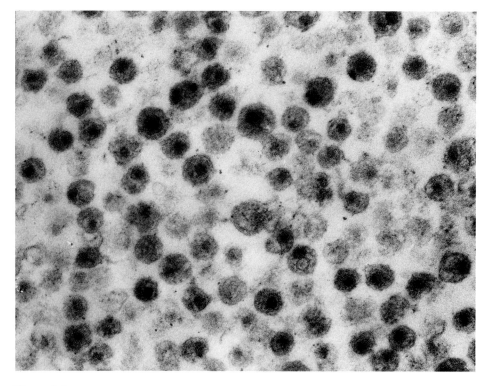

Figure 3.3.
Visna virus particles purified by cesium chloride density gradient centrifugation.
×70,000 (courtesy of Dr. Joe E. Coward)

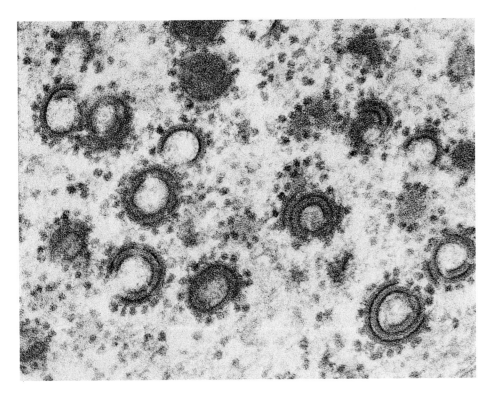

Figure 3.4.
Intracytoplasmic lamellar structures in sheep testes cell inoculated with visna virus.
× 100,000 (courtesy of Dr. Joe E. Coward)

PHYSICOCHEMICAL PROPERTIES

Visna and maedi viruses are readily inactivated by lipid solvents, meta-periodate, ethanol, phenol, formaldehyde, oxidized spermine, and trypsin (30, 67). Virus maintained in 1% sheep serum loses 90% of its infectivity after 4 months at 4°C, 9 days at 20°C, 24 to 30 hours at 37°C, and 10 to 15 minutes at 50°C (64, 67). Viral infectivity is relatively stable between pH 5.1 to 10 (64). Visna virus can withstand several cycles of rapid freezing and thawing as well as sonication (70); and it is unaffected by exposure to RNAse or DNAse (57). When irradiated with ultraviolet light, visna virus has resistance similar to that of avian oncornaviruses (67).

Although red blood cells from many different species have been tried, neither visna nor maedi virus has been found to cause hemagglutination; hemadsorption has not been seen in infected-cell monolayers (67). Purified visna virions, however, are capable of inhibiting the hemagglutination of influenza virus (6).

Nucleic Acid

The predominant nucleic acid species present in visna virions is a rapidly sedimenting (60–70 S), single-stranded RNA with a molecular weight of 10×10^6 to 12×10^6 daltons (3, 20, 24, 26). This high molecular weight

59

RNA contains long stretches of polyadenylic acid (15). It cosediments with the 60 to 70 S RNA extracted from Rous sarcoma virus (RSV) (20).

When 70 S visna virus RNA is heated to 80°C for 2 minutes, subunits are released that comigrate in polyacrylamide gel electrophoresis with the subunits of RSV RNA (20). The molecular weight of these subunits is 2.8×10^6 daltons indicating that there may be three or four subunits in the 70 S genome. Visna virus 70 S RNA can be completely dissociated into 35 S subunits by brief incubation at 37°C in 2.5×10^{-4} M EDTA (20). Denaturation of 66 S visna RNA (prepared from virus harvested every 2 hours) by heat, urea, or dimethylsulfoxide (DMSO) also produces a 36 S subunit (4).

Low molecular weight species (4–7 S) have been observed in rate zonal sedimentation studies of RNA extracted from visna virions (26, 34). In electrophoretic analysis, however, only a single low molecular weight RNA species migrating at 4 S (20) could be resolved; 5, 7, 18, and 28 S species such as those present in RSV were not detected.

Electron microscopic observations of visna virus RNA using the Kleinschmidt technique have been described (13). Visna virions disrupted by exposure to 0.05 or 0.1% sodium dodecyl sulfate (SDS) release an internal nucleic acid component in the form of rings or short curvilinear rods. Addition of DMSO to SDS-treated virus particles causes uncoiling of the rings and produces a heterogeneous population of single, unbranched filaments up to 9.3 μm long; these strands are similar to those observed in 60 to 70 S RNA recovered from glycerol velocity gradients. Prolonged exposure to DMSO causes denaturation of the viral RNA into short fragments with a mean length of 3.2 μm. The visna virus genome appears to consist of a molecule 9.3 μm long, which is composed of subunits and assumes a coiled configuration within the virus particle.

DNA Polymerase Activities

Visna, maedi, and PPV particles contain DNA polymerase activities similar to those found in oncornaviruses and primate syncytial virus (12, 33, 35, 49, 50, 58, 59). The product of the endogenous polymerase reaction is DNA, as shown by its resistance to RNAse and alkali digestion; its sensitivity to DNAse; and its density after centrifugation in cesium sulfate solutions (49).

The DNA produced by the visna virus polymerase reaction is synthesized in a two-step reaction; initial transcription of single-stranded DNA bound to template RNA is followed by the formation of double-stranded DNA (21). The second reaction is blocked by actinomycin D. The double-stranded DNA product represents only 5 to 10% of the viral genome. The single-stranded DNA made in the presence of actinomycin D contains sequences complementary to almost the entire viral genome.

Visna virus DNA polymerase has been separated into three enzymatically active polypeptides (32). The three enzymes differ in their pH optimum, sensitivity to N-ethylmaleimide, rate of catalytic reaction, and template preference. Polymerase I has a molecular weight of approximately 125,000 and appears similar to DNA polymerase of oncornaviruses.

Visna DNA polymerase activity is not inhibited by antisera directed against the polymerase of avian myeloblastosis virus (AMV), the Schmidt–Rupin strain of RSV or Rauscher murine leukemia virus (43, 44).

Proteins

The proteins of visna, maedi, zwoegerziekte, and PPV resemble one another (19). They appear to contain at least 15 polypeptides, of which one is phosphorylated and two or three glycosylated (19, 41). The carbohydrate-containing proteins are believed to be surface components of the virus (41). Like RSV, the bulk of total visna virion protein is in small polypeptides. The major polypeptide has a molecular weight of 25,000 to 30,000 daltons (19). However, they have distinctive small molecular weight polypeptides and a pattern of glycosylation that differs from that found in RSV particles (1936).

Intracellular Events in Viral Replication

Relatively little is known about the site and mode of synthesis of virus specific components in infected cells. Viral antigen detected by immunofluorescence remains confined to the cytoplasm of infected cells (25, 72).

Visna and maedi virus multiplication is inhibited by 5-bromodeoxyuridine when it is added 1 to 2 hours after infection (68). Actinomycin D added to visna-infected cell cultures as late as 24 hours after inoculation also interferes with virus multiplication (68). These effects suggest that a DNA intermediate was involved in viral replication. Such a virus specific DNA intermediate or provirus has been demonstrated in visna virus-infected SCP cells (22). Furthermore, the visna genome appears integrated into host cell DNA in a manner similar to that observed with oncornaviruses (22).

RELATIONSHIP TO ONCORNAVIRUSES (TABLE 3.1)

Takemoto and Stone reported that murine tissue cultures (AL/N and BALB/c) develop foci of altered spindle-shaped cells 3 to 4 weeks after exposure to either visna virus or PPV (62). Visna virus or PPV was "rescued" from the cultures by cocultivation with normal sheep testicular cells. When X-irradiated 3-week-old mice were inoculated with visna virus- or PPV-transformed AL/N cells, they developed fibrosarcomas. Although these observations have not as yet been confirmed and the presence of a latent oncornaviruses in the AL/N and BALB/c cells has not been fully excluded, the findings indicate that the sheep progressive pneumonia viruses may have oncogenic potential under special circumstances.

No serologic cross reactivity has been demonstrated between sheep PPV and several RNA tumor viruses. Antiserums to murine leukemia viruses and RSV fail to neutralize visna and maedi viruses (74). Ether-treated visna

TABLE 3.1 / Comparative Features of Sheep Progressive Pneumonia Viruses and Oncornaviruses

Similarities	*Differences*
Disease after long incubation period	Chronic inflammatory disease in sheep
Size and morphology of virion	Cytolysis in cell cultures
Maturation by budding from cell membrane	Prominent cell-fusing activity
60 to 70 S single-stranded RNA genome	Intracytoplasmic laminated structures
RNA-dependent DNA polymerase	Lack of antigenic relationship to RNA tumor viruses
Replication involving a DNA intermediate	Lack of nucleic acid sequence homology to representative RNA tumor viruses

virions do not give precipitates in gel diffusion test with group specific antiserums prepared against avian leukosis-sarcoma, murine leukemia-sarcoma, hamster leukemia-sarcoma, feline leukemia, mouse mammary tumor, or simian mammary tumor viruses (42). Furthermore, there appears to be no significant sequence homology between the nucleic acids of Rauscher murine leukemia and mouse mammary tumor viruses and those of visna and maedi viruses (23). Therefore, although visna and maedi viruses may utilize the same mode of intracellular replication as oncornaviruses, they are not serologically related and have distinctive nucleic acid genomes.

HOST RANGE

One other virus may be related to the PPV. This agent was isolated from cattle with persistent lymphocytosis; its ultrastructural appearance and syncytia-inducing properties are very much like the PPV (2, 76).

Whether infection with this group of agents is limited to sheep and other grazing animals remains to be answered. One would suspect that certain chronic pulmonary diseases of man may be due to similar viral agents. The histologic changes seen in lymphoid interstitial pneumonia most closely match the findings in the progressive viral pneumonia of sheep (31). Encephalitis and inflammation in subependymal regions and meninges have been reported in a patient with lymphoid interstitial pneumonia (27). It may be possible to detect infectious agents related to the PPV in tissues from patients with chronic pulmonary or neurologic disease by using methods currently being applied in the search for viruses in human tumors.

REFERENCES

1. August, M. D., and Harter, D. H. (1974). Visna virus-induced fusion of continuous simian kidney cells. *Arch. Gesamte Virusforsch. 44*, 92–101.
2. Boothe, A. D., and van der Maaten, M. J. (1974). Ultrastructural studies of a visna-like syncytia-producing virus from cattle with lymphocytosis. *J. Virol. 13*, 197–204.

3. Brahic, M., Tamalet, J., and Chippaux-Hyppolite, C. (1971). Virus visna: Isolement d'une molécule d'acide ribonucleique de haut poids moléculaire. *C. R. Acad. Sci. [D] (Paris) 272*, 2115–2118.

4. Brahic, M., Tamalet, J., Filippi, P., and Delbecchi, L. (1973). The high molecular weight RNA of visna virus. *Biochimie 55*, 885–891.

5. Bunge, R. P., and Harter, D. H. (1969). Cytopathic effects of visna virus in cultured mammalian nervous tissue. *J. Neuropathol. Exp. Neurol. 28*, 185–194.

6. Compans, R. W., and Harter, D. H. (1967). Unpublished observations.

7. Coward, J. E., Harter, D. H., Hsu, K. C., and Morgan, C. (1972). Ferritin-conjugated antibody labeling of visna virus. *Virology 50*, 925–930.

8. Coward, J. E., Harter, D. H., and Morgan, C. (1970). Electron microscopic observations of visna virus-infected cell cultures. *Virology 40*, 1030–1038.

9. Creech, G. T., and Gochenour, W. S. (1936). Chronic progressive pneumonia of sheep, with particular reference to its etiology and transmission. *J. Agric. Res. 52*, 667–679.

10. DeBoer, G. F. (1970). Zwoegerziekte, een persisterende virusinfectie bij schapen. Thesis, University of Utrecht, Utrecht, Drukkerij.

11. Duran-Reynals, F., Jungherr, E., Cuba-Caparo, A., Rafferty, K. A., Jr., and Helmboldt, C. (1958). The pulmonary adenomatosis complex in sheep. *Ann. N.Y. Acad. Sci. 70*, 726–742.

12. Filippi, P., Brahic, M., Tamalet, J., and Delbecchi, L. (1972). L'ADN polymerase ARN dépendante du virus visna. Etude des produits de la réaction. *C. R. Acad. Sci. [D] (Paris) 275*, 1567–1570.

13. Friedmann, A., Coward, J. E., Harter, D. H., Lipset, J. S., and Morgan, C. (1974). Electron microscopic studies of visna virus ribonucleic acid. *J. Gen. Virol. 25*, 93–104.

14. Georgsson, G., and Pálsson, P. A. (1971). The histopathology of maedi. A slow, viral pneumonia of sheep. *Pathol. Vet. 8*, 63–80.

15. Gillespie, D., Takemoto, K. K., Robert, M., and Gallo, R. C. (1973). Polyadenylic acid in visna virus RNA. *Science 179*, 1328–1330.

16. Gudnadóttir, M., and Kristinsdóttir, K. (1967). Complement-fixing antibodies in sera of sheep affected with visna and maedi. *J. Immunol. 98*, 663–667.

17. Gudnadóttir, M., and Pálsson, P. A. (1966). Host-virus interaction in visna infected sheep. *J. Immunol. 95*, 1116–1120.

18. Gudnadóttir, M., and Pálsson, P. A. (1967). Transmission of maedi by inoculation of a virus grown in tissue culture from maedi-affected lungs. *J. Infect. Dis. 117*, 1–6.

19. Haase, A. T., and Baringer, J. R. (1974). The structural polypeptides of RNA slow viruses. *Virology 57*, 238–250.

20. Haase, A. T., Garapin, A. C., Faras, A. J., Taylor, J. M., and Bishop, J. M. (1974). A comparison of the high molecular weight RNAs of visna virus and Rous sarcoma virus. *Virology 57*, 259–270.

21. Haase, A. T., Garapin, A. C., Faras, A. J., Varmus, H. E., and Bishop, J. M. (1974). Characterization of the nucleic acid product of the visna virus RNA dependent DNA polymerase. *Virology 57*, 251–258.

22. Haase, A. T., and Varmus, H. E. (1973). Demonstration of a DNA provirus in the lytic growth of visna virus. *Nature 254*, 237–239.

23. Harter, D. H., Axel, R., Burny, A., Gulati, S., Schlom, J., and Spiegelman, S. (1973). The relationship of visna, maedi and RNA tumor viruses as studied by molecular hybridization. *Virology 52*, 287–291.

24. Harter, D. H., and Choppin, P. W. (1967). Cell fusing activity of visna virus particles. *Virology 31*, 279–288.

25. Harter, D. H., Hsu, K. C., and Rose, H. M. (1967). Immunofluorescence and cytochemical studies of visna virus in cell culture. *J. Virol. 1*, 1265–1270.

26. Harter, D. H., Schlom, J., and Spiegelman, S. (1971). Characterization of visna virus nucleic acid. *Biochim. Biophys. Acta 240*, 435–441.

27. Jefferson, M., Riddoch, D., and Smith, W. T. (1971). Fatal encephalopathy complicating lymphoid interstitial pneumonia. *J. Neurol. Neurosurg. Psychiatry 34*, 341–347.
28. Karl, S. C., and Thormar, H. (1971). Antibodies produced by rabbits immunized with visna virus. *Infect. Immun. 4*, 715–719.
29. Kennedy, R. C., Eklund, C. M., Lopez, C., and Hadlow, W. J. (1968). Isolation of a virus from the lungs of Montana sheep affected with progressive pneumonia. *Virology 35*, 483–484.
30. Kremzner, L. T., and Harter, D. H. (1970). Antiviral activity of oxidized polyamines and aldehydes. *Biochem. Pharmacol. 19*, 2541–2550.
31. Liebow, A. A. (1968). New concepts and entities in pulmonary disease. In *The Lung*, International Academy of Pathology Monograph No. 8 (A. A. Liebow and D. E. Smith, eds.), pp. 332–365. Williams and Wilkins, Baltimore.
32. Lin, F. H., Genovese, M., and Thormar, H. (1973). Multiple activities of DNA polymerase from visna virus. *Prep. Biochem. 3*, 525–539.
33. Lin, F. H., and Thormar, H. (1970). Ribonucleic acid-dependent deoxyribonucleic acid polymerase in visna virus. *J. Virol. 6*, 702–704.
34. Lin, F. H., and Thormar, H. (1971). Characterization of ribonucleic acid from visna virus. *J. Virol. 7*, 582–587.
35. Lin, F. H., and Thormar, H. (1972). Properties of maedi nucleic acid and the presence of ribonucleic acid- and deoxyribonucleic acid-dependent deoxyribonucleic acid polymerase in the virions. *J. Virol. 10*, 228–233.
36. Lin, F. H., and Thormar, H. (1974). Substructures and polypeptides of visna virus. *J. Virol. 14*, 782–790.
37. Lopez, C., Eklund, C. M., and Hadlow, W. J. (1971). Tissue culture studies of the virus of progressive pneumonia, a slow infectious disease of sheep. *Proc. Soc. Exp. Biol. Med. 138*, 1035–1040.
38. Malmquist, W. A., Krauss, H. H., Moulton, J. E., and Wandera, J. G. (1972). Morphologic study of virus-infected lung cell cultures from sheep pulmonary adenomatosis (Jaagsiekte). *Lab. Invest. 26*, 528–533.
39. Marsh, H. (1923). Progressive pneumonia in sheep. *J. Am. Vet. Med. Assoc. 15*, 458–473.
40. Mehta, P. D., and Thormar, H. (1974). Neutralizing activity in isolated serum antibody fractions from visna-infected sheep. *Infect. Immunol. 10*, 678–680.
41. Mountcastle, W. E., Harter, D. H., and Choppin, P. W. (1972). The proteins of visna virus. *Virology 47*, 542–545.
42. Nowinski, R. C., Edynak, E., and Sarkar, N. H. (1971). Serological and structural properties of Maron-Pfizer monkey virus isolated from the mammary tumor of a rhesus monkey. *Proc. Natl. Acad. Sci. U.S.A. 68*, 1608–1612.
43. Nowinski, R. C., Watson, K. T., Yaniv, A., and Spiegelman, S. (1972). Serological analysis of the deoxyribonucleic acid polymerase of avian oncornaviruses. II. Comparison of avian deoxyribonucleic acid polymerases. *J. Virol. 10*, 959–964.
44. Parks, W. P., Scolnick, E. M., Ross, J., Todaro, G. J., and Aaronson, S. A. (1972). Immunological relationships of reverse transcriptases from ribonucleic acid tumor viruses. *J. Virol. 9*, 110–115.
45. Pautrat, G., Tamalet, J., Chippaux-Hyppolite, C., and Brahic, M. (1971). Etude de la structure du virus Visna en microscopie électronique. *C. R. Acad. Sci. [D] (Paris) 273*, 653–655.
46. Pette, E., Mannweiler, K., and Palacios, O. (1961). Die Visnakrankheit der Schafe. Beitrag zum Problem der virusbedington Granulomencephalomyelitis. *Z. Neurol. 182*, 635–651.
47. Ressang, A. A., DeBoer, G. F., and deWijn, C. G. (1968). The lung in zwoegerziekte. *Pathol. Vet. 5*, 353–369.
48. Ressang, A. A., Stamm, F. C., and DeBoer, G. F. (1966). A meningoleucoencephalomyelitis resembling visna in Dutch zwoeger sheep. *Pathol. Vet. 3*, 401–411.

49. Schlom, J., Harter, D. H., Burny, A., and Spiegelman, S. (1971). DNA polymerase activities in virions of visna virus, a causative agent of a "slow" neurological disease. *Proc. Natl. Acad. Sci. U.S.A. 68*, 182–186.
50. Scolnick, E., Rands, E., Aaronson, S. A., and Todaro, G. J. (1970). RNA-dependent DNA polymerase activity in five RNA viruses: divalent cation requirements. *Proc. Natl. Acad. Sci. U.S.A. 67*, 1789–1796.
51. Sigurdardóttir, B., and Thormar, H. (1964). Isolation of a viral agent from the lungs of sheep affected with maedi. *J. Infect. Dis. 114*, 55–60.
52. Sigurdsson, B., Grimsson, H., and Pálsson, P. A. (1952). Maedi, a chronic progressive infection of sheep's lung. *J. Infect. Dis. 90*, 233–241.
53. Sigurdsson, B., and Pálsson, P. A. (1958). Visna of sheep. A slow, demyelinating infection. *Br. J. Pathol. 39*, 519–528.
54. Sigurdsson, B., Pálsson, P. A., and Grimsson, H. (1957). Visna, a demyelinating transmissible disease of sheep. *J. Neuropathol. Exp. Neurol. 16*, 389–403.
55. Sigurdsson, B., Pálsson, P. A., and Tryggvadóttir, A. (1953). Transmission experiments with maedi. *J. Infect. Dis. 93*, 166–175.
56. Sigurdsson, B., Pálsson, P. A., and van Bogaert, L. (1962). Pathology of visna. Transmissible demyelinating disease in sheep in Iceland. *Acta Neuropathol. (Berl.) 1*, 343–362.
57. Sigurdsson, B., Thormar, H., and Pálsson, P. A. (1960). Cultivation of visna virus in tissue culture. *Arch. Gesamte Virusforsch. 10*, 368–381.
58. Stone, L. B., Scolnick, E., Takemoto, K. K., and Aaronson, S. A. (1971). Visna virus: A slow virus with an RNA dependent DNA polymerase. *Nature 229*, 257.
59. Stone, L. B., Takemoto, K. K., and Martin, M. A. (1971). Physical and biochemical properties of progressive pneumonia virus. *J. Virol. 8*, 573–578.
60. Takemoto, K. K., Aoki, T., Garon, C., and Sturm, M. M. (1973). Comparative studies on visna, progressive pneumonia and Rous sarcoma viruses by electron microscopy. *J. Natl. Cancer Inst. 50*, 543–547.
61. Takemoto, K. K., Mattern, C. F. T., Stone, L. B., Coe, J. E., and Lavelle, G. (1971). Antigenic and morphological similarities of progressive pneumonia virus, a recently isolated "slow virus" of sheep, to visna and maedi viruses. *J. Virol. 7*, 301–308.
62. Takemoto, K. K., and Stone, L. B. (1971). Transformation of murine cells by two "slow viruses"; visna virus and progressive pneumonia virus. *J. Virol. 7*, 770–775.
63. Terpstra, C., and DeBoer, G. F. (1973). Precipitating antibodies against maedi-visna virus in experimentally infected sheep. *Arch. Gesamte Virusforsch. 43*, 53–62.
64. Thormar, H. (1960). Stability of visna virus in infectious tissue culture fluid. *Arch. Gesamte Virusforsch. 10*, 501–509.
65. Thormar, H. (1961). An electron microscope study of tissue cultures infected with visna virus. *Virology 14*, 463–475.
66. Thormar, H. (1963). The growth cycle of visna in monolayer cultures of sheep cells. *Virology 19*, 273–278.
67. Thormar, H. (1965). A comparison of visna and maedi viruses. I. Physical, chemical and biological properties. *Res. Vet. Sci. 6*, 117–129.
68. Thormar, H. (1965). Effect of 5-bromodeoxyuridine and actinomycin D on the growth of visna virus in cell cultures. *Virology 26*, 36–43.
69. Thormar, H. (1966). A study of maedi virus. In *Third International Conference on Lung Tumours in Animals, Univ. Perugia, 1965* (L. Sereri, ed.), pp. 393–402. Perugia, Italy.
70. Thormar, H. (1966). Physical, chemical and biological properties of visna virus and its relationship to other animal viruses. In *Slow, Latent, and Temperate Virus Infections*, N.I.N.D.B. Monograph No. 2, pp. 335–340. Washington, D.C.
71. Thormar, H. (1967). Cell-virus interactions in tissue cultures infected with visna and maedi viruses. *Curr. Top. Microbiol. Immunol. 40*, 22–32.
72. Thormar, H. (1969). Visna and maedi virus antigen in infected cell cultures

studied by the fluorescent antibody technique. *Acta Pathol. Microbiol. Scand. 75,* 296–302.

73. Thormar, H., and Cruickshank, J. G. (1965). The structure of visna virus studied by the negative staining technique. *Virology 25,* 145–148.

74. Thormar, H., and Helgadóttir, H. (1965). A comparison of visna and maedi viruses. II. Serological relationship. *Res. Vet. Sci. 6,* 456–465.

75. Thormar, H., and Pálsson, P. A. (1967). Visna and maedi-two slow infections of sheep and their etiological agents. In *Perspectives in Virology,* Vol. 5 (M. Pollard, ed.), pp. 291–304. Academic Press, New York.

76. Van Der Maaten, M. J., Boothe, A. D., and Seger, C. L. (1972). Isolation of a virus from cattle with persistent lymphocytosis. *J. Natl. Cancer Inst. 49,* 1649–1657.

Discussion / Chapter 3

Dr. Mims initiated the discussion by asking why a virus, such as visna, which has a conventional cycle of 1 to 2 days and which is detectable in the animal within a few weeks, causes the disease years later. This prompted Dr. Weiss to comment that in Germany the related disease, progressive pneumonia, is rather common, but that it rarely occurs in a coincidence with encephalitis. Therefore it is likely that the answer lies in the extraneural events and that in visna, as in progressive pneumonia, the extraneural infection proceeds at a relatively rapid pace, and under certain circumstances it may affect the central nervous system and produce a slow encephalitis.

Dr. Bloom inquired whether visna virus transformed nonsheep cells *in vitro*. Dr. Harter responded that Takemoto did report such a transformation. He cautioned, however, that Takemoto's results were not subjected then to the type of scrutiny that would now be required in order to establish the absence of an endogenous tumor virus in the cell lines that the investigator used for transformation. Moreover, these cell lines are no longer available; therefore, the unsuccessful attempts to reproduce transformation, such as those of Thormar, did not strictly repeat what Takemoto has reported.

Dr. Dickinson suggested that the best control for the types of studies Dr. Dubois–Dalcq described might be normal, uninfected animals, whose brain tissue was damaged by manifestly toxic chemicals, such as hexachlorophene. Although this has not yet been done, responded Dr. Dubois–Dalcq, the work is now being planned. Dr. Choppin criticized the use of "complete" and "infectious" virus particles, on the basis of their ultrastructural appearance. He pointed out that the infectious particle might be the one shown in Dr. Dubois–Dalcq's pictures as the "intermediate step." The particles constituting the majority of those seen under electron microscope need not necessarily be complete, but may in fact be degradation products. For example, in the case of RNA tumor viruses, whose infectivity rate is very high, there are changes in the nucleic acids through degradation. What is seen ultrastructurally is not the complete particles, but the degraded ones. It is important, therefore, to be cautious about concluding what *the* infectious agent is, when one views the morphology alone.

Dr. Gajdusek asked Dr. Harter to express an opinion about the relationship between the foamy viruses of primates, which are members of the subgroup of oncorna viruses that does not produce transformation, and the visna subgroup. Dr. Harter replied that this relationship is yet to be established, because there are at present no immunologic studies to suggest such a relationship.

Comment/ Chapter 3
Monique Dubois-Dalcq

Dr. Harter demonstrated for us the structure of visna virus. I would like to elaborate this subject by pointing out the difference in size between the budding virus and the complete virus (Fig. 3A.1). The buds are almost twice the size of the complete virus. Serial sections reveal occasionally a cross-sectional view of the buds, which may falsely appear as detached virus. In reality, however, the majority of particles are not detached and we have hypothesized that the truly detached units have a very short life span and become quickly converted into the complete virus with its dense core. The development of a complete virus involves an intermediate stage during which the dense material appears in a crescent, but is later rearranged in its final form of dense core. Not all of these steps have become apparent and, somewhere in this process, a certain quantity of membrane material disappears.

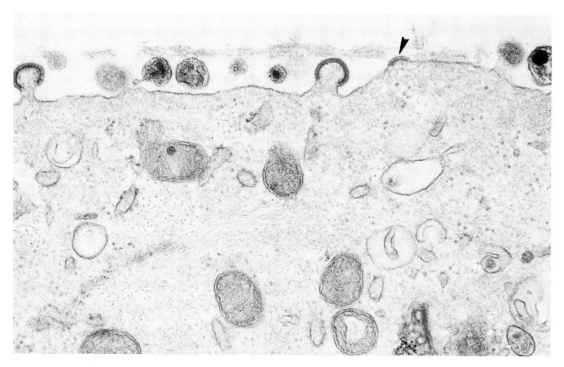

Figure 3A.1.
Thin section of sheep choroid plexus cell 7 days after inoculation. This productive cell has one small (arrow) and two larger crescent buds. The left one is attached to the cell only by a narrow cytoplasmic neck. Along the cell, several viral particles, apparently detached from the cell, are pleomorphic in size and structure. Note that the small particle with a central core is approximately half the size of the adjacent viral bud. Larger particles contain two dense cores of membrane fragments. ×60,000.

Figure 3A.2.
Note difference in size and structure between the visna viral bud and the bud of a type C endogenous virus found in a mouse cell line (inset). In the case of visna, the dense crescent material, corresponding to the nucleoprotein material, is closely apposed to the plasmalemma which is covered with discrete surface projections. In contrast the hemicrescent of the type C bud is not so close to the unit membrane. ×135,000

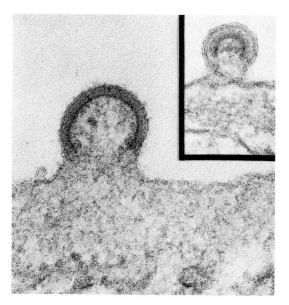

Figure 3A.2 illustrates the difference between the budding visna virus and that of type C particles in a RNA tumor virus of the mouse.

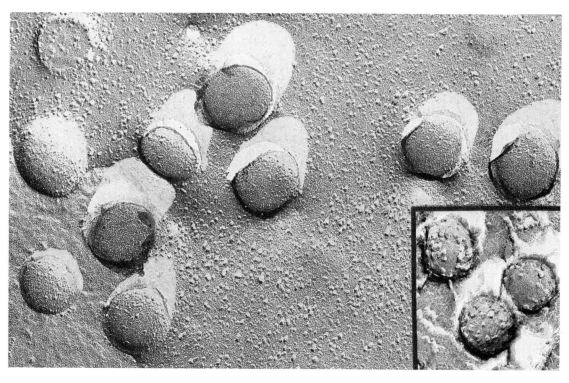

Figure 3A.3.
Replica of freeze-fractured plasmalemma of sheep choroid plexus cells infected with visna virus. Several viral buds are identified on this inner membrane leaflet characterized by numerous 85 A intramembranous particles. Few of them, if any, are present on the viral buds. In the inset, the true outer surface of viral buds has been revealed after deep etching. They are covered with subunits which are of irregular size (10–20 nm) and space. ×120,000

The mechanism and structure of budding can be better examined by the freeze etching technique. This technique permits cleaving of the inner and outer leaflet of the membrane by fracturing these membranes in the cold under conditions of high vacuum. Thus the inside of the membrane becomes visible. Figure 3A.3 provides a panoramic view of the inside of such a membrane. In contrast to pictures of thin sections, which reveal only few buds, this technique permits a simultaneous view of many buds.

Comment/Chapter 3
G. Petursson

Dr. Harter has given a very good, complete description of the general properties of visna virus, referring briefly to the disease process and the problems of pathogenesis. Some of the work on the pathogenesis of Visna currently being carried out at our institute in collaboration with G. Georgsson, P. A. Pálsson, H. Panitch, and N. Nathanson defines the role of immunologic responses of visna-infected sheep in the pathogenesis of the disease. In the early days of these investigations, M. Gudnadóttir and P. A. Pálsson infected a group of 24 sheep with visna virus and reported that the preclinical incubation period varied from 3 months to 8.5 years. Two of the animals were killed close to the end of their normal lifespan without ever developing signs of the disease. The infection is slow indeed. If animals are studied during this silent incubation period, however, the development of pathologic changes is not seen to be very slow after all. As early as 2 weeks after intracerebral injection, some animals display pleocytosis of the cerebrospinal fluid (CSF). In most animals, this reaches a maximum 1 month later and then slowly decreases in an irregular manner. The majority of the sheep continued to have elevated CSF cell counts during the first year of infection.

Infectious virus can be readily isolated from the CSF during the first month of infection but not later. Isolation of the virus is possible for 2 weeks after infection, and from the buffy coat of at least 25% of the animals throughout the course of the disease. Virus isolation can be accomplished in spite of increasing titers of neutralizing antibodies.

Complement-fixing antibodies are first detected approximately 1 month after infection, and their titer increases rapidly and remains at a level of approximately 1:250. The neutralizing activity appears about 2 months after infection and reaches an average level of 1:120. In addition, low complement-fixing antibodies against myelin basic protein was found in some sheep before infection with visna virus, but it did not increase during the first 9 months of infection.

Successful virus isolation from blood, CSF, and a number of organs and tissues was accomplished by inoculating homogenates into sheep choroid plexus cells and by establishing plasma clot explants of tissues and their cocultivation with permissive choroid plexus cells from healthy sheep. Although the efficiency of these methods is comparable, the homogenates proved, somewhat unexpectedly, to be most effective. The results clearly indicate that we are dealing with low amounts of infectious virus in the tissues of infected sheep. Therefore, simultaneous use of more than one method increases isolation rates. Blind passage also markedly increases the yield.

Choroid plexus is most likely to yield the virus with other tissues of the central nervous system being a close second in frequency. Spleen, lymph nodes, lungs, and the buffy coat are relatively good sources of infectious virus. On the other hand, we failed to isolate the virus from plasma in more than 200 attempts.

In the circulating blood, the virus is associated with mononuclear cells. There is, however, some cell-free infectious virus at least early in the infection. Thus virus can be isolated from cell-free supernatant of CSF and from tissue homogenates 1 month after infection.

In order to analyze the antibody response, we partitioned the antibodies in terms of immunoglobulin classes by sucrose density gradient ultracentrifugation, Sephadex gel filtration, treatment with 2-mercaptoethanol, DEAE–cellulose ion exchange chromatography, and specific antisera against the different sheep immunoglobulin classes. There is no evidence of antibody activity in the IgM class even as early as 2 months after infection. Neither was there any antibody activity detected in the IgG_2 or the IgA immunoglobulin classes. Complement-fixing and virus-neutralizing antibodies are found in the IgG_1 immunoglobulin class. It is highly probable that these two types of antibodies are directed against different virus antigens.

Obviously, it is possible to apply classical and conventional methods to the study of pathophysiology of Visna. Many aspects of this problem can then be solved without resorting to some exotic means of inquiry.

PART II
CONVENTIONAL AGENTS

CHAPTER 4
Borna, the Disease — A Summary of Our Present Knowledge

H. LUDWIG / H. BECHT

INTRODUCTION

Borna, a viral disease of horses and sheep, has been known for more than 150 years. The clinical picture was first described in 1813 as "Hitzige Kopfkrankheit der Pferde," and the name *borna* derives from a town in Saxony where the disease was first described. The clinical picture is characterized by incoordination and sensory loss. The incubation period varies between a few weeks and several months. After the onset, the disease progresses gradually and is usually fatal. Recovery has been recorded in about 5% of clinically manifest cases (10, 28).

HOST RANGE

The experimental animal of choice is the rabbit (16, 28). In this species, the incubation period lasts for 2 to 6 weeks after an intracerebral (i.c.) infection, and the resulting disease is fatal in about 1 week.

Several other species of animals are susceptible to experimental infection (Table 4.1), but the incubation periods and the expression of symptoms vary greatly and are much less distinct than in rabbits (28). In neonatal rats and adult hamsters, the infection tends to be subclinical and not associated with antibody production, although antigen and infectious virus are found in the brain tissue (1,17).

In our studies, particular interest has focused on the tree shrew (*Tupaia glis*) as an experimental animal because of its primatelike brain and its defined social behavior (24). Tree shrews were infected i.c. with brain suspension of diseased rabbits. After 4 to 7 weeks, the animals exhibited tremendous hyperactivity for 1 week after which they developed various types of pareses and had a severely altered behavior pattern. One or two weeks later most of the animals began recovering and have been well now for 2 years or more. After clinical recovery, however, the animals appeared to be slightly drowsy. During the observation period, they had serum antibodies against the virus. The animals killed 23 months after

TABLE 4.1 / Borna Disease in Naturally and Experimentally Infected Animals

Host Species	Incubation Period	Disease	Pathology	Antibody Response[a]	Virus or Antigen in Brain	References
NATURAL						
Horse	Weeks to months	Lethal	Encephalomyelitis	?	+	23
Sheep	6–7 wks.	Lethal	Encephalomyelitis	?	+	22
EXPERIMENTAL						
Horse	4 wks.	Lethal	Encephalomyelitis	?	+	7, 25
Sheep	6–7 wks.	Lethal	Encephalomyelitis	?	+	3
Rhesus monkey	7–14 wks.	Lethal	Encephalomyelitis	?	?	13
Tree shrew	4–7 wks.	Not Lethal	Encephalomyelitis	+ (CF, ID)	+	11
Rabbit	2–6 wks.	Lethal	Encephalomyelitis	+ (CF, ID, FA)	+	11, 21, 24
Hamster	?	None	—	— (CF)	+	2
Guinea pig	1–13 mos.	Lethal	Encephalomyelitis	?	?	13
Rat (adult)	(Weeks to months)	(Lethal)	Encephalomyelitis	+ (CF, ID)	+	11, 25
Rat (newborn)	?	None	—	— (CF)	+	15
Mouse	(5–18 weeks)	(Lethal)	?	?	?	13
Chicken	5–8 wks.	Lethal	Encephalomyelitis	+ (ID)	+	11, 26

[a] CF, Complement-fixation test; ID, immunodiffusion test; FA, fluorescence antibody test.

recovery from the clinical illness harbored the virus in their brains. This was demonstrated by i.c. inoculation of tree shrew brain suspensions into rabbits which subsequently died from borna disease (23).

HISTOPATHOLOGY

In spite of the absence of any clinical symptoms, the histologic examination of the tree shrew's brain revealed the typical picture of borna encephalitis (7) corresponding to that in the natural host, that is, inflammation, particularly of the gray matter, with perivascular lymphocytic infiltration, and in some cases also mild meningitis (20). Acidophilic, intranuclear inclusions, the so-called Joest–Degen bodies, are seen infrequently; they are mainly located in the ganglia of the Ammon's horn (11). Our observations (26), as well as those of others (21), demonstrated by immunofluorescence that the inclusion bodies consist of accumulations of virus specific antigens. Electron microscopic examination reveals that the inclusions represent closely packed granules of about 18 nm, surrounded by a microfibrillar capsule (4).

In infected rabbits, intracytoplasmic viruslike aggregates were detected by electron microscopy in microglia, mesenchymal cells, and the neurons. There is no evidence, however, that they have an etiologic relationship to the disease (1, 9).

VIRUS SPECIFIC ANTIGENS AND ANTIBODIES IN ANIMALS

Specific antigen can be readily demonstrated in brain extracts by classic serologic procedures, such as complement-fixation (25) or immunodiffusion (12). There is no cross reaction with antibodies against the visna–maedi, sheep leukosis, and subacute sclerosing panencephalitis viruses.

In the diseased rabbits, antibodies were demonstrable not only in the serum, but also in the cerebrospinal fluids (CSF). In three tested cases serum complement-fixing titers were identical with those in the CSF. There was also CSF pleocytosis of 200 to 300 cells/mm³. More than 90% of these cells were lymphocytes; therefore, it is likely that antibodies were produced locally rather than passively diffused from the serum (13).

CULTIVATION OF BORNA VIRUS IN VITRO

Studies of the structure of the virus have been hampered by the unavailability of an appropriate *in vitro* system for virus production and quantitative analysis. First attempts at propagation of the virus by alternating passages in embryonated chicken eggs and rabbit brains were made by Rott and Nitzschke (19). The chicken embryos did not die; however, they could not serve as an indicator system. The first attempts at infecting tissue cultures were made in 1967 when Daubney (5) reported that the virus multiplied in monkey kidney cells. More recently, Mayr and Danner (14) and we (12) demonstrated infectious virus in explants of brains of infected rabbits.

Presence of intracellular antigen in the explants was demonstrable by immunofluorescence. Since the antigen was also present in the subcultures, it is reasonable to conclude that synthesis of virus specific antigen took place *in vitro*. This was demonstrated convincingly when green monkey kidney (GMK) cells cocultivated with infected rabbit brain cells were found to contain borna virus antigens (12). One line of GMK cells, infected by cocultivation, has been kept in culture for more than 2 years and has undergone 120 passages. When extracts of these cells were injected i.c. into rabbits, the animals died after having exhibited typical symptoms of borna disease. Their brains contained specific complement-fixing antigen. Cell-free culture medium inoculated into 6-week-old rabbits had an LD_{50} titer of $10^{-1.5}$, whereas the cell-associated infectivity titers reached values of 10^{-5} to 10^{-7}. This indicated that at most only small amounts of the virus were released into the medium.

There is no evidence of a cytopathic effect in borna virus-infected monkey cells, either by direct microscopy or cytologic examination of cells stained with Giemsa or hematoxylin–eosin solution or by electron microscopy of ultrathin sections.

ANTIGENS

Virus specific antigens were demonstrated by immunofluorescence in the persistently infected cells. They had the appearance of dustlike spots or solid circular areas of various diameters in the nucleus. Some approached in size that of the nucleolus. The number of antigen-containing cells varied between 20 and 80%. Brilliant fluorescence was also seen when cerebrospinal fluid was used in place of serum in the indirect technique. When unfixed cells were stained by the indirect procedure there was no fluorescence of the cell membrane. Cytoplasm of the infected cells did not exhibit definite staining reactions (Fig. 4.1).

The antigen produced in GMK cells is apparently identical with the soluble antigen present in the brain material. Precipitation lines of identity formed in agar when extracts from brains of infected rabbits, an infected horse, infected tree shrews, or extracts of persistently infected GMK cells were diffused against immune sera obtained from rabbits, rats, chickens, or tree shrews (12) (Fig. 4.2).

Molecular weight of the antigens in the persistently infected cells was derived by an indirect immunoprecipitation assay with S^{35}-methionine-labeled extracts of the cells. Polyacrylamide gel analyses of the precipitates

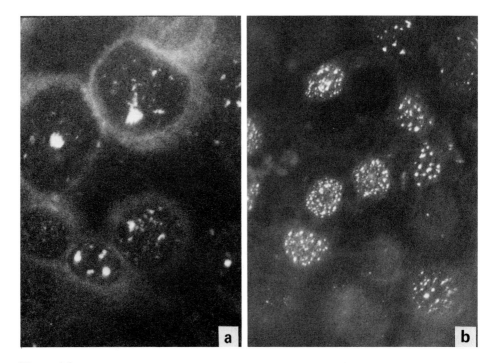

Figure 4.1.
Localization of borna virus specific antigen in infected GMK cells by the indirect fluorescence antibody technique. Cells treated with a specific antiserum (a) and with cerebrospinal fluid (b) from the same rabbit were overlaid with goat fluorescein conjugated antiglobulin serum.

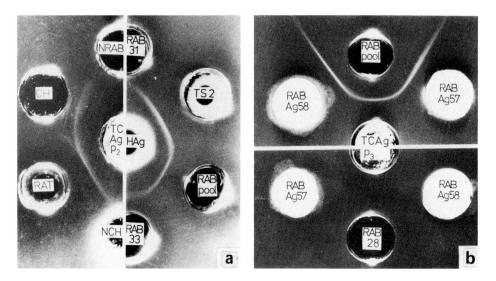

Figure 4.2.
Immunodiffusion test with extracts from infected tissue culture and brain material.
a. TCAgP$_2$ is the passage of two of the infected GMK cells; HAg is the brain
material of a horse that died of borna disease; RAB 31, RAB 33, and RAB pool are
sera of infected rabbits; convalescent sera of a rat (RAT), a tree shrew (TS), and
a chicken (CH) are noted; NCH is the normal chicken serum; and NRAB is the
normal rabbit serum.
b. RABAg 57 and RABAg 58 are the extracts from diseased rabbits that had been
inoculated with infectious rabbit brain suspension, and RAB 28 is the serum of
a rabbit inoculated with normal rabbit brain suspension. For other labels see **(a)**.
[From Ludwig *et al.* (12).]

revealed two specific peaks corresponding to molecular weights of about
40,000 and 22,000, respectively. The same radioactivity peaks appeared in
the gels when purified nuclei of infected cells were used as the source of
antigen (18) (Fig. 4.3).

CHARACTERIZATION OF VIRUS

After titration in rabbits revealed the presence of infectious virus in GMK
cells, we attempted unsuccessfully to purify the cell-associated virus by
different types of gradient centrifugation. Therefore, we tried to isolate
the virus by affinity chromatography. Cell extracts were filtered through a
column of antibody-coated agarose beads, and the retained material was
eluted by high ionic concentrations. The concentrated eluate had a high
titer of complement-fixing antigen and contained viruslike particles when
examined by electron microscopy (Fig. 4.4). The particles were spherical
with a diameter of 50 to 60 nm and seemed to have spikelike projections
on their surface. Their size was in agreement with the estimates obtained
from filtration studies of infected brain suspension (6). Moreover, many
smaller, corelike particles with a diameter of 20 to 25 nm were visible in
the preparations. It is uncertain whether these particles represent the causa-

tive agent of borna disease. Formation of artifacts during the purification procedure, which employed high salt concentrations, must be taken into consideration, and the remote possibility that this type of a particle is merely a passenger virus of rabbit origin cannot be excluded.

When material prepared from the medium of infected H^3-labeled uridine GMK cells was run into a sucrose gradient, a radioactive peak appeared at density of about 1.2 g/ml; it could not be seen with a H^3-thymidine label or material from uninfected cells (Fig. 4.5). This may indicate that infected cells produce an RNA-containing particle, whose viral nature and etiologic significance will have to be established in future experiments.

Figure 4.3.
Polyacrylamide gel electro-phoresis of radioimmune pre-cipitates. Extracts from S^{35}-methionine labeled cells were mixed with borna virus specific serum and precipitated with anti-rabbit globulin of the sheep. Extracts from whole cells (a) of the infected (closed circles) and uninfected (open circles) culture and from nuclei of the infected (b) and uninfected (c) cells.

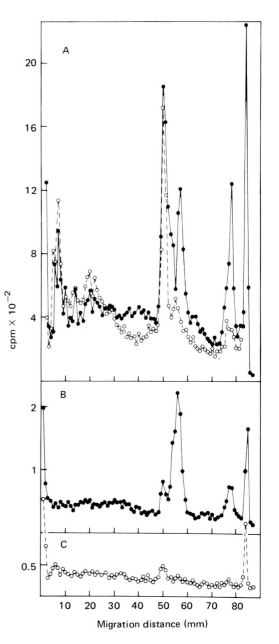

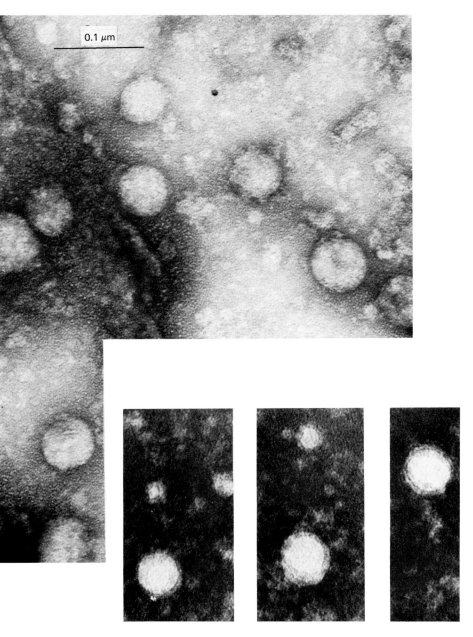

Figure 4.4.
Electron microscopy of virus structures obtained by affinity chromatography.
Negative staining was done with uranyl acetate. Inset: staining was done with
phosphotungstic acid.

CONCLUSION

In our opinion, borna disease should be considered a slow virus infection
(22) of the central nervous system. It is native to horses, in which it apparently has a long incubation period (weeks to months), has a relentless
progression, and is fatal in about 5% of cases.

Figure 4.5.
Sucrose gradient density centrifugation of radioactive material obtained from the medium of labeled GMK cells. Borna virus infected **(a)** and uninfected **(b)** H^3-thymidine labeled GMK cells; infected **(c)** and uninfected **(d)** H^3-uridine labeled cells.

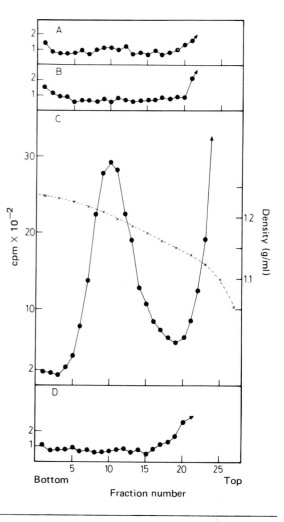

REFERENCES

1. Anzil, A. P. (1972). Transmission expérimentale du virus de l'encéphalomyélite de Borna: Etude ultrastructurale de la maladie du lapin et étude analytique de l'infection du hamster. *Ann. Inst. Pasteur Lille 123*, 537–544.

2. Anzil, A. P., Blinzinger, K., and Mayr, A. (1973). Persistent Borna virus infection in adult hamsters. *Arch. Ges. Virusforschung 40*, 52–57.

3. Beck, A., and Frohboese, H. (1926). Die enzootische Encephalitis des Schafes. Vergleichende experimentelle Untersuchungen über die seuchenhafte Gehirnrückenmarksentzündung der Pferde und Schafe. *Arch. Wiss. Prakt. Tierhk. 54*, 84–110.

4. Blinzinger, K., and Anzil, A. P. (1973). Large granular nuclear bodies (Karyosphaeridia) in experimental Borna virus infection. *J. Comp. Pathol. 83*, 589–596.

5. Daubney, R. (1967). Viral encephalitis of equines and domestic ruminants in the Near East, part II. *Res. Vet. Sci. 8*, 419–439.

6. Elford, W. J., and Galloway, I. A. (1933). Filtration of the virus of Borna disease through graded collodium membranes. *Br. J. Exp. Pathol. 14*, 196–205.

7. Frese, K. (1976). Personal communication.

8. Galloway, I. A. (1930). Borna disease. In *System of Bacteriology in Relation to Medicine.* Privy Council, H.M.S.O. London.

9. Hager, M., and Rott, R. (1972). Licht- und elektronenmikroskopische sowie virologische Untersuchungen über die Borna'sche Encephalitis. *Tagung Osterr. Arb. Neuropathol. Salzburg.*

10. Heinig, A. (1969). Die Borna'sche Krankheit der Pferde und Schafe. In *Handbuch der Virusinfektionen bei Tieren* (H. Röhrer, ed.), Vol. 4, pp. 83–148. VEB Fischer Verlag, Jena.

11. Joest, E., and Degen, H. (1909). Über eigentümliche Kerneinschlüsse der Ganglienzellen bei der enzootischen Gehirn-Rückenmarksentzündung der Pferde. *Z. Inf. Krankh. Haustiere 6*, 348–356.

12. Ludwig, H., Becht, H., and Groh, L. (1973). Borna disease (BD), a slow virus infection; Biological properties of the virus. *Med. Microbiol. Immunol. (Berl.) 158*, 275–289.

13. Ludwig, H., and Koestner, A. (1974). Unpublished data.

14. Mayr, A., and Danner, K. (1972). *In vitro* Kultivierung von Borna-Virus über Gehirn-Explantate infizierter Tiere. *Zentralbl. Veterinaermed. [B] 19*, 785–800.

15. Nicolau, S., and Galloway, I. A. (1927). Preliminary note on the experimental study of enzootic encephalomyelitis (Borna disease). *Br. J. Exp. Pathol. 8*, 336–341.

16. Nicolau, S., and Galloway, I. A. (1928). Borna disease and enzootic encephalomyelitis of sheep and cattle. *Priva Council Medical Research Council Special Report*, Series 121, pp. 7–90.

17. Nitzschke, E. (1963). Untersuchungen über die experimentelle Bornavirus-Infektion bei der Ratte. *Zentralbl. Veterinaermed. [B] 10*, 470–527.

18. Pauli, G. Personal communication.

19. Rott, R., and Nitzschke, E. (1958). Untersuchungen über die Züchtung der Virus der Borna'schen Krankheit im bebrüteten Hühnerei unter verschiedenen Bedingungen. *Zentralbl. Veterinaermed. [B] 5*, 629–633.

20. Seifried, O., and Spatz, H. (1930). Die Ausbreitung der encephalitischen Reaktion bei der Borna'schen Krankheit der Pferde und deren Beziehung zu der Encephalitis epidemica, der Heine-Medinschen Krankheit und der Lyssa der Menschen. Eine vergleichend-pathologische Studie. *Z. Gesamte Neurol. Psychiat. 124*, 317–382.

21. Shadduck, J. A., Danner, K., and Dahme, E. (1970). Fluoreszenzserologische Untersuchungen über Auftreten und Lokalisation von Borna-Virusantigen in Gehirnen experimentell infizierter Kaninchen. *Zentralbl. Veterinaermed. [B] 17*, 453–459.

22. Sigurdsson, B. (1954). Rida, a chronic encephalitis of sheep with general remarks on infections which develop slowly and some of their special characteristics. *Br. Vet. J. 110*, 341–354.

23. Sprankel, H., and Ludwig, H. (1976). Unpublished data.

24. Sprankel, H., and Richards, A. (1976). Nicht produktives Verhalten von tupaia glis DIARD 1820 im raumzeitlichen Bezug. Eine qualitative Analyse. *Z. für Säugetier Kd 41*, 77–101.

25. Sprockhoff, H. v. (1954). Untersuchungen über die Komplement-bindungsreaktion bei der Borna'schen Krankheit. *Zbl. Vet. Med. 1*, 494–530.

26. Wagner, K., Ludwig, H., and Paulsen, J. (1968). Fluoreszenzserologischer Nachweis von Borna-Virus Antigen. *Berl. Munch. Tieraerztl. Wochenschr. 81*, 395–396.

27. Walther, A. (1899). Die Gehirnrückenmarksentzündung bei Schafen. *Ber. Vet. Wes. Sachsen. 44*, 80.

28. Zwick, W. (1939). Borna'sche Krankheit und Encephalomyelitis der Tiere. In *Handbuch der Viruskrankheiten*, Vol. 2 (E. Gildenmeister, E. Haagen, and O. Waldmann eds.), pp. 252–354. Fischer, Jena.

29. Zwick, W., and Seifried, O. (1925). Übertragbarkeit der seuchenhaften Gehirn-Rückenmarksentzündung des Pferdes (Borna'sche Krankheit) auf kleine Versuchstiere (Kaninchen). *Berl. Munch. Tieraerztl. Wochenschr. 41*, 129–132.

30. Zwick, W., Seifried, O., and Witte, J. (1926). Experimentelle Untersuchungen über die seuchenhafte Gehirn-und Rückenmarksentzündung der Pferde (Borna'sche Krankheit). *Z. Infekt. Krankh. Haustiere 30*, 43–136.

31. Zwick, W., Seifried, O., and Witte, J. (1927). Weitere Untersuchungen über die seuchenhafte Gehirn-Rückenmarksentzündung der Pferde (Borna'sche Krankheit). *Z. Infekt. Krankh. Haustiere 32*, 150–179.

CHAPTER 5
Borna Disease: Patterns of Infection

KURT DANNER

INTRODUCTION

Cultivation of borna virus *in vitro* (5, 8, 9, 10, 11) and infectivity titration through immunofluorescence (12) made extensive laboratory studies with this agent possible. Borna virus has a wide host range *in vivo* and a comparatively wide spectrum of cell cultures susceptible to it (Table 5.1). Borna antigen can be detected through immunofluorescence (2) in the nuclei of infected cells 2 or 3 days after inoculation (Fig. 5.1). On the third or fourth day, fluorescence is noted also in the cytoplasm (Fig. 5.2). The virus spreads slowly from cell to cell and thus forms distinct fluorescent microplaques. Titration is easily accomplished by counting these foci between the fifth and tenth day after infection. There is no need for an overlayer of, for example, methyl cellulose (4).

TABLE 5.1 / Cell Spectrum of Borna Virus

Primary Cells	Established Cell Lines
SHEEP	RABBIT
Kidney (adult and fetal)	RK 13
Testes (fetal)	MA 111
Skin (fetal)	HAMSTER
Brain (fetal)	BHK 21
BOVINE	DOG
Testes (adult and fetal)	MDCK
PIG	MONKEY
Kidney (adult)	CV-1
DOG	Vero
Kidney (infantile)	Rita
HORSE	AGMK
Kidney (fetal)	
RABBIT	
Kidney (infantile)	
Brain (infantile)	
Spleen (infantile)	
HUMAN	
Kidney (fetal)	
CHICK EMBRYO	
Fibroblasts	
Brain	

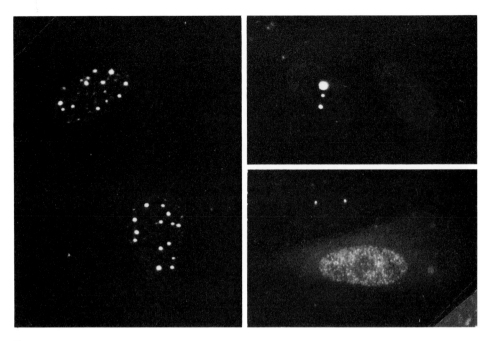

Figure 5.1.
Early fluorescence in the nuclei of borna virus infected cells (2 to 4 days after inoculation).

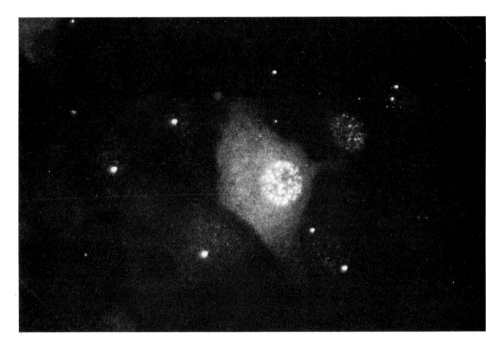

Figure 5.2.
A microplaque 6 days after infection with borna virus (immunofluorescence).

DETECTION

Infectious virus cannot usually be detected before the fourth day after infection of cell cultures and often appears even later. Its concentration rises slowly and depends on the nutritional status of the cultured cells. Infectious virus is strongly cell associated and is therefore never present in the supernatant culture medium. Figure 5.3 depicts a typical growth curve of borna virus in CV-1 cells and demonstrates the slow rise in its concentration, the dependence of virus growth on cell nutrition, and the limited virus yield from the infected cells, which approximate 1/10 infectious unit (I.U.) per antigen bearing cell. The optimal incubation temperature is 36°C; at 40°C, there is no virus replication.

CHARACTERISTICS

Infected cells can be readily subcultured in AGMK (African Green Monkey Kidney) (5) or RK-13 (Rabbit Kidney) (13) cells, in which the virus has been carried for 150 cell passages. Each of these virus-infected cells is infective, but cell extracts have only minimal infectivity. Therefore, purification of the virus is difficult. However, limited studies in our laboratory have revealed certain physicochemical properties of the virus. Its replication in CV-1 cells is unaltered by the presence of 100 μg/ml IUdR or BUdR but is completely inhibited by 5 μg/ml of 6-azauridine and is enhanced by 0.1 μg/ml of actinomycin D. Thus it reacts like a paramyxovirus (16) and apparently contains RNA. Enhancement of growth by actinomycin may be

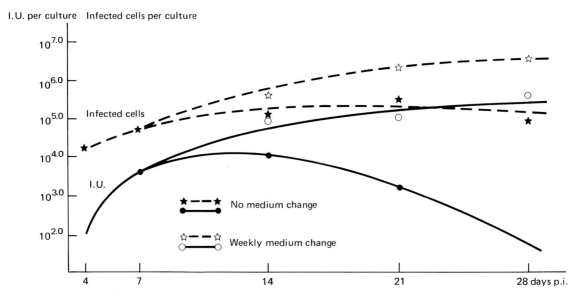

Figure 5.3.
Growth curve of borna virus in CV-1 cells after infection with 10^4 I.U. per culture bottle. No virus was detectable in the culture medium. Number of infected cells was determined by counting the fluorescing cells on coverslips in Leighton tubes.

due to inhibition of interferon synthesis as has been suggested for measles virus (7). Virus infectivity passes 100-nm filters in a low percentage of 0.1%; but 99.5% is held back by 450-nm filters. The virus has a density of about 1.18 g/cm³ in cesium chloride gradient. It is sensitive to chloroform treatment.

REPLICATION

In view of the cell association of borna virus and the wide cell range *in vitro*, it is likely that *in vivo* borna virus also replicates by cell-to-cell passage in a variety of cell types rather than only in neurons as has been assumed (18). The neurons, however, are the only cells that develop large nuclear inclusion bodies (17). Regardless of the site of entry, borna virus must reach its target organ, the central nervous system, and presumably does so slowly by the cell-to-cell spread. The disease does not express itself until a sufficiently large number of cells becomes infected.

CONCLUSIONS

In view of the failure of virus release from the infected cells, it is unlikely that there is a viremic phase (6). Yet, there is antibody response, and this is probably due to attrition of some infected cells and consequent release of viral antigen. The antibodies, of course, cannot inhibit virus spread because of its cell-to-cell passage, and therefore they do not interfere with persistence of the virus. Absence of cytolysis may be explained by a lack of virus specific surface antigens.

Future studies will have to address themselves to other defense mechanisms, such as interferon, and to the influence of temperature on the

TABLE 5.2 / Patterns of Borna Virus Infections

| Infection Type | Clinical Course | CNS | | Antibodies in Serum | Species |
		Positive Histology	Virus Recovery		
Acute-	Death After 4 to 20 Days	+	+	+/−	Horse, rabbit (18)
	Recovery "Auto-sterilization"	−	−	−	Horse, sheep, rabbit (14)
Subacute	Persistent infection	+	+	+	Chicken, tree shrew (5)
Chronic	Chronic-recurrent	+	+	+/−	Horse (3), rat (5)
Slow	Slowly progressing	+	+	?	Rat (15, 19)
Tolerant	No illness	−	+	−	Hamster (1), rat (15)

replication of borna virus and the role either may play in pathogenesis of the disease. In any studies of pathogenesis of borna, it must be remembered that the infection takes different courses (Table 5.2) and varies with the species and age of the animals, as well as the dose of the inoculum.

REFERENCES

1. Anzil, A. P., Blinzinger, K., and Mayr, A. (1973). Persistent Borna virus infection in adult hamsters. *Arch. Virusforsch. 40*, 52–57.
2. Danner, K., and Mayr, A. (1973). Fluoreszenzserologische Untersuchungen über das Auftreten von Borna-Virusantigen in Zellkulturen aus Gehirnexplantaten infizierter Kaninchen. *Zentralbl. Veterinaermed. [B] 20*, 497–508.
3. Goerttler, V. (1941). Ein bemerkenswerter Fall von Bornascher Krankheit. *Berl. Munch. Tierarztl. Wochenschr. 11*, 138–139.
4. Heubeck, D. (1976). Studien über die Züchtung von Borna-Virus in Zellkulturen. Vet. Med. Dissertation, München.
5. Ludwig, H., Becht, H., and Groh, L. (1973). Borna disease (BD), a slow virus infection. Biological properties of the virus. *Med. Microbiol. Immunol. (Berl.) 158*, 275–289.
6. Matthias, D. (1953). Beitrag zum Infektionsmodus der Bornaschen Krankheit der Pferde. *Arch. Exp. Veterinaermed. 7*, 313–318.
7. Matumoto, M. (1966). Multiplication of measles virus in cell cultures. *Bacteriol. Rev. 30*, 152–176.
8. Mayr, A. (1972). Borna virus: A new model for slow virus research. *Ann. Inst. Pasteur Lille 123*, 545–552.
9. Mayr, A., and Danner, K. (1971). Cultivation of Borna virus in cell cultures. 2nd Int. Congr. Virol., Budapest, June 27–July 3.
10. Mayr, A., and Danner, K. (1972). Production of Borna virus in tissue culture. *Proc. Soc. Exp. Biol. Med. 140*, 511–515.
11. Mayr, A., and Danner, K. (1972). In-vitro-Kultivierung von Borna-Virus über Gehirn-Explantate infizierter Tiere. *Zentralbl. Veterinaermed. [B] 19*, 785–800.
12. Mayr, A., and Danner, K. (1974). Züchtung und Titrierung von Borna-Virus in Zellkulturen aus Organen fötaler Lämmer. *Zentralbl. Veterinaermed. [B] 21*, 131–137.
13. Mayr, A., and Danner, K. (1974). Persistent infections caused by Borna virus. *Infection 2*, 64–69.
14. Nicolau, S., and Galloway, I. A. (1930). L'encéphalo-myélite expérimentale (maladie de Borna). *Ann. Inst. Pasteur Lille 45*, 457–523.
15. Nitzschke, E. (1963). Untersuchungen über die experimentelle Bornavirus-Infektion bei der Ratte. *Zentrolbl. Veterinaermed. [B] 10*, 470–527.
16. Phillips, L. A., and Bussell, R. H. (1974). The nucleic acid of canine distemper virus: effects of 6-azauridine and actinomycin D on viral replication, and the incorporation of uridine into virions. *Am. J. Vet. Res. 35*, 821–824.
17. Sprockhoff, H. von. (1957). Über das Vorkommen der Joest-Degen'schen Einschluβkörper bei Bornavirus-infizierten Kaninchen, Meerschweinchen und Ratten verschiedenen Alters. *Mh. Tierheilk. 9*, 129–142.
18. Zwick, W. (1939). Bornasche Krankheit und Enzephalomyelitis der Tiere. In *Handbuch der Viruskrankheiten*, Vol. 2 (E. Gildemeister, E. Haagen, and O. Waldmann, eds.). Fischer-Verlag, Jena.
19. Zwick, W., Seifried, O., and Witte, J. (1929). Weitere Beiträge zur Erforschung der Bornaschen Krankheit des Pferdes. *Arch. Wiss. Prakt. Tierheilk. 59*, 511–545.

Discussion / Chapters 4–5

Dr. Wecker challenged the contributors to convince him that borna is in fact a slow virus disease, since it develops acutely and has a relatively short incubation period. Dr. Ludwig replied that it was the persistence of the virus and antibodies against it and the localization of the infection to one organ system that made it comparable to the slow virus infections. Furthermore, in the natural infection of horses, the incubation period seems to be prolonged, lasting for months and perhaps even years. The problem with estimating the incubation period is that it is difficult to decide retrospectively when an animal had become infected. Dr. Petursson added that an important aspect of what is usually accepted as slow virus infections is the relentless progression of the disease to death. He asked therefore whether there were any recoveries of borna-infected animals. Dr. Ludwig replied that in the natural disease a small proportion of the infected animals apparently do recover. The experimentally infected rabbits usually die of the progressive disease. The experimentally infected tree shrews developed typical clinical symptoms of borna with characteristic paresis, but all of them recovered.

Dr. Mims inquired whether neutralizing antibodies were found in borna and whether there was viral antigen on cell surfaces. Dr. Ludwig replied that indirect immunofluorescence techniques failed to detect such antigen in unfixed, live cells. Dr. Danner added that in his attempts to neutralize the virus, only serum of animals inoculated by perenteral injection of cell culture gave evidence of plaque reduction. This happened, however, only with the undiluted serum, whereas diluted sera gave no effect, even if they contained high levels of complement-fixing antibodies. Since the sera had not been inactivated, they probably all contained complement.

The discussion now turned to the nature of borna virus, and Dr. Schäfer asked whether it was a budding virus. Although there was no definite answer to this question, Dr. Rott described his electron microscopic observations of borna-infected rabbit brains, in which he noted particles with a diameter of about 20 to 30 nm in the cytoplasm, but he had no evidence that these particles were in fact related to the etiologic agent. Although he saw no budding, he allowed the possibility that the particles were crystalline arrays that might acquire an envelope through the process of budding. Dr. Wecker did not accept this readily, because he pointed out that the titers of the cell-bound virus were approximately 10,000-fold higher than those of the free virus. Therefore, this would indicate that the virus matured within the cell and that, it ought to be seen as it acquired its envelope through the process of budding. Yet, it was not seen! Thus the question of budding was not resolved satisfactorily.

Dr. Wecker then posed the question of passive immunization and directed it not only to the borna investigators, but also to those working with visna. He wondered whether an experimental animal might be protected by serum containing antibodies against these viruses. Dr. Ludwig replied that this had not been done, but there was speculation that since the experimental disease was transmitted only by intracerebral inoculation it was unlikely that passively transmitted antibodies would protect. Dr. Dickinson, alluding to his long-term observations of scrapie animals, wondered whether rabbits inoculated peripherally, rather than intra-cerebrally, with borna virus have been observed long enough to demonstrate encephalitis, since it may have a very long incubation period. Dr. Danner replied that such long-term observations had not yet been completed.

Dr. Katz criticized the many questions about classification of particular diseases as slow virus infections or not slow virus infections. He pointed out that the older definitions might be too restrictive and that one thing that might emerge from such discussions as this would be a redefinition of a slow virus infection. Once the mechanisms that are involved are better understood, such infections would then be defined in terms of some basic processes and not the somewhat crude characteristic of the incubation period. When that happens, many diseases with an unusual host–parasite relationship may be classified as slow virus infections. Dr. Choppin supported this view and suggested that a given infection may be slow in one host and fast in another.

The remainder of the discussion addressed itself to the question whether borna and visna were immunopathologic diseases. Dr. Mims stated that newborn hamsters tended to develop a persistent infection, but not disease, whereas adults developed a lethal disease. Therefore he wondered whether histologic examination of the horse and the sheep might indicate stigmata of immunopathology. Dr. Weiss replied that there was lymphocytic infiltration in the cases of visna in the brain and maedi in the lungs; therefore he took it as an indication of an immunologic event. Dr. Johnson agreed, but cautioned that mere presence of mononuclear cells may not be an indication that they were there primarily. He suggested an experiment involving immunosuppressed adult animals, to see if they could be rendered tolerant of the infection and made to behave like the neonates.

Dr. Johnson continued by citing some of the experiments in his laboratory with the visna virus. In American sheep inoculated by intracerebral injection of the fetuses or the neonates, he and his colleagues have not yet observed any clinical disease, but the time interval of 2 years has not been long enough on the visna incubation period time scale. However, these clinically healthy animals do have abnormalities noted on histopathologic examination of the brain. Their white matter exhibits patchy areas of pleomorphic mononuclear cells around the blood vessels in a pattern reminiscent of that described in Icelandic sheep early in the incubation period before there is demyelination. Neither immunofluorescence techniques nor electron microscopic examination revealed any evidence of visna virus in the tissues. Moreover infectivity tests of tissue cultures also have been negative. It appeared therefore that the disease was progressing in the absence of infectious virus, viral antigen, or viral particles. On the other hand, explants of such brains gave 100% virus recovery, and the virus has been identified serologically as visna virus. It appears therefore that in these animals there is either an extraordinarily small amount of virus, which therefore escapes detection, or a sudden burst of viral replication *in vitro*. The latter alternative suggested to Dr. Johnson the intriguing possibility that the virus may have become integrated into the cell as a provirus. If that were, in fact, the case, it might be one mechanism of slow infections.

CHAPTER 6
Progressive Multifocal Leukoencephalopathy*

RICHARD T. JOHNSON / OPENDRA NARAYAN
LESLIE P. WEINER / JOHN E. GREENLEE

INTRODUCTION

Progressive multifocal leukoencephalopathy (PML) is a subacute demyelinating disease apparently resulting from the selective destruction of oligodendrocytes by papovaviruses. The pathology and pathogenesis of PML are distinct from those of the other slow infections of the human nervous system. Kuru and Creutzfeldt–Jakob disease appear to be caused by obligate "slow viruses" that produce noninflammatory degenerative disease in primate brains and that fail to produce cytopathic infections in cell cultures. Subacute sclerosing panencephalitis (SSPE) results from a defective measles virus infection that causes a diffuse indolent inflammatory disease of the brain in otherwise normal children. In contrast, PML is a noninflammatory demyelinating process, and the pathogenesis appears to be related not to uniqueness or defectiveness of the viruses but to defects in the host immune response. The viruses associated with this disease are not human pathogens in the usual sense but cause disease almost exclusively in patients with disorders affecting their immune response or in patients given immunosuppressive drugs to maintain organ transplants or to treat other illness (41, 42).

Although a rare disease, PML is the first human demyelinating disease in which viruses have been consistently identified and, therefore, has implications for studies of multiple sclerosis, the most common human demyelinating disease. Furthermore, the viruses recovered from PML are of interest, since they are the first agents of the simian virus 40 (SV40)–polyoma group related to human disease, and both serotypes isolated from PML have proved to be oncogenic in hamsters. Finally, the methodology employed in the identification of agents in PML is germane, because identification of the viral agents can now be performed by immunofluorescence and electron microscopic agglutination methods. Thus, in this disease, it has been feasible to devise rapid methods to study a slow infection.

* Supported by grants from the U. S. Public Health Service (NC-1-43266 and NS-08838).

CHARACTERISTICS

Over 100 cases of PML have been reported, and the majority have been associated with malignant proliferative diseases including lymphosarcoma. Chronic and acute myelogeneous leukemia, carcinomatosis, tuberculosis, and sarcoidosis account for the majority of the remaining cases. In addition, three cases have been reported in patients receiving immunosuppressive therapy after renal allografts (20, 21, 50), and one has been described in a patient receiving large doses of immunosuppressive drugs for systemic lupus erythematosus (44). In a small number of patients, no predisposing disease has been evident, but in these cases where immunologic studies have been carried out, abnormalities of the cell-mediated immune response have usually been found (23).

The neurologic manifestations of PML may begin at any time during the course of the underlying disease process. The patient develops multifocal neurologic signs, such as paralysis, mental deterioration, visual loss, sensory abnormalities, and ataxia, which follow a progressive course and usually lead to death in less than 1 year. The patients remain afebrile and rarely experience headache. The cerebrospinal fluid is normal. One patient has been described who survived for 5 years with two periods of apparent remission (17). One of our patients, after an initial rapid period of deterioration, stabilized for almost 2 years, and this period of survival was associated with an extraordinary increase in antibody against the papovavirus that had been isolated from an earlier brain biopsy (44).

The pathologic changes consist of multifocal patches or plaques of demyelination throughout the white matter with subcortical areas most prominently affected. These plaques become confluent producing large multilobulated areas of demyelination. These demyelinated foci show a relative sparing of axis cylinders and a loss of oligodendrocytes and myelin sheaths. The oligodendrocytes surrounding the foci are often enlarged and contain large intranuclear inclusion bodies. Within the lesions, the astrocytes are enlarged, often containing bizarre mitotic figures, multiple nuclei, or multilobulated nuclei. In the original histologic description of the disease, the authors describe these "bizarre gigantic forms with unequivocal mitosis" as "suggesting neoplastic cells" (1).

The presence of inclusion bodies and the association with underlying diseases known to lead to defects in immune response led Richardson (31) and Cavanagh et al. (9) to postulate that PML might have a viral etiology despite the chronic afebrile course and the lack of inflammatory changes within either the brain or cerebrospinal fluid. In 1965, ZuRhein and Chou (49) reported electron microscopic studies of the oligodendrocyte inclusions in which they found large numbers of particles resembling papovaviruses. Extraction and negative staining of these particles indicated a size and capsid structure of papovaviruses of the simian virus 40 (SV40)–polyoma group (18). ZuRhein's subsequent review of numerous cases showed a remarkable consistency of these particles in the inclusion bodies and along the endoplasmic reticulum of the oligodendrocytes. Virions were only rarely found within astrocytes (48).

In contrast, similar papovaviruslike virions have not been convincingly associated with other human diseases or found in normal brains. Papovaviruslike particles were reported in cell cultures derived from human brain tissue (25), and particles with the diameter of papovaviruses have been reported in a human brain biopsy and a human choroid plexus tumor (2, 39). However, in a subsequent study of choroid plexus tumors similar particles have been shown to be glycogen granules by histochemical staining (6). Thus, it has only been in PML that these viruses have been seen in extraordinary quantities, have been extracted to demonstrate their capsomere structure, and have been found in the appropriate cells to explain the demyelinating process (19).

VIRUS ISOLATIONS FROM PROGRESSIVE MULTIFOCAL LEUKOENCEPHALOPATHY

Initial attempts to isolate viruses from brain tissue of patients with PML inoculating cell cultures, small laboratory rodents, and embryonated eggs were unsuccessful, and the inoculation and long-term holding of primates induced no disease (11, 15, 32, 49). However, during the last 4 years, multiple virus isolations have been successful.

Initial isolation of a new human papovavirus was made by Padgett *et al.* (27) by inoculating a homogenate of brain from a patient dying with PML complicating Hodgkin's disease onto cultures derived from human fetal brain. These primary cultures contain populations of both large flattened cells, thought to represent astrocytes, and small dense cells called spongioblasts, thought to represent the neuronal and glial precursor cells (36). The virus caused cytopathology only in the spongioblasts. This agent, termed JC virus, has now been isolated from five cases of PML in that laboratory as well as individual cases in several other laboratories (8, 12, 41, 46).

Another virus indistinguishable from SV40 was isolated in our laboratory from brains of two patients with PML (44). Initial isolations were made by fusion of cultured cells derived from the brains of the patients with primary cultures of African green monkey kidney cells. Subsequently, from one case this agent was reisolated by the inoculation of homogenates of the brain onto cultures of human fetal brain (43).

A third papovavirus distinct from the JC and SV40 viruses has also been isolated from man, but this agent has not been associated with PML. This virus, called BK, was originally recovered by Gardner *et al.* (13) from the urine of a patient following a renal allograft. Subsequently, BK virus has been isolated from urines of other patients receiving immunosuppressive drugs after renal allografts or for cancer chemotherapy and from urines of children with Wiskott–Aldrich syndrome (10, 30, 38). Takemoto reported recovery of BK virus from a brain tumor, as well as from the urine of a child with Wiskott–Aldrich syndrome (38), but the etiologic relationship of this virus to the tumor or to any disease in man is still in doubt.

Cell culture susceptibilities are different among these three agents. The JC virus has been found to cause cytopathic effect only in cultures of human fetal glial cells containing spongioblasts, and this cytopathology may be sufficiently subtle to necessitate electron microscopic monitoring of cultures (46). No replication of JC virus has been demonstrated in a number of human cells, African green monkey kidney cells, rabbit kidney cells, or mouse cells (41). In contrast, the SV40 viruses from PML and BK viruses cause cytopathic change in a variety of primate cells, although SV40 from PML replicates optimally in monkey cells, and BK virus replicates optimally in human cells (24, 37).

The tissue culture isolation of viruses from patients with PML have proved laborious. Production and maintenance of primary cultures of human fetal glial cells is difficult, and the cytopathology induced by JC virus, even after long periods of time, is subtle. In the initial studies that recovered SV40, the use of cells of simian origin raised the specter that isolates might represent laboratory contaminants or even recombinants with simian viruses latent in cell cultures. Therefore, other methods of recovery and identification have been sought.

VIRAL ANTIGENIC RELATIONSHIPS AND STUDIES OF DISTRIBUTION IN MAN

The JC, SV40 (PML), and BK viruses all resemble SV40 structurally. The tumor (T) antigen produced by each of these three viruses cross reacts by fluorescent antibody staining with antibodies to SV40 T antigen. Electron microscopic agglutination studies show that the three viruses share capsid antigens (28). Hyperimmune sera show some cross reaction of hemagglutinating, fluorescing, and neutralizing antibodies (37, 45). The JC and BK viruses have particle-associated hemagglutinin similar to that of polyoma virus, which is not found in SV40 or in the SV40 viruses isolated from PML.

Sera of some rabbits 10 days after a single intravenous inoculation of virus have been found to contain antibody that reacts only with the homologous virus (28). These monospecific antisera permit direct identification of agents in PML by fluorescent antibody staining (Fig. 6.1) and electron microscopic agglutination (Fig. 6.2). The latter method employs the treatment of the brain tissue with detergent (Freon-113) and direct observation of negatively stained particles with the electron microscope. Preparations are incubated overnight with the monospecific sera, and antibody attachment to virus particles in the case of antibody excess, or agglutination of particles, in the case of antigen excess is observed with the electron microscope (29). This method can differentiate among SV40, JC, and BK viruses. Utilizing fluorescent antibody and/or electron microscopic agglutination methods, brain tissues of 18 patients with PML have been studied in our laboratory. The JC virus has been identified in 13 patients, SV40 in two, and three specimens were inadequate for electron microscopic agglutina-

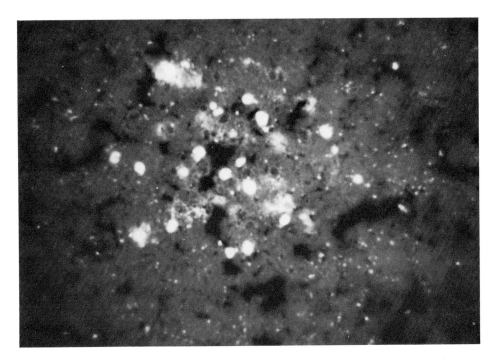

Figure 6.1.
Section of brain of patient with PML. Stained with antiserum against JC virus and fluorescein-labeled anti-rabbit immunoglobulin. A focus of cells in white matter show specific nuclear fluorescence. ×200

tion. No tissues have been studied where virions were abundant and could not be identified.

Epidemiologic, serologic studies have demonstrated antibodies to JC and BK viruses only in humans. Antibodies to BK virus have been found in the majority of persons in early childhood (14, 35), and antibodies to JC virus have been found in a majority of adolescents or adults (26). However, a recent study of isolated populations demonstrated some groups with a high prevalence of JC antibodies and not BK antibodies or vice versa (5). In contrast, antibody to SV40 in man is primarily dependent on exposure to monkeys or to contaminated vaccines. Approximately 20% of persons in age groups having risk of exposure to contaminated, killed poliovirus vaccines have neutralizing antibody to SV40. However, some non-monkey reservoir for SV40 has been suggested by the finding of antibody in 2 to 4% of humans who had little or no contact with monkeys and who were bled prior to dispensing of contaminated vaccines or were born after the vaccines were cleared of SV40 (33).

ONCOGENIC PROPERTIES

The JC, SV40, and BK viruses are oncogenic in hamsters, and each has been shown to produce brain tumors. The JC virus is unique in that it is more oncogenic after intracerebral (i.c.) than extraneural inoculation and

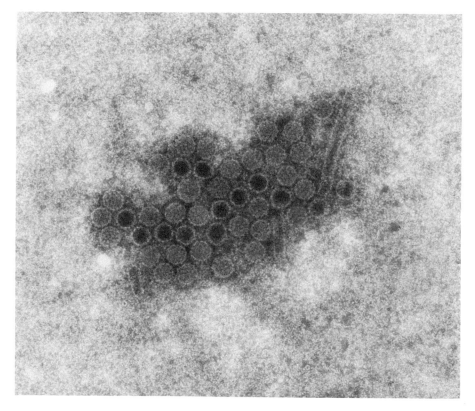

Figure 6.2.
Agglutination of virions extracted from brain with diluted antiserum against JC
virus. A latticework of antibody molecules can be seen between particles. Stained
with phosphotungstic acid. ×130,000

in producing cerebral and cerebellar tumors that resemble gliomas (40).
The SV40 strains from PML produce undifferentiated sarcomas after subcutaneous inoculation and choroid plexus papillomas after i.c. inoculation
similar to tumors induced by other strains of SV40. The BK virus appears
to be the least oncogenic of the three. Only a small number of tumors have
been induced in hamsters with this virus (34), but they are similar to
those induced by SV40 virus, including choroid plexus papillomas after i.c.
inoculation (16).

The possible relationship of these agents in human oncogenesis deserves
further investigation. The neoplastic appearance of astrocytes within the
lesions of PML has long raised speculation regarding the potential cerebral
oncogenic properties of these viruses in man (19, 45, 48), and recently a
patient with multifocal gliomas associated with PML lesions has been
described (7). Nevertheless, cryostat-sectioned tissues from PML lesions
stained with fluorescent antibodies for T antigen have consistently been
negative, but this is also true of the majority of sections of SV40-induced
tumors in hamsters (3). However, cells from the brain of one patient
(Patient 1, Ref. 44) have been maintained in culture, and these cultured
cells express T antigen and contain infectious SV40 DNA (22). Unfortu-

nately, fresh brain tissue from PML cases is seldom available to establish such cultures.

Another possible relationship of these papovaviruses to human cerebral neoplasms was suggested by isolating BK virus from a brain tumor of a child with Wiskott–Aldrich syndrome (38), but unfortunately cells from the tumor were not successfully cultured to stain for T antigen, and blood was not examined to determine whether this child with viruria had a concomitant viremia contaminating the tumor. Weiss et al. (47) have grown cells from brain tumors and reported SV40 T antigen in cells grown from two of seven meningiomas. However, we have carried out similar studies of 31 cerebral tumors, including eight meningiomas, and have failed to detect T antigen in any cultured tumor cells (4).

CONCLUSIONS

The primate papovaviruses serologically related to SV40 represent an unusual group of agents. They cause frequent infections in man, as shown in serologic studies, yet they display little virulence. To date, only SV40 and JC virus have been related to disease, and this disease, PML, seems limited to persons with immunologic deficits. The BK virus, the most widespread of these agents, has not been clearly related to any disease, although tissues from patients with PML complicating renal allografts have not been studied to determine the possible role of BK virus in demyelinating disease in this specific situation.

Progressive multifocal leukoencephalopathy appears to result from the lytic infection of oligodendrocytes causing demyelination and the relatively nonpermissive infection of astrocytes causing bizarre hyperplasia and, in one instance, possible tumor formation. However, the pathogenesis of extraneural infection with these papovaviruses is unknown. The JC and SV40 viruses must replicate in extraneural sites in man, yet they have not been identified in other tissues. However, remarkably few specimens of extraneural tissue have been available for studies. It is unknown whether the virus after childhood infection remains latent in the body and is activated in the brain or in extraneural tissues with dissemination to the brain or whether the occasional patient who develops PML is one of that minority who escape childhood infection with JC virus but have their first encounter after being immunologically crippled by some other disease. Finally, the ubiquity of these agents, their demonstrated effects on human astrocytes in PML, and their oncogenic properties in hamsters all make them prime suspects as etiologic agents in human cerebral neoplasms.

REFERENCES

1. Astrom, K. E., Mancall, E. L., and Richardson, E. P., Jr. (1958). Progressive multifocal leuko-encephalopathy. *Brain 81*, 93–111.
2. Bastian, F. O. (1971). Papova-like virus particles in human brain tumor. *Lab. Invest. 25*, 169–175.

3. Becker, L. E., Narayan, O., and Johnson, R. T. (1975). Demonstration of papovavirus tumor antigen in brain tumors. *J. Neuropathol. Exp. Neurol. 34*, 95.

4. Becker, L. E., Greenlee, J. E., and Narayan, O. (1975). Unpublished observations.

5. Brown, P., Tsai, T., and Gajdusek, D. C. (1975). Seroepidemiology of human papovaviruses: The discovery of virgin populations and some unusual patterns of antibody prevalence among remote peoples of the world. *Am. J. Epidemiol.*, in press.

6. Carter, L. P., Beggs, J., and Waggener, J. D. (1972). Ultrastructure of three choroid plexus papillomas. *Cancer 30*, 1130–1136.

7. Castaigne, P., Rondot, P., Escourolle, R., Ribadeau Dumas, J.-L., Cathala, F., and Hauw, J.-J. (1974). Leucoencephalopathie multifocale progressive et "gliomes" multiples. *Rev. Neurol. 130*, 379–392.

8. Cathala, F., Hauw, J.-J., and Escourolle, R. (1973). Isolement et etude ultrastructurale d'un virus de type Papova non neutralisé par le sérum de référence anti-SV40 au cours de la leucoencéphalopathie multifocale progressive. *C. R. Acad. Sci. [D] (Paris) 276*, 1081–1084.

9. Cavanagh, J. B., Greenbaum, D., Marshall, A. H. E., and Rubinstein, L. J. (1959). Cerebral demyelination associated with disorders of the reticuloendothelial system. *Lancet ii*, 525–529.

10. Coleman, D. V., Gardner, S. D., and Field, A. M. (1973). Human polyomavirus infection in renal allograft recipients. *Br. Med. J. 3*, 371–375.

11. Dolman, C. L., Furesz, J., and Mackay, B. (1967). Progressive multifocal leukoencephalopathy. Two cases with electron microscopic and viral studies. *Can. Med. Assoc. J. 97*, 8–12.

12. Field, A. M., Gardner, S. D., Goodbody, R. A., and Woodhouse, M. A. (1974). Identity of a newly isolated polyomavirus from a patient with progressive multifocal leukoencephalopathy. *J. Clin. Pathol. 27*, 341–347.

13. Gardner, S. D., Field, A. M., Coleman, D. V., and Hulme, B. (1971). New human papovavirus (BK) isolated from urine after renal transplantation. *Lancet i*, 1253–1257.

14. Gardner, S. D. (1973). Prevalence in England of antibody to human polyomavirus (BK). *Br. Med. J. i*, 77–78.

15. Gibbs, C. J., Jr., Gajdusek, D. C., and Alpers, M. P. (1969). Attempts to transmit subacute and chronic neurological diseases to animals. *Add. Ach. Allerg. 36*, 519–552.

16. Greenlee, J. E., and Narayan, O. (1976). Unpublished observations.

17. Hedley-Whyte, E. T., Smith, B. P., Tyler, H. R., and Peterson, W. P. (1966). Multifocal leukoencephalopathy with remission and five year survival. *J. Neuropathol. Exp. Neurol. 25*, 107–116.

18. Howatson, A. F., Nagai, M., and ZuRhein, G. M. (1965). Polyma-like virions in human demyelinating brain disease. *Can. Med. Assoc. J. 93*, 379–386.

19. Johnson, R. T., Narayan, O., and Weiner, L. P. (1974). The relationship of SV40-related viruses to progressive multifocal leukoencephalopathy. In *Mechanisms of Virus Disease* (W. S. Robinson and C. F. Fox, eds.), pp. 187–197. W. A. Benjamin, Menlo Park, California.

20. Legrain, M., Graveleau, J., Brion, S., Mikol, J., and Kuss, R. (1974). Leucoencephalopathie multifocale progressive apres transplantation renale. *J. Neurol. Sci. 23*, 49–62.

21. Manz, H. J., Dinsdale, H. B., and Morrin, P. A. F. (1971). Progressive multifocal leukoencephalopathy after renal transplantation. *Ann. Intern. Med. 75*, 77–81.

22. Narayan, O. (1975). Unpublished observations.

23. Narayan, O., Penney, J. B., Jr., Johnson, R. T., Herndon, R. M., and Weiner, L. P. (1973). Etiology of progressive multifocal leukoencephalopathy. Identification of papovavirus. *N. Engl. J. Med. 289*, 1278–1282.

24. Narayan, O., and Weiner, L. P. (1974). Biological properties of two strains of

simian virus 40 isolated from patients with progressive multifocal leukoencephalopathy. *Infect. Immun. 10*, 173–179.

25. Oyanagi, S., ter Meulen, V., Muller, D., Katz, M., and Koprowski, H. (1970). Electron microscopic observations in subacute sclerosing panencephalitis brain cell cultures: Their correlation with cytochemical and immunocytological findings. *J. Virol. 6*, 370–379.

26. Padgett, B. L., and Walker, D. L. (1973). Prevalence of antibodies in human sera against JC virus, an isolate from a case of progressive multifocal leukoencephalopathy. *J. Infect. Dis. 127*, 467–470.

27. Padgett, B. L., Walker, D. L., ZuRhein, G. M., and Eckroade, R. J. (1971). Cultivation of papova-like virus from human brain with progressive multifocal leukoencephalopathy. *Lancet i*, 1257–1260.

28. Penney, J. B., Jr., and Narayan, O. (1973). Studies of the antigenic relationships of the new human papovaviruses by electron microscopy agglutination. *Infect. Immun. 8*, 299–300.

29. Penney, J. B., Jr., Weiner, L. P., Herndon, R. M., Narayan, O., and Johnson, R. T. (1972). Virions from progressive multifocal leukoencephalopathy: rapid serological identification by electron microscopy. *Science 178*, 60–62.

30. Reese, J. M., Reissig, M., Daniel, R. W., and Shah, K. V. (1975). The occurrence of BK virus and BKV-specific antibodies in the urine of patients receiving chemotherapy for malignancy. *Infect. Immun. 11*, 1375–1381.

31. Richardson, E. P., Jr. (1961). Progressive multifocal leukoencephalopathy. *N. Engl. J. Med. 265*, 815–823.

32. Schwerdt, P. R., Schwerdt, C. E., Silverman, L., and Rubinstein, L. J. (1966). Virions associated with progressive multifocal leukoencephalopathy. *Virology 29*, 511–514.

33. Shah, K. V. (1972). Evidence for an SV40-related papovavirus infection of man. *Am. J. Epidemiol. 95*, 199–206.

34. Shah, K. V., Daniel, R. W., and Strandberg, J. D. (1975). Sarcoma in a hamster inoculated with BK virus, a human papovavirus. *J. Natl. Cancer Inst. 54*, 945–950.

35. Shah, K. V., Daniel, R. W., and Warszawski, R. (1973). High prevalence of antibodies to BK, an SV40-related papovavirus, in residents of Maryland. *J. Infect. Dis. 128*, 784–787.

36. Shein, H. M. (1967). Transformation of astrocytes and destruction of spongioblasts induced by a simian tumor virus SV40 in cultures of human fetal neuroglia. *J. Neuropathol. Exp. Neurol. 26*, 60–76.

37. Takemoto, K. K., and Mullarkey, M. F. (1973). Human papovavirus, BK strain: Biological studies including antigenic relationship to simian virus 40. *J. Virol. 12*, 625–631.

38. Takemoto, K. K., Rabson, A. S., Mullarkey, M. F., Blaese, R. M., Garon, C. F., and Nelson, D. (1974). Isolation of papovavirus from brain tumor and urine of a patient with Wiskott–Aldrich syndrome. *J. Natl. Cancer Inst. 53*, 1205–1207.

39. Vernon, M. L., Horta-Barbosa, L., Fuccillo, D. A., Sever, J. L., Baringer, J. R., and Birnbaum, G. (1970). Creutzfeldt–Jakob disease: Virus-like particles and nucleoprotein filaments in two brain biopsies. *Lancet i*, 964–966.

40. Walker, D. L., Padgett, B. L., ZuRhein, G. M., Albert, A. E., and Marsh, R. F. (1973). Human papovavirus (JC): Induction of brain tumors in hamsters. *Science 181*, 674–676.

41. Walker, D. L., Padgett, B. L., ZuRhein, G. M., Albert, A. E., and Marsh, R. F. (1974). Current study of an opportunistic papovavirus. In *Slow Virus Diseases* (W. Zeman and E. H. Lennette, eds.), pp. 49–58. Williams and Wilkins, Baltimore.

42. Weiner, L. P., Herndon, R. M., and Johnson, R. T. (1973). Viral infections and demyelinating diseases. *N. Engl. J. Med. 288*, 1103–1110.

43. Weiner, L. P., Herndon, R. M., Narayan, O., and Johnson, R. T. (1972). Further

studies of a simian virus 40-like virus isolated from human brain. *J. Virol. 10,* 147–149.

44. Weiner, L. P., Herndon, R. M., Narayan, O., Johnson, R. T., Shah, K., Rubinstein, L. J., Preziosi, T. J., and Conley, F. K. (1972). Isolation of virus related to SV40 from patients with progressive multifocal leukoencephalopathy. *N. Engl. J. Med. 286,* 385–390.

45. Weiner, L. P., and Narayan, O. (1974). Virologic studies of progressive multifocal leukoencephalopathy. *Prog. Med. Virol. 18,* 229–240.

46. Weiner, L. P., Narayan, O., Penney, J. B., Jr., Herndon, R. M., Feringa, E. R., Tourtellotte, W. W., and Johnson, R. T. (1973). Papovavirus of JC type in progressive multifocal leukoencephalopathy. *Arch. Neurol. 29,* 1–3.

47. Weiss, A. F., Portmann, R., Fischer, H., Simon, J., and Zang, K. D. (1975). Simian virus 40-related antigens in three human meningiomas with defined chromosome loss. *Proc. Natl. Acad. Sci. U.S.A. 72,* 609–613.

48. ZuRhein, G. M. (1969). Association of papova-virions with a human demyelinating disease (progressive multifocal leukoencephalopathy). *Prog. Med. Virol. 11,* 185–247.

49. ZuRhein, G. M., and Chou, S. M. (1965). Particles resembling papova viruses in human cerebral demyelinating disease. *Science 148,* 1477–1479.

50. ZuRhein, G. M., and Varakis, J. (1974). Progressive multifocal leukoencephalopathy in a renal-allograft recipient. *N. Engl. J. Med. 291,* 798.

100

Discussion / Chapter 6

Dr. Koprowski inquired about an hypothesis to explain the isolation of SV40-PML virus from two cases and demonstration of JC virus (JCV) in 12 other cases of the same disease. Dr. Johnson replied that he had no hypothesis, but noted that the two patients with SV40-PML did not have neoplasms. Both were immunosuppressed—one because of therapy for lupus erythematosus and the other because of some inborn defect of the immune system. Of the other 12, most had neoplastic diseases and shorter courses than the two patients from whom SV40-PML was isolated.

Dr. Bloom wondered whether the SV40-PML virus caused transformation, and Dr. Johnson replied that in one, as yet unconfirmed, report there had been some transformation of mouse fibroblasts and that Dr. Walker transformed hamster kidney cells with the BK virus (BKV). Dr. Bloom further wondered whether these viruses are neurotropic and therefore exhibit this kind of specificity. Dr. Johnson replied that JCV has remarkable specificity, but that the other viruses did not. In reply to Dr. Bloom's question whether there was a particular cell type that was predominantly or exclusively involved in the PML, Dr. Johnson identified the oligodendrocytes as the primary targets, because they become lysed in this disease, whereas the astrocytes appear to be transformed, or at least altered, in their morphology. The neurons, on the other hand, are spared. This led Dr. Bloom to speculate that the slow turnover time of specific cells in the central nervous system may be responsible for the slow manifestations of such diseases. Dr. Johnson then commented that the brain was a heterogeneous population of cells that had different embryologic origins and that even the neurons themselves differed in their susceptibility to infections.

Dr. Choppin wondered about the epidemiologic evidence among people who had been inoculated inadvertently with the SV40 virus in the polio vaccine, and Dr. Johnson replied that there has not yet been a case of PML, or for that matter any other unusual disease, among these individuals now observed for some 20 years. Dr. Choppin pointed out that if one of them were immunosuppressed for some reason, such a disease may be triggered, but Dr. Johnson replied that, to his knowledge, such immunosuppression had not yet occurred. Dr. Koprowski, on the other hand, felt that it was unlikely that this population would provide cases of PML, because the children were vaccinated after the neonatal age. He stated that in laboratory experiments one could produce tumors with SV40 virus only if newborn animals were inoculated. Inoculation of SV40 into adult rhesus monkeys, in which this virus is endemic, produced no disease and no tumors. But Dr. Choppin pointed out that induction of PML need not necessarily be comparably age dependent.

Dr. Mims then commented about BKV, which is regarded as a human polyoma virus, because it is found in the urine of patients with renal transplants, who are being immunosuppressed. Why not administer this virus to primates and determine what its effect might be? Dr. Walker responded that apparently BKV had been put into some monkeys, but no disease has yet been reported, and no examination of the urine for BKV has yet been made. Dr. Gajdusek reported that in his laboratory eight of the specimens identified as JCV, concentrated from frozen brain material, were inoculated into primates. Thus far no evidence of disease has been detected. These studies are still preliminary, and no serologic or other data are available.

The question of transformation of cells by the PML viruses came under scrutiny of several discussants next. Dr. Wechsler wanted to know what evidence there was that such transformation did take place within the PML lesions in the brain and whether there was any evidence of *in vitro* transformation of tissue cultures. Dr. Johnson summarized the evidence by listing the presence of viral deoxyribonucleic acid in cell cultures derived from PML brains, presence of T antigen within the cells and their ability to grow through many passages in the laboratory. By these criteria they appeared to be transformed. They did not contain virions, or viral antigens, as one might expect in a lytic infection. Dr. Bloom countered that mere presence of T antigen and the cells' ability to grow for a number of passages does not indicate transformation. Dr. Koprowski responded that the criteria for transformation are not sufficiently precise, but if the cells exposed to the SV40-PML virus change their characteristics so that after the exposure they need much less serum for growth than do the original cells, they grow in soft agar, and they are immortal, this could be taken as the best possible evidence of transformation. Such cells obviously cannot be put into an isologous host; therefore, the definitive test of their transformation can never be carried out.

Dr. ter Meulen now turned the discussion to the host who gets PML. He wondered, in view of the very small percentage of patients who get this disease among a large group of immunosuppressed individuals, whether genetic predisposition played a role. In addition, Dr. Rott wondered whether there was any evidence of immunopathology in PML. But Dr. Johnson doubted it, in view of the fact that it is the immunosuppressed individual who is subject to this disease.

Comment/Chapter 6
D. L. Walker

Dr. Johnson raised some interesting points. The first is in regard to the cause of progressive multifocal leukoencephalopathy (PML). Are all three of the papovaviruses etiologically involved? If so, how many cases are due to SV40, how many to JC virus (JCV), and how many, if any, to BK virus (BKV)? The answer can only come from continued study of cases of PML, but unfortunately they are relatively rare, and it is difficult to get the tissues before the neuropathologist has immersed them in formalin. To date, in 21 cases of PML in which the virus in the lesions has been identified, 19 have been found to be JCV and two were SV40. BKV has not yet been found in PML brain tissue.

A major difficulty in understanding the pathogenesis of PML has been the lack of an animal model. There is hope, however, for the development of such a model in the recent work at David, California, by D. H. Gribble et al. (1). They examined and did careful autopsies on 400 monkeys and found lesions similar to those of human PML in the central nervous systems of eight animals. Oligodendrocytes containing intranuclear inclusions were found by electron microscopy to contain intranuclear virion-like particles that sometimes were in crystalloids. The abnormal oligodendrocytes were not quite as abundant as in human PML, but in the main the disease appeared similar to human PML. Three of the eight monkeys had underlying lymphomas, one had a chronic hemolytic anemia, two had chronic shigellosis, and two had giant cell pneumonia. Thus at least some of them probably had some immunologic impairment. Seven of the monkeys were *Macacca mulatta* and one was *Macacca speciosa*. Only two had been recognized as having neurologic disease prior to autopsy.

The observations of Gribble et al. (1) are exciting in that they may fortell the development of an animal model for PML. This is of importance because we have been unsuccessful in causing significant disease in primates with JCV in several experiments. In collaboration with investigators at the primate laboratory operated by Litton Bionetics, JCV has been inoculated into newborn rhesus monkeys by multiple routes in two experiments. In one of these experiments, a course of immunosuppression was initiated 2 years after the original inoculation, but after an additional year (a total of 3 years) the monkeys were still free of any indication of PML-like disease. In collaboration with other investigators, JCV has also been inoculated into newborn marmosets and adult owl monkeys by multiple routes. The observation time for the marmosets and owl monkeys has been less than 1 year, and they have not shown any signs of disease. In view of the high degree of species specificity characteristic of the papovaviruses, it may be very difficult to produce an animal model of PML using JCV.

In the absence of a useful animal model, gaining information about the pathogenesis of PML will have to depend upon large, prospective, long-term studies of patients under immunosuppression after kidney transplants or under therapy for Hodgkin's disease or chronic lymphocytic leukemia. The cost and effort involved in this will be large. We have initiated such studies on a small scale, and would like to know such simple things as whether PML developed in the 75% of persons who were infected with JCV long before their immunosuppression or in the 25% who had not been infected prior to immunosuppression. It may be that rather than a reactivation of a latent JCV infection, PML is the result of a primary infection with JCV in a person who is unlucky enough to encounter the virus while under immuno-suppression.

An area of interest regarding these new human papovaviruses is the question of their epidemiology. So far, there is no evidence for a reservoir, other than the human population, for JCV or BKV. In fact, for JCV we have considerable evidence from serologic surveys of animals that this is a strictly human virus. Serologic surveys show that JCV and BKV infect most children early in life, but we know essentially nothing about the characteristics of the primary infections or about the routes of transmission among children. It seems most likely that the viruses are excreted in urine and feces and enter by the respiratory or intestinal route, but at present this is mainly an hypothesis.

Dr. Johnson discussed cells susceptible to JCV. It is a puzzling and frustrating fact that in spite of much effort we have not been able to get JCV to multiply in cells other than spongioblasts in human fetal glial cell cultures. We have reasoned that if JCV infects children by the respiratory or intestinal route, multiplies, and is ex-creted in urine or feces, it must surely multiply fairly efficiently in cells other than fetal spongioblasts. However, extensive testing of human fetal intestine, lung, kid-ney, liver, spleen, and amnion cells plus VERO and CV-1 cells, and less extensive testing of many other cells, has not revealed a useful permissive cell. We have also tried to modify cells by treatment with IUdR and BUdR but without success in ob-taining productive infection.

Even in the human fetal spongioblasts in fetal glial cell cultures, JCV multiplies very slowly. Our calculations indicate that the multiplication cycle can be no shorter than 24 hr, and it is probably considerably longer than 24 hr.

A point of interest brought up by Dr. Johnson is the oncogenicity of JCV, BKV, and the SV40 isolated from PML. When inoculated into newborn hamsters by the intracerebral, intraperitoneal, or subcutaneous route, JCV is highly oncogenic. It seems especially oncogenic in the brain where it causes tumors in about 80% of animals. We then anticipate that JCV would be efficient in transforming hamster cells *in vitro.* This has not turned out to be the case, for reasons we do not under-stand. On the other hand, Dr. Billie Padgett has recently found that JCV does seem to transform human fetal brain cells *in vitro.* The evidence for transformation is that some cells exposed to JCV will continue to multiply in serial subculture long after uninoculated cultures die out; that they will multiply in medium of reduced serum content in which normal cells die; and that about 90% of transformed cells contain T antigen. BKV seems to be significantly less oncogenic than JCV in hamsters, but it does transform hamster cells *in vitro.* In view of the oncogenic tendencies of these viruses, it is important to examine the possibility that they may have a role in causing human tumors. Several laboratories are already engaged in a search for evidence of the presence of BKV, JCV, or SV40 genome in cells from various human tumors.

In summary, newly recognized human papovaviruses that are widely distributed in the human population occur in JCV and BKV. JCV is the virus usually found in PML. We know little about the pathogenesis of PML, but the recent report of PML in rhesus monkeys offers some hope of an animal model that may help clarify patho-genesis. We have much to learn about the natural cycles of these viruses and about their disease-producing potential, including their possible role in human tumors.

REFERENCE

1. Gribble, D. H., Haden, C. C., Schwartz, L. W., and Hendrickson, R. V. (1975). Spontaneous progressive multifocal leukoencephalopathy (PML) in macaques. *Nature 254*, 602–604.

CHAPTER 7
Subacute Sclerosing Panencephalitis

MICHAEL KATZ

INTRODUCTION

Subacute sclerosing panencephalitis (SSPE) has been described "originally" on a number of occasions (6, 32), but two people primarily credited with the classic description of this disease are Dawson (13) and van Bogaert (7). Clinically, the condition begins with subtle intellectual deterioration, with a gradual appearance of incoordination and other motor abnormalities, proceeding to myoclonic jerks, sustained myoclonus, coma, and death. The course of the disease has varied from a few months to a few years. Victims of SSPE have been primarily children, but a rare adult, usually in the third decade of life, has developed this disease. The diagnosis is made on clinical grounds, supported by the classic electroencephalographic abnormality, known as burst-suppression pattern, and an increase in the IgG fraction of gamma globulin of the cerebrospinal fluid. Dawson's contribution to the understanding of SSPE was his description of the intranuclear, eosinophilic Cowdry type-A inclusion bodies, which he saw in the neurons and oligodendroglial cells. Van Bogaert reported the sclerosing pattern in the white matter of the brain. The critical observation of structures resembling paramyxovirus nucleocapsids in the brains of patients with SSPE by Bouteille *et al.* (8) and Telez-Nagel and Harter (34) pointed the way to identification of a specific pathogen. As a consequence of these ultrastructural observations, Connoly *et al.* (12) identified unusually high levels of measles antibodies in all patients with SSPE whom he studied. Of note is the fact that these antibodies against all known antigenic determinants of measles are manyfold higher than those in the general population. Finally, in this indirect search for a pathogenic agent, Connoly *et al.* (12), Freeman *et al.* (14), ter Meulen *et al.* (27), and later others, using measles antibody in an immunofluorescence test, reported presence of an antigen reacting with these antibodies in the neurons and glial cells of brains of patients with SSPE (Fig. 7.1).

MEASLESLIKE VIRUSES IN SSPE PATIENTS

In spite of the force of circumstantial evidence pointing to the involvement of measles or a measleslike virus, the infectious agent could not be isolated directly. Its eventual "rescue" depended on establishment of tissue cultures

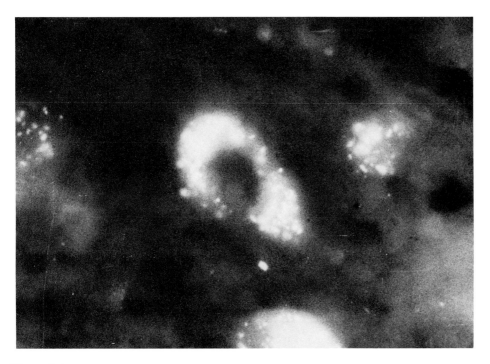

Figure 7.1.
Section of human brain treated with measles antibody in direct fluorescence microscopy. Antigen reacting with the antibody is seen in the cytoplasm.

from fresh brain explants of patients with SSPE, available from brain biopsies and early (usually under 6 hr) autopsies. Cell cultures, thus established, grew to confluent monolayers and were susceptible to serial passage. During the process of such passage, many of these cultures tended to develop syncytia and giant cells, morphologically resembling the type of cytopathic effect induced by measles virus. Moreover, as was first reported by Baublis and Payne (4), such cultures contained measles antigen and, as reported by Katz *et al.* (20), structures resembling paramyxovirus nucleocapsids which were identical in appearance to those observed in the brain tissues themselves. Nevertheless, no infectious virus could be found either in the supernatant or in a mixture of disrupted cells. It was not until such cells were either cocultivated (16, 31) or fused (3) with human or simian permissive cells that infectious virus was finally isolated.

Although this viral rescue was accomplished in several laboratories and from several different patients—and it could be achieved repeatedly in each instance—there were also brain cell cultures from patients with SSPE that never yielded an infectious virus, even though they were characterized by the same kind of viral "footprints" as those in the cells that did yield infectious virus (Table 7.1). On the basis of this observation, Katz and Koprowski (19) hypothesized that the pathogenic effect of the virus did not depend on such a late genomic function as production of infectious virus, but on an earlier function contemporaneous with the synthesis of the fusion factor and the consequent syncytiogenic effect.

107

TABLE 7.1 / Characteristics of Brain Cells in Cultures Derived from SSPE Patients[a]

Cells	Morphologic pattern	Detection of measleslike antigen by immuno-fluorescence	Detection of nucleocapsids by electron microscopy[b]	Isolation of infectious virus
JAC	Many syncytia and multinucleated giant cells	60% of giant cells, occasional single cells	10%	Yes
LEC	Many syncytia and multinucleated giant cells	60% of giant cells, occasional single cells	10%	Yes
ROB	Many syncytia, moderate number of multinucleated giant cells	10% of giant cells, rare single cells	10%	No
MCG	No syncytia, occasional multinucleated giant cells	Rare giant cells	5%	No
MOS	Moderate syncytia, rare multinucleated giant cells	Rare single cells	0	No
WES	No syncytia, occasional multinucleated giant cells	Negative	5%	No
MCL	No syncytia, occasional multinucleated giant cells	Negative	0	No
STO	No syncytia, occasional multinucleated giant cells	Negative	0	No

[a] From Katz and Koprowski (19).
[b] 200 cells examined.

Location of Cause of SSPE

Given the isolated virus and, by now, a fairly extensive group of patients, the question that had to be asked was whether the cause of SSPE resided in the virus or in the host. On epidemiologic grounds, it would be difficult to ascribe this disease to an infection with a variant of measles virus, because if this were the case, one would expect to see geographic clusters of SSPE, rather than the seemingly spontaneous, individual, random instances adding up to estimated incidence of one in a million. It is true that Brody and Detels (9) reported some rural predominance of this disease, but it suggested to them not so much clustering, as a possible zoonotic origin of the viral agent or at least a coupling of the measles virus with a zoonotic agent that might give rise to SSPE.

If, on the other hand, the disease results from an unusual genetic predisposition of the host, then one would expect SSPE, rare as it is, to show at least some familial tendency. None has been observed. If there is no indication of a common source outbreak to suggest infection with a variant of the virus and no familial tendency to suggest an inherited abnormality of the host, then one might consider the possibility that the viral variant develops after the individual has been infected with a conventional virus, or that the host's defense mechanisms become abnormal after conception.

Differences in Measleslike Viruses

There appear to be some differences among the various measles-like viruses rescued from patients with SSPE and also between each of these isolates and the "conventional" measles virus. In our own studies (24), this comparison was conducted with a wild strain of measles virus, the Woodfolk strain, and the attenuated Edmonston strain. We noted differences in several characteristics. The SSPE virus did not reach as high a titer as did the wild or attenuated measles virus; in tissue culture, its antigen as seen by immunofluorescence tended to fill densely intranuclear inclusion bodies, and its nucleocapsids tended to fill the nucleus. There was also a considerable difference in the susceptibility of SSPE virus to 6-azauridine, which inhibited its growth more readily than it did the wild measles virus (26).

Recent attempts to establish genetic relatedness of SSPE and measles viruses, based on competition–hybridization experiments, also showed some differences. Using the LEC, JAC, WSO, and Mantooth SSPE viruses and the Woodfolk, attenuated Edmonston, and Braxator measles viruses, Hall and ter Meulen (15) showed that all seven were genomically 100% homologous. However, all four of the SSPE viruses contained an additional 10% genetic information.

Albrecht and Schumacher (2) testing the viruses for heat sensitivity noted that some SSPE viruses were more sensitive than others and all were more sensitive than the measles viruses Albrecht tested. Payne and Baublis (30) reported that several SSPE virus strains had a decreased reactivity with the neutralizing antibody in comparison with measles virus. This was true whether the antibody was prepared against SSPE or measles virus.

Besides these differences determinable *in vitro*, there appeared to be differences in the behavior of the viruses when they were introduced into animals. These viruses tend to be encephalitogenic early after rescue, in that they cause encephalitis without adaptation to the brain. In contrast, measles virus has to be adapted by serial passage in the brain before it can induce encephalitis in experimental animals. When the SSPE viruses cause encephalitis in experimental animals, they do it without provoking a humoral antibody response. On the other hand, when measles virus is injected intracerebrally (i.c.) into these animals it does provoke an antibody response, even if it causes no neurologic disease.

Evaluation of other SSPE strains has revealed some similarities to those characteristics we observed, but it has also revealed some differences. It is not important at present to consider those in detail; the point is that these differences are evidence of the variability of measles viruses.

In making such a comparison among virus strains, it is important to bear in mind that we are dealing with a virus capable of a gradual change in the laboratory setting, so that certain features of the virus may reflect the passage history, rather than some primordial characteristics of the agent in nature. What does seem to be common, however, or even universal, in SSPE is that the agents isolated from the brains tend to be neurotropic for animals, without adaptation (25), and that pools of such agents tend to contain a large number of morphologically defective viral particles (29). Moreover, the SSPE viral isolates tend to be highly cell associated, which is the probable basis of the relatively lower titers of the SSPE viruses grown in tissue culture and of the cases of nonproductive infections with some of these agents.

IMMUNOLOGIC ABNORMALITIES

Investigations of the SSPE patients for evidence of immunologic abnormalities have of necessity been conducted after development of the disease. With respect to humoral immunity, SSPE patients were shown in one study to have an increased level of IgG, approximately 1.5 times normal, normal levels of IgA and IgM, but perhaps markedly elevated levels of IgE (5). The high titers of antibodies against measles are unique in SSPE patients; levels of antibodies against other viral agents are not unusually high (23). Moreover, these patients tend to respond normally to antigenic stimulation with, for example, *Brucella*, pneumococcal polysaccharide, diphtheria toxoid, tetanus toxoid, typhoid vaccine, and others (5). The question about functional capacity of the specific IgG in SSPE patients was raised by Payne and Baublis (30), who found that the specific measles antibody of SSPE patients tended to have lower avidity for the antigen, then the antibody produced in normal, post-measles subjects. The specific anti-measles IgG in the cerebrospinal fluid of patients with SSPE appears to be produced by restricted clones of lymphocytes (36).

Evaluation of cell mediated immunity (CMI) in SSPE has given variable results. Kreth *et al.* (22) found no evidence of any impairment in nine SSPE patients. Ahmed *et al.* (1) also found essentially normal CMI responses in SSPE patients by testing for the presence of lymphocytotoxins, K lymphocytes, and MIF. Likewise, Blaese and Hofstrand (5) reported no abnormalities of CMI in the SSPE patients they studied. These patients had a normal rejection pattern of skin allografts, normal proportion of T lymphocytes, normal response to DNCB, and normal lymphokine responses.

These direct results are supported indirectly by the failure in two investigations to document any response of a number of SSPE patients to treatment with transfer factor (18). There is a report of a successful therapy with transfer factor in one SSPE patient (35), but this has not been duplicated elsewhere and there has not been a follow-up.

Two studies suggested that there was failure of delayed hypersensitivity skin response to live and killed measles viruses in SSPE patients (17). In view of the difficulties with interpretation of the skin test and problems with the preparation of measles antigen for such tests, the significance of these findings must await elaboration. Steele *et al.* (33) reported inhibition by SSPE sera of lymphocytotoxicity in cells infected with measles virus. Ahmed *et al.* (1) described an inhibitor of CMI, which they believe to be an immune complex, circulating in plasma of most patients they studied with SSPE. These results await confirmation.

ANIMAL MODEL SYSTEM

Since it has not been possible to study natural history of SSPE until the disease has declared itself and therefore the true slow nature of the infection has never been observed, it would be desirable to have an animal model system wherein such studies could be conducted. Unfortunately, no satisfactory system has yet been developed. In the first place, all of the animal transmission experiments that succeeded have depended on i.c. injection of the agent, and second, most of them produced a relatively acute disease. The fact that, except for suckling rodents, the infection could not be induced in any of intact postneonatal animals by the inoculation of cell-free virus has been of particular interest. Only cell-associated virus has been able to cause encephalitis in these animals, and it has done so without provoking any antibody response (25). It is reasonable to interpret these results as indicative of a cell-to-cell spread of the virus within the central nervous system (CNS).

Two sets of experiments in hamsters have come perhaps closest to reproduction of the human disease. Wear and Rapp (37) used suckling hamsters born to measles-immune mothers and inoculated them i.c. with a hamster-adapted strain of measles virus. When these infected animals were given cyclophosphamide, they developed a chronic CNS disease. Unfortunately, neither histologic nor serologic studies were made of these animals. Byington and Johnson (11) succeeded in establishing first a productive infection and later a disease associated with high antibody levels, when they inoculated weanling, rather than suckling, hamsters with a hamster-adapted SSPE virus. All of the animals developed an acute encephalitis, but in some it was followed by a chronic neurologic disease. Nearly 3 months after the inoculation, brains of these animals yielded cell-associated virus by the technique of cell cocultivation.

PATHOGENESIS OF SSPE

Since there is no explanation for the pathogenesis of SSPE, hypotheses abound. One holds that the defective virus infection is the key to the pathogenesis and that owing to the slowness of the spread of the infection and a continual, albeit minute, release of antigen from the cells that die, the patient becomes hyperimmunized and hence develops the very high antibody levels. However, the apparently intact humoral and cellular immune mechanisms fail to eliminate the virus and abolish the infection. This probably happens because the virus spreads by cell-to-cell transfer and cannot be neutralized by the antibodies. Moreover, the virus specific antibodies may block viral expression at the cell membrane and prevent the immunocompetent lymphocytes from recognizing the infected cells (28).

The basis for the defectiveness of the virus may be if mutation within the host, after the original infection, or at least a change in viral tropism that need not be genetically determined. An alternative is that some extraneous event alters the virus–host relationship. One of such possible events

111

might be a second viral infection. This concept was suggested by Barbanti-Brodano *et al.* (3), when they observed, through the electron microscope structures resembling papova virions in cell cultures established from an SSPE brain explant. It has not been possible to identify the virus or to develop a biologic test for its presence.

Hypotheses attempting to implicate failure of CMI suggest as did Burnett (10) that the patient may have a specific tolerance for the measles virus or, as has been proposed by others, that the basic immune system is intact, but that it is inhibited from expressing itself (1). It is also possible, of course, that the immune system is primarily impaired.

In the end, a satisfactory explanation of pathogenesis of SSPE must account for its development after a presumably normal measles infection in a presumably normal host, through a process that either affects the virus itself or the host response. It is important to bear in mind that a change in the one can influence the other.

REFERENCES

1. Ahmed, A., Strong, D. M., Sell, K. W., Thurman, G. B., Knuolsen, R. C., Wiston, R. Jr.; Grace, W. R. (1974). Demonstration of a blocking factor in the plasma and spinal fluid of patients with subacute sclerosing panencephalitis, *J. Exp. Med. 139,* 902–924.
2. Albrecht, P., and Schumacher, H. P. (1972). Markers for measles virus. I. Physical properties. *Arch. Ges. Virusforsch. 36,* 23–35.
3. Barbanti-Brodano, G., Oyanagi, S., Katz M., Koprowski, H. (1970). Presence of two different viral agents in brain cells of patients with subacute sclerosing panencephalitis. *Proc. Soc. Exp. Biol. Med. 134,* 230–236.
4. Baublis, J. V., and Payne, R. E. (1968). Measles antigen and syncytiom formation in brain cell cultures from subacute sclerosing panencephalitis (SSPE). *Proc. Soc. Exp. Biol. Med. 129,* 543–597.
5. Blaese, R. M., and Hofstrand, H. (1975). Immunocompetence of patients with SSPE (abstract). *Arch. Neurol. 32,* 494–495.
6. Bodechtel, G., and Guttman, E. (1931). Diffuse encephalitis mit sklerosierender entzündung des hemispherenmarkes. *A. Ges. Neurol. Psychiatr. 133,* 601–619.
7. Bogaert, L. van (1945). Une leuco-encephalite sclerosante subaigue. *J. Neurol. Psychiatry 8,* 101–120.
8. Bouteille, M., Fontaine, D., Vedrenne, C. L., Delarve, J. (1965). Sur un cas d'encephalite subaigue a inclusions. Etude anatomoclinique et ultrastructurale. *Rev. Neurol. (Paris) 113,* 454–458.
9. Brody, J. A., and Detels, R. (1970). Subacute sclerosing panencephalitis: A zoonosis, following aberrant measles. *Lancet ii,* 500–501.
10. Burnett, F. M. (1968). Measles as an index of immunological function. *Lancet ii,* 610–613.
11. Byington, D., and Johnson, K. P. (1972). Experimental subacute sclerosing panencephalitis in hamster: Correlation of age with chronic inclusion-cell encephalitis. *J. Infect. Dis. 126,* 18–26.
12. Connoly, J. H., Allen, I. V., Hurwitz, L. J., Millar, J. H. D. (1967). Measles virus antibody and antigen in subacute sclerosing panencephalitis. *Lancet i,* 542–544.
13. Dawson, J. R. (1933). Cellular inclusions in cerebral lesions of lethargic encephalitis. *Am. J. Pathol. 9,* 7–16.
14. Freeman, J. M., Magoffin, R. L., Lennette, E. H., Herndon, R. M. (1967). Addi-

tional evidence of the relation between subacute inclusion-body encephalitis and measles virus. *Lancet ii,* 129–131.

15. Hall, W., and Meulen V. ter (1974). Biochemical comparison of SSPE and measles viruses (abstract W1), p. 46. *Proceedings of Third International Congress of Virology, Madrid.*

16. Horta-Barbosa, L., Fuccillo, D. A., London, W. T., Jabbour, J. T., Zeman, W., Sever, D. L. (1969). Isolation of measles virus from brain cell cultures of two patients with subacute sclerosing panencephalitis. *Proc. Soc. Exp. Biol. Med. 132,* 272–277.

17. Jabbour, J. T., Roane, J. A., and Sever, D. L. (1969). Studies of delayed dermal hypersensitivity in patients with SSPE. *Neurology 19,* 929–932.

18. Käckell, Y. M., Grob, P. J., Kreth, W. H., *et al.* (1975). Transfer factor therapy in patients with subacute sclerosing panencephalitis. *J. Neurol. 21,* 1–11.

19. Katz, M., and Koprowski, H. (1973). The significance of failure to isolate infectious viruses in cases of subacute sclerosing panencephalitis. *Arch. Ges. Virusforsch. 41,* 390–393.

20. Katz, M., Oyanagi, S., and Koprowski, H. (1969). Subacute sclerosing panencephalitis: Structures resembling myxovirus neuclocapsids in cells cultured from brains. *Nature 222,* 888–890.

21. Koprowski, H., Barbanti-Brodano, G., and Katz, M. (1970). Interactions between papova-like virus and paramyxovirus in human brain cells: A hypothesis. *Nature 225,* 1045–1047.

22. Kreth, H. W., Käckell, Y. M., and Meulen, V. ter (1974). Cellular immunity in SSPE patients. *Med. Microbiol. Immunol. (Berl.) 160,* 191–199.

23. Meulen, V. ter, Enders-Ruckle, G., Müller, D., Joppich, G. (1969). Immunbiological microscopic and studies on encephalitis. III. Subacute progressive panencephalitis; virology and immunhistology. *Acta Neuropathol. (Berl.) 12,* 244–259.

24. Meulen, V. ter, Katz, M., Käckell, Y. M., *et al.* (1972). Subacute sclerosing panencephalitis: *In-vitro* characterization of viruses isolated from brain cells in culture. *J. Infect. Dis. 126,* 11–17.

25. Meulen, V. ter, Katz, M., and Käckell, Y. M. (1973). Properties of SSPE virus: Tissue culture and animal studies. *Ann. Clin. Res. 5,* 293–297.

26. Meulen, V. ter, Leonard, L. L., Katz, M., and Lennette, E. H. (1972). The effect of 6-azauridine upon subacute sclerosing panencephalitis virus in tissue cultures. *Proc. Soc. Exp. Biol. Med. 140,* 1111–1115.

27. Meulen, V. ter, Müller, D., and Joppich, G. (1967). Fluorescence microscopy studies of brain tissue from a case of subacute progressive encephalitis. *Ger. Med. 12,* 438–441.

28. Oldstone, M. B. A. Role of antibody in regulating virus persistence modulation of viral antigen expression on the cell plasma membrane and analysis of cell lysis. In *The Development of Host Defenses* (M. Cooper and D. Dayton, eds.), Raven Press, New York. (In Press)

29. Oyanagi, S., Muelen, V. ter, Katz, M., Koprowski, H. (1971). Comparison of subacute sclerosing panencephalitis and measles viruses, and electron microscope study. *J. Virol. 7,* 176–187.

30. Payne, F. E., and Baublis, J. V. (1973). Decreased reactivity of SSPE strain of measles virus with antibody. *J. Infect. Dis. 127,* 505–511.

31. Payne, F. E., Baublis, J. V., and Itabashi, H. H. (1969). Isolation of measles virus from cell cultures of brain from a patient with subacute sclerosing panencephalitis. *N. Engl. J. Med. 281,* 585–589.

32. Pette, H., and Döring, G. (1939). Über eine einheimische Panencephalomyelitis vom Character der Encephalitis Japonica. *Dtsch. A. Nervenheilk. 149,* 7–44.

33. Steele, R. W., Fuccillo, D. A., Hensen, S. A., *et al.* (1976). Specific inhibitory factors of cellular immunity in children with SSPE. *J. Pediatr. 88,* 56–62.

34. Tellez-Nagel, I., and Harter, D. H. (1966). Subacute sclerosing panencephalitis. I. Clinicopathological, electron microscopic and virological observations. *J. Neuropathol. Exp. Neurol. 25,* 560–581.

35. Vandvik, B., Froland, S. S., Hoyeraal, H. M., Stien, R., Degre, M. (1973). Immunological features of a case of subacute sclerosing panencephalitis treated with transfer factor. *Scand. J. Immunol. 2,* 367–374.

36. Vandvik, B., and Norrby, E. (1963). Oligoclonal IgG antibody response in the CNS to different measles virus agents in SSPE. *Proc. Natl. Acad. Sci. U.S.A. 70,* 1060–1063.

37. Wear, D. J., and Rapp, F. (1971). Latent measles virus infection of the hamster CNS. *J. Immunol. 107,* 1593–1598.

Comment/Chapter 7
Edwin H. Lennette

Dr. Katz's discussion is a very concise and lucid exposition on the value of a genome rescue on the resolution of the etiology of a disease. Using this approach, we have uncovered a potential candidate for inclusion in the slow virus disease family, namely, rubella. Recently, there have been two studies describing a hitherto unreported late complication of congenital rubella viral infection that becomes manifest as a chronic progressive panencephalitis.

In one study, comprised of three patients, motor and mental deterioration characteristic of subacute sclerosing panencephalitis developed in all three during the second decade of life. Attempts to isolate a virus from brain biopsy of one patient at age 22 were negative.

In the other study, involving a single male patient, progressive dementia began when the patient was 8 years old and a chronic progressive panencephalitis developed at the age of 12. Material from a brain biopsy taken at the age of 11 yielded a rubella virus. The virus was isolated by cocultivation of the trypsinized brain tissue with CV-1 cells. Culture of the trypsinized brain tissue showed no cytopathic effects, but at third passage indirect staining with fluorescent antibody revealed occasional cells containing rubella antigen. When this culture was cocultured with BSC-1 cells and serially passaged with these cells, the presence of rubella virus was confirmed by indirect fluorescent antibody staining and by refractoriness of the cultures to infection with an ECHO virus. The rubella antibody titer in the serum of this patient was 1:256 by the complement fixation method and 1:8196 by the hemagglutination inhibition test. The hemagglutination inhibiting antibody titer in the cerebrospinal fluid was 1:128. The hemagglutinating antibody in the serum and in the cerebrospinal fluid was determined to be of the IgG class. The hemagglutination inhibiting antibody titers to measles virus were 1:8 in the serum and less than 1:2 in the spinal fluid.

As was the case with the RV strain of rubella virus in one of our previous studies, viral particles of the present rubella virus strain were more readily seen in BHK 21 cells of other species, despite the high concentration of antigen stained by fluorescent antibody in the latter. Unlike the RV strain, however, the virus from this patient was not seen to bud from the cell surface. This may be a reflection of a low virus concentration. Alternatively, this may imply inability of the present virus to replicate at the cell surface, which would thus afford protection to the infected cell not only against neutralizing antibody but also against the action of cytolytic antibody or cytotoxic lymphocytes on cell membranes.

In summary, this study, together with other evidence in the current literature, indicates that rubella virus should be added to the growing list of viral agents involved in slow infections of the central nervous system.

CHAPTER 8
A Concept of Virus-Induced Demyelinating Encephalomyelitis Relative to an Animal Model

A. KOESTNER / S. KRAKOWKA

INTRODUCTION

Demyelination has been recognized as the principal lesion in many encephalopathies of man and animals. Multiple sclerosis (MS) is perhaps the best known of these demyelinating diseases. Demyelination has also been described, however, as the most prominent lesion in copper deficiency and visna in sheep, as well as in several so-called degenerative diseases of the central nervous system (CNS) in man, such as subacute sclerosing panencephalitis (SSPE), Schilder's disease, neuromyelitis optica, and the various leukodystrophies. Whereas the leukodystrophies are recognized as inherited degenerative disorders, there is no evidence of a genetic basis for other primary demyelinating diseases in man. A turning point in our understanding of the mechanisms of demyelination came when the occasional neurologic complications after rabies vaccination (Pasteur treatment) were recognized as demyelinating encephalopathies and correctly linked to the injection of rabbit spinal cord material contained within the vaccine. The postvaccinal disease was reproduced experimentally in animals by injection of heterologous or autologous spinal cord alone or in combination with Freund's complete adjuvant. This induced disease has been thoroughly explored and is well known as experimental allergic encephalomyelitis (EAE). The basic mechanism underlying EAE is a cell-mediated immune response of the host to myelin basic protein.

The discovery by Sigurdsson and his co-workers (30, 31, 32) that visna in sheep is a demyelinating disease caused by a viral agent suggested that viruses can cause demyelination of the CNS. Subacute sclerosing panencephalitis, which is related to measles virus (5, 7, 9, 11) and other subacute diseases of viral etiology involving the CNS, have pointed the way to a consideration of MS as a viral disease (10, 26).

Canine distemper virus (CDV) is a paramyxovirus closely related to measles virus. Both viruses may produce a subacute encephalitis following acute illness. In canine distemper, demyelinating encephalomyelitis may appear several weeks or months after recovery from the acute infection [acute MS of dogs (29) and SSPE of dogs (34)]. Encephalitis may also develop in any dog without any antecedent acute clinical illness. There is a variant of the disease in aged or immunized dogs, referred to as old dog encephalitis (20).

Intracytoplasmic and intranuclear inclusion bodies typical of distemper virus infection have been detected in glial cells within demyelinated lesions (1), which occur primarily in the white matter of the cerebellum, brain stem, and spinal cord and have a periventricular localization. The inclusions contain distemper virus antigen, as demonstrated by immunofluorescence, and paramyxovirus nucleocapsids, as seen by electron microscopy (27, 35).

Because of the morphologic similarities of CDV-associated demyelination to SSPE and perhaps also to MS, canine distemper may be a useful model for studies of paramyxovirus-induced demyelinating encephalitis (15).

VIRUS CELL INTERACTIONS IN VITRO

Interactions of CDV with neuroectodermal cells were studied in canine cerebellar explant cultures (12, 33). It was demonstrated that infected glial cells continued to replicate. Two weeks after the infection, essentially all cells had CDV inclusion bodies, which contained viral antigen and aggregates of viral nucleocapsids (Fig. 8.1). Maturation of virus through budding was noted (Fig. 8.2).

Cultures infected with CDV before myelination failed to myelinate. Cultures myelinated at the time of infection demyelinated slowly. It was

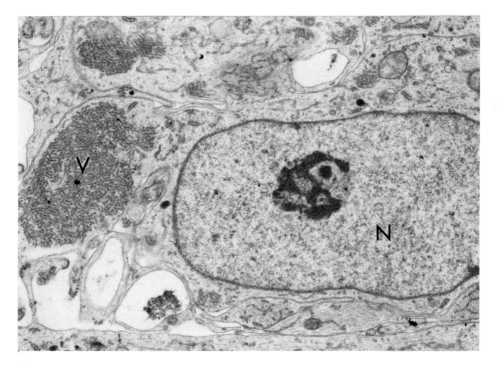

Figure 8.1.
Astrocyte in cerebellar explant culture infected with canine distemper virus. Intra-cytoplasmic aggregates of viral nucleocapsids (V) are illustrated. Uranyl acetate and lead citrate. N, nucleus. ×15,000

Figure 8.2.
Budding of CDV particles (arrow) are lining projecting cellular membranes of an infected glial cell in tissue culture. Uranyl acetate and lead citrate. ×57,500

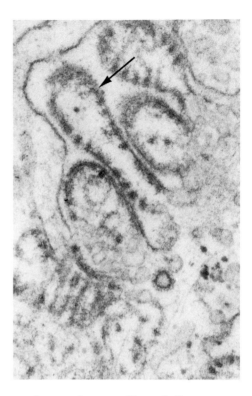

concluded that infection of cerebellar explant cultures affected the process of myelinization perhaps indirectly by impeding the function of glial cells responsible for myelin synthesis and maintenance.

AUTOIMMUNE REACTIONS

Autoimmune reactions have been investigated extensively in Experimental allergic encephalomyelitis (EAE). EAE can be transmitted to syngeneic hosts by sensitized lymphocytes obtained from animals with EAE (19). Although serum will not transmit the disease to animals, it will demyelinate cerebellar explant cultures. This reaction is complement dependent. Similar antibody activity has been observed with sera from patients with MS, particularly when the specimens were obtained during an exacerbation of the disease (3, 4).

Sera of dogs affected with distemper-associated demyelinating encephalitis also possess this type of demyelinating activity (13, 14). Addition of convalescent sera to explant cultures of canine cerebellum results in myelin destruction within 32 to 48 hr. When the serum is replaced with normal medium, the cultures remyelinate within 2 weeks. Not all such sera, however, demyelinate the cultures, and some sera from unaffected dogs can also cause demyelination. This inconsistency suggests that perhaps factors other than antimyelin antibodies affect myelin in tissue culture and that during the course of distemper encephalitis different classes of antibodies may prevail at various times. Some of them may interfere with complement activation that is essential for *in vitro* demyelination.

118

In order to resolve some of these problems, sera were examined for antibody activity against myelin (16). For this purpose, sera were collected from histopathologically confirmed cases of naturally occurring distemper with demyelinating encephalitis. Control sera were obtained from randomly selected healthy dogs and from gnotobiotic dogs. They were tested by the microtiter complement-fixation, complement-fixation inhibition, and indirect immunofluorescence methods. Complement-fixing immunoglobulin M antibodies and non-complement-fixing immunoglobulin G antibodies were found in 97% of the sera of CDV infected dogs. In comparison, only 28% of control sera contained these antibodies with a mean antibody titer significantly lower ($p < 0.05$) than that of the distemper group. It was further demonstrated that sera of animals not reacting with myelin in the complement-fixation test always had noncomplement-fixing antibody titers against myelin. This suggests an explanation for the inability of some sera to demyelinate explant cultures. When the complement-fixation test was compared with the immunofluorescence test, good correlation was demonstrated, although the complement-fixation test was more sensitive. The results of these tests indicate that immune mechanisms may play an important pathogenetic role in demyelination associated with canine distemper infection.

ESTABLISHMENT OF AN EXPERIMENTAL MODEL FOR CANINE DISTEMPER-INDUCED DEMYELINATION

Delineation of pathogenetic events in any naturally occurring disease is hampered by the uncertainty of the time of onset of the infection, influence of intercurrent disease, treatment, and the unavailability of animals for study during the early stages of the disease. It became apparent during the studies of canine distemper that an experimental model was essential. Previous attempts to produce demyelinating encephalomyelitis by infecting dogs with available isolates of CDV were unsuccessful. Only a small percentage of animals (2 to 3% in some experiments) developed demyelination, whereas the remaining dogs died of acute respiratory infection (2). Experience with SSPE suggested that only certain specific virus isolates or strains may be effective. Reculard and Guillon (8, 28) caused demyelination in a large percentage of dogs with a special virus strain used in the production of canine distemper vaccines. We succeeded in inducing demyelinating encephalomyelitis in a large number of dogs, using a CDV isolate originally obtained from a natural case of encephalitis and passaged through the brains of gnotobiotic pups. After several trials, the R252 virus was isolated by cocultivation with Vero cells.

BIOLOGIC PROPERTIES OF THE R252 CANINE DISTEMPER VIRUS ISOLATE

The R252 CDV in contrast to other widely studied distemper virus strains, such as Snyder-Hill and Onderstepoort, does not produce a fatal respiratory infection but causes demyelinating encephalomyelitis in 47% of animals after an incubation period of 45 to 60 days (13–15, 22, 23). In tissue culture, intracellular R252 virus accumulates more slowly than the other strains. Immunofluorescence studies indicate that the rate of spread of R252 virus infection within the monolayers of Vero cells is intermediate between the rapid Snyder-Hill and the slow Onderstepoort strains. The R252-virus infected cells develop characteristics immunofluorescent cytoplasmic inclusions (6), which initially stain homogeneously but later appear as nonfluorescent bodies surrounded by a fluorescent ring. Such a pattern is seen only in the late stages of Snyder-Hill infection and never in Onderstepoort infections. The three strains cannot be distinguished immunologically by the neutralization test (6).

EFFECT OF THE VIRUS ON GNOTOBIOTIC PUPS

The effect of the virus upon the natural host was tested in gnotobiotic dogs in order to avoid the effects of colostrum-derived immunity and complication of secondary bacterial infections (22, 23). Animals were inoculated at 4 weeks of age; animals inoculated at younger ages often died of an acute infection. Various routes of infection were tested. Most effective were the intracerebral inoculation and contact exposure. The infected animals fell into three groups based upon the effect of the virus. Group 1 consisted of 11 dogs all of which developed encephalitis after an incubation period of 20 to 45 days, which was characterized by focal demyelination. There was no perivascular cuffing. The lesions contained inclusion bodies. All of the animals died within 6 days and exhibited a sustained lymphopenia throughout the course of the disease. Group 2 consisted of five animals that developed a subacute demyelinating encephalitis and a transient lymphopenia. The clinical course was prolonged, and all dogs were alive at the termination of the experiments 12 weeks after infection. The lesions were multifocal and associated with perivascular cuffs of lymphoid and mononuclear cells. Viral inclusion bodies were demonstrated. Two of these animals showed improvement and remission during the observation period. The 19 dogs in Group 3 had an asymptomatic CDV infection and no CNS lesions. They did, however, demonstrate transient lymphopenia.

All of the affected animals had lesions in predilection sites corresponding to those seen in naturally occurring distemper virus encephalitis. Demyelinated patches were found in the cerebellar folia, medulla oblongata, and spinal cord. The optic tract was often extensively affected. Electron microscopy revealed naked, intact axons surrounded by astrocytic processes (Fig. 8.3). Numerous macrophages containing breakdown products of myelin were also noted. Extracellular edema was prominent in areas of demyelination. Intracytoplasmic nucleocapsids were demonstrated in glial cells and in lymphocytes, but they did not line the cellular membranes. This pattern was reminiscent of the one observed in SSPE and in cases of MS where paramyxoviruses were found in glial cells within the lesions (27).

Figure 8.3.
Demyelinated axons (A) in cerebellum of dog experimentally infected with R252 CDV, 11 weeks after infection. Demyelinated axons are intact and surrounded by astrocytic processes (arrow). Uranyl acetate and lead citrate. ×11,500

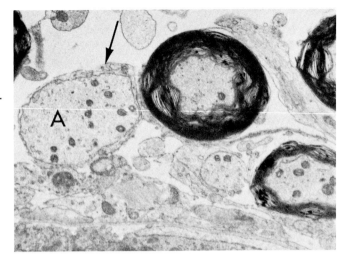

IMMUNE RESPONSES IN EXPERIMENTALLY INFECTED DOGS

In five of seven dogs in Group 1, thymus glands could not be demonstrated grossly; in the remaining two, the glands weighed approximately 5 g. Dogs in Groups 2 and 3 had thymuses weighing between 5 and 27 g (21).

Lymphocyte function was tested by phytomitogen stimulation *in vitro* and skin allograft rejection *in vivo*. Infection with R252 CDV resulted in a depression of peripheral blood lymphocyte mitogen response as measured by tritiated thymidine incorporation for up to 10 weeks after inoculation (17). Although that effect coincided with the appearance of viral antigen in leukocytes, it persisted after the virus was no longer detectable by immunofluorescence. Although all infected dogs had a decreased mitogen reactivity, there was no significant delay in graft rejection in comparison with controls. This study suggested that the suppression of immune function during the course of CDV infection is incomplete and that perhaps a small number of sensitized T lymphocytes is sufficient to stimulate macrophages to reject skin allografts.

All animals were monitored throughout the course of this experiment for their antibody response to CNS myelin and viral antigens (16, 18). The antimyelin response differed among the three groups but was consistent within each group. Dogs of Group 3 produced the highest antibody titers with a peak at 3 weeks and a slow decrement thereafter. In contrast, acutely affected dogs of Group 1 showed little or no antibody activity against myelin. Persistently infected dogs of Group 2 were intermediate in antibody response (16). This pattern of activity was also discernable in the complement-fixing and serum neutralization assays for CDV antibodies (18). The possibility was considered that the CNS myelin and viral proteins share common antigens and that these similar antibody response patterns reflecting this cross reactivity. In order to test this possibility, sera from dogs previously immunized with Keyhole Limpet Hemocyanin (KLH) and subsequently infected with CDV were examined by absorption experiments. Absorption of sera with CNS myelin removed antimyelin activity, whereas antibody titers to CDV and KLH were unaffected. In addition, sera from normal gnotobiotic dogs hyperimmunized with either CNS myelin or CDV failed to cross react in either complement-fixing or viral neutralization tests (18). These studies made the possibility of cross reactivity between virus and myelin unlikely.

ENZYME ACTIVITIES ASSOCIATED WITH THE DEMYELINATING PHASE OF CANINE DISTEMPER

This study was concerned with the enzymatic processes responsible for the initiation of demyelination, which are still poorly understood. White matter from which myelin has been lost as a consequence of MS and SSPE in man and swayback in sheep contains abnormally low amounts of the myelin lipids, cholesterol, galactolipid, and ethanolamine plasmalogen. Each of these myelin components must be catabolized or removed from the brain. Plasmalogenase (1-alk-1′-enyl-2-acyl-sn-glycero-e-phosphorylethanolamine alk-1′-enyl hydrolase) initiates the catabolism of ethanolamine plasmalogen by hydrolysis of its vinyl ether linkage to release a fatty aldehyde. The enzyme is located in white matter. An elevation of plasmalogenase activity has been found in partially demyelinated white matter resulting from MS in a human patient and avitaminosis B_{12} in monkeys, suggesting a common catabolic mechanism in demyelination caused by apparently unrelated factors. We have demonstrated that plasmalogenase activity is 67% higher in the brains of dogs with demyelination resulting from canine distemper than in brains of age-matched control dogs (24). Plasmalogenase activity was also significantly higher in the CSF of distemper dogs than in the CSF of healthy controls. The finding that plasmalogenase activity in demyelinating diseases was highest in the tissues with the least severe demyelination suggests that plasmalogenase acts early in the process of demyelination. The elevation of plasmalogenase activity and loss of plasmalogen that occurs in other demyelinating diseases supports the hypothesis that plasmalogenase is part of a common catabolic mechanism of demyelination.

When rabbit serum containing antimyelin antibody (titer 1:256) was injected intracerebrally into rats, a 45% elevation of plasmalogenase activity over uninoculated control brain levels was detected at 3 days and a 100% elevation at 6 days after innoculation. Plasmalogenase levels returned to normal levels 9 days after injection. Control rats receiving normal serum had a moderate but transient elevation of plasmalogenase (up to 25%) attributable to trauma of injection.

Three proteolytic enzymes were also tested: β-glucuronidase and acid and neutral proteinases (25). The first objective of this study was the determination of the activities of acid and neutral proteinase and β-glucuronidase in the cerebellum of dogs with distemper-associated demyelination in comparison to normal dogs. The second objective was evaluation of the source and significance of the enzyme changes found in demyelinated tissue. This was attempted (a) by comparing the content of these enzymes in isolated lymph node lymphocytes with the enzyme changes in severely demyelinated tissue, (b) by measuring these enzyme activities in canine glial monolayer cultures infected with CDV or exposed to myelinotoxic serum and comparing them with the levels of activity in uninfected and unexposed control cultures, and (c) by assessing the activities of these enzymes during early and late cerebral infarction and comparing any enzyme changes with enzyme changes previously demonstrated in areas of demyelination.

Specific enzyme activity was higher in the cerebellum of dogs with distemper-associated demyelination than in age-matched controls. The highest elevation corresponded with the most severely cerebellar demyelination. The direct effect of distemper virus and serum on these enzymes was tested in canine glial monolayers. Virus infection resulted in lower enzyme activity in cells concomitant with the appearance of cellular lesions. There was a relative increase of β-glucuronidase activity in the medium suggesting that distemper virus released preformed lysosomal enzymes. Serum obtained from dogs with distemper-associated demyelination that had previously demyelinated cerebellar explants also decreased activities of all three enzymes *in vitro*.

The three enzymes were also measured in gerbil brains at various time intervals following unilateral cerebral infarction to determine whether processes other than demyelination resulted in an increase of enzyme activity. Uncomplicated ischemic necrosis (24 hr after infarction) had no detectable effect. Invasion of macrophages 10 days after infarction resulted in a fivefold increase of acid proteinase and a 15-fold increase of β-glucuronidase activities over the control values but caused no change in neutral proteinase activity (25).

It was concluded that the increased activity of acid proteinase and β-glucuronidase in demyelinated tissue probably results from macrophages ingestion of the damaged tissue. Neutral proteinase may be more specifically involved in the demyelinating process, since it is partially located within myelin and can degrade the myelin basic protein.

CONCLUSIONS

The importance of the agent and immune response of the host must both be considered in forming an hypothesis on the pathogenesis of this disease.

The Agent

Guillon and Reculard (8, 28) tested in dogs the effect of distemper virus infection, immunosuppression, and infusion of immune serum on the development of demyelinative encephalitis. After several trials with different virus isolates, they noted that the nature of the virus was the most important variable. Only one of the five isolates available for testing produced encephalitis. In our experiments, only two viral isolates, the French isolate and the R252 isolate, were capable of producing demyelinative encephalomyelitis in gnotobiotic pups. Other distemper virus strains, the Snyder-Hill strain and the Lederle vaccine strain, produced fatal acute respiratory disease, but no demyelination.

Similarly, only some isolates of measles virus cause encephalitis in experimental animals and the same has been observed for SSPE viruses. So far, no laboratory data are available that would define neurotropism from a virologic point of view. It has been shown in other virus systems that defective interfering virus particles play an important role in establishing virus persistency. Such defective interfering particles have also been described for measles virus, and the same seems to be true for SSPE virus, since isolation of infectious virus from brain material can only be achieved by cell fusion. This phenomenon reactivates infectious virus. It is not known at what stage of SSPE virus replication the defect occurs in the CNS and how the defect is biochemically defined. However, ultrastructural studies of SSPE brain material and distemper encephalitis have revealed that infected brain cells are loaded with nucleocapsids, but the typical budding process of the paramyxoviruses has never been observed in such material. This suggests that virus budding is inhibited and virus particles are probably not found. The analysis of the virus-host relationship in these CNS diseases will certainly contribute toward the understanding of the pathogenic processes.

Immune Mechanisms

The presence of circulating myelin specific autoantibodies in experimentally infected dogs early during the course of infection and perhaps preceding clinical disease by 2 to 3 weeks suggests that such antibodies participate in the process of demyelination. It seems significant that circulating antibodies in the presence of complement are capable of demyelinating cerebellar explant cultures and that this capability is shared by lymphocytes obtained from animals with EAE where immune mechanisms have been definitely established as the pathogenetic factor. It is very likely that distemper sensitized lymphocytes, which play a major role in EAE, contribute to the further development of demyelinating lesions.

The immunosuppressive activity of the distemper virus may be an important factor in establishing a permanent infection. How the persistence of this infection is maintained is still unknown. Immunologic mechanisms (antiviral antibodies or sensitized lymphocytes) may exert a regulatory role on the production of free infectious virus in the brain and thus promote a cell-associated infection.

Reactivation of latent infection by either reinfection with the same virus or antigenically similar viruses, immunosuppression, or yet unknown mechanisms may trigger relapses as they occur in MS. The model described will be used to investigate these aspects of demyelinating encephalomyelitis.

REFERENCES

1. Appel, M. J. G. (1969). Pathogenesis of canine distemper. *Am. J. Vet. Res. 30,* 1167.
2. Appel, M. J. G., and Gillespie, J. J. (1972). Canine distemper virus. *Virol. Monogr. 11,* 1–96.
3. Bornstein, M. B., Appel, S. H., and Murray, M. R. (1961). The application of tissue culture to the study of experimental allergic encephalomyelitis. *J. Neuropathol. Exp. Neurol. 20,* 141–157.
4. Bornstein, M. B. (1963). A tissue culture approach to demyelinative disorders. *Natl. Cancer Inst. Monogr. 11,* 197–214.
5. Chen, T. T., Watanabe, I., Zeman, W., and Mealey, Jr., J. (1969). Subacute sclerosing panencephalitis: Propagation of measles virus from brain biopsy in tissue culture. *Science 163,* 1193–1194.
6. Confer, A. W., Kahn, D. E., Koestner, A., and Krakowka, S. (1975). Biological properties of a canine distemper virus isolate associated with demyelinating encephalitis. *Infect. Immun. 11,* 835–844.
7. Connolly, J. H., Allen, I. V., Hurwitz, L. H., and Millar, J. H. (1967). Measles-virus antibody and antigen in subacute sclerosing panencephalitis. *Lancet i,* 542–544.
8. Guillon, J. C., and Reculard, P. (1970). L'encéphalite de la maladie de carré du chien, modéle expérimentale pour la neuropathologie humaine. *Bull. Acad. Vet. Fr. 43,* 293–298.
9. Horta-Barbosa, L., Fuccillo, D. A., Sever, J. L., and Zeman, W. (1969). Subacute sclerosing panencephalitis: Isolation of measles virus from a brain biopsy. *Nature 221,* 974.
10. Iwasaki, Y., Koprowski, H., Müller, D., ter Meulen, V., and Käckell, Y. M. (1973). Morphogenesis and structure of a virus in cells cultured from brain tissue from two cases of multiple sclerosis. *Lab. Invest. 28,* 494–500.
11. Katz, M., Rorke, L. B., Masland, W. S., Koprowski, H., and Tucker, S. H. (1968). Transmission of an encephalitogenic agent from brains of patients with subacute sclerosing panencephalitis to ferrets. *N. Engl. J. Med. 279,* 793–798.
12. Koestner, A., and Long, J. F. (1970). Ultrastructure of canine distemper virus in explant tissue cultures of canine cerebellum. *Lab. Invest. 23,* 196–201.
13. Koestner, A., Long, J. F., Jacoby, R. O., Olsen, R. G., and Shadduck, J. A. (1970). Canine distemper as a model of parainfectious demyelinating encephalopathy. *Proc. VI Int. Congress Neuropathol. (Paris),* p. 837.
14. Koestner, A., McCullough, B., Krakowka, G. S., Long, J. F., and Olsen, R. G. (1974). Canine distemper. A virus-induced demyelinating encephalomyelitis. In *Slow Virus Diseases* (W. Zeman and E. H. Lennette, eds.), pp. 86–101. Williams & Wilkins, Baltimore.
15. Koestner, A. (1975). Animal model of human disease. Animal model: Distemper associated demyelinating encephalomyelitis. *Am. J. Pathol. 78,* 361–364.
16. Krakowka, S., McCullough, B., Koestner, A., and Olsen, R. G. (1973). Myelin-specific autoantibodies associated with central nervous system demyelination in canine distemper infection. *Infect. Immun. 8,* 819–827.
17. Krakowka, S., Cockerell, G., and Koestner, A. (1975). Effects of canine distemper virus infection on lymphoid function in vitro and in vivo. *Infect. Immun. 11,* 1069–1078.
18. Krakowka, S., Olsen, R., Confer, A., Koestner, A., and McCullough, B. (1975). Serologic response to canine distemper viral antigens in gnotobiotic dogs infected with R252 canine distemper virus. *J. Infect. Dis.* in press. 132: 384–392.
19. Levine, S. (1970). Allergic encephalomyelitis: Cellular transformation and vascular blockade. *J. Neuropathol. Exp. Neurol. 29,* 6–20.

20. Lincoln, S. D., Gorham, J. R., Ott, R. L., and Hegreberg, G. A. (1971). Etiologic studies on old dog encephalitis. *Vet. Pathol. 8*, 1–8.
21. McCullough, B., Krakowka, S., and Koestner, A. (1974). Experimental canine distemper virus-induced lymphoid depletion. *Am. J. Pathol. 74*, 155–166.
22. McCullough, B., Krakowka, S., Koestner, A., and Shadduck, J. (1974). Demyelinating activity of canine distemper virus isolates in gnotobiotic dogs. *J. Inf. Dis. 130*, 343–350.
23. McCullough, B., Krakowka, S., and Koestner, A. (1974). Experimental canine distemper virus-induced demyelination. *Lab. Invest. 31*, 216–222.
24. McMartin, D. N., Horrocks, L. A., and Koestner, A. (1972). Enzyme activities associated with the demyelinating phase of canine distemper. II. Plasmalogenase. *Acta Neuropathol. (Berl.) 22*, 288–294.
25. McMartin, D. N., Koestner, A., and Long, J. F. (1972). Enzyme activities associated with the demyelinating phase of canine distemper. I. Beta-glucuronidase, acid and neutral proteinases. *Acta Neuropathol. (Berl.) 22*, 275–287.
26. Prineas, J. (1972). Paramyxovirus-like particles associated with acute demyelination in chronic relapsing multiple sclerosis. *Science 178*, 760–763.
27. Raine, C. S. (1972). Viral infections of nervous tissue and their relevance to multiple sclerosis. In *Multiple Sclerosis* (F. Wolfram, G. W. Ellison, J. G. Stevens, and J. M. Andrews, eds.), p. 91. Academic, New York, London.
28. Reculard, P., and Guillon, J. C. (1972). Étude expérimerimentale de quelques souches du virus de la maladie de carré du chien. Identification et définition de souches variantes. *Ann. Inst. Pasteur Lille 123*, 477–487.
29. Scherer, H. J. (1944). *Vergleichende Pathologie des Nervensystems der Saügetiere*, p. 282. Georg Thieme, Leipzig.
30. Sigurdsson, B., Pálsson, P. A., and Grímsson, H. (1957). Visna, a demyelinating transmissible disease of sheep. *J. Neuropathol. Exp. Neurol. 16*, 389–403.
31. Sigurdsson, B., and Pálsson, P. A. (1958). Visna of sheep. A slow, demyelinating infection. *Br. J. Exp. Pathol. 39*, 519–528.
32. Sigurdsson, B., Thormar, H., and Pálsson, P. A. (1960). Cultivation of visna virus in tissue culture. *Arch. Gesamte Virusforsch. 10*, 368–381.
33. Storts, R. W., Koestner, A., and Dennis, R. A. (1968). The effects of canine distemper virus on explant tissue cultures of canine cerebellum. *Acta Neuropathol. 11*, 1–14.
34. Van Bogaert, L., and Innes, J. R. M. (1962). Subacute diffuse sclerosing encephalitis in the dog. In *Comparative Neuropathology* (Innes and Saunders, eds.), p. 394. Academic, New York.
35. Wisniewski, H. M., Raine, C. S., and Kay, W. J. (1972). Observations on viral demyelinating encephalomyelitis. Canine distemper. *Lab. Invest. 26*, 589.

Comment / Chapter 8
Monique Dubois-Dalcq

It is worth illustrating a morphologic technique for the study of cells in productive and resistant infections. We have used surface replica technique, which provides a simple means for looking at the outer surface of cells as they grow on coverslips. Figure 8A.1 illustrates Vero cells in productive SSPE infection. Only the infected cells have surfaces that seem to be covered with granular strands. These strands appear 2 days after infection and begin to increase in numbers and thickness until they eventually become more convoluted. Immunoperoxidase method, in which reaction products of the peroxidase can be visualized on the surface replica, allows recognition of viral antigenic sites.

When virus is produced, the changes on the surface are even more extensive in the giant cells (Fig. 8A.1). In contrast, a chronically infected cell line (Fig. 8A.2) exhibits an entirely different budding process. Ninety percent of the infected cells show surfaces covered by elongated projections that do not appear like the normal cellular projections in infected cells. It is important to realize that underneath each of the elongated ridges there is a nucleocapsid. It appears that these ridges can be

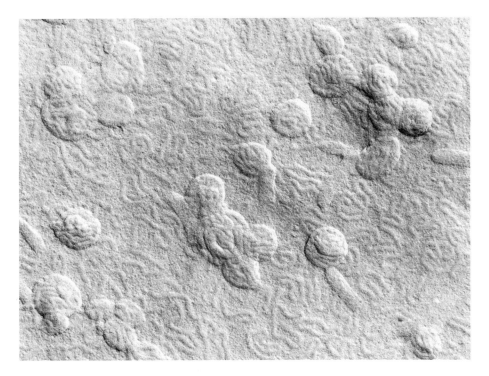

Figure 8A.1.
Vero cells inoculated with the Halle strain of SSPE virus. The surface of giant cells is covered with twisted ridges which have been shown to bear specific viral antigenic sites (1). Round-shaped viral buds or particles are present on the cell surface, isolated or in groups. The spacing between ridges is smaller on the viral buds than on the adjacent membrane.

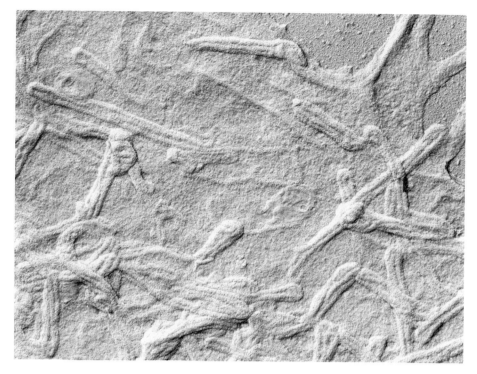

Figure 8A.2.
Human prostate cells chronically infected with the Mantooth strain of SSPE virus. Scattered straight ridges are seen on the membrane. Many elongated processes bear long ridges, often hairpin-shaped.

as long as 5 μm and can be extremely rigid. If this is true, then the nucleocapsids beneath these ridges are likely to be very rigid also and may, therefore, be prevented from entering the viral bud. This may explain, perhaps, the reason for the many defective, empty viral particles in cells chronically infected with SSPE viruses.

REFERENCES

1. Dubois-Dalcq, M., and Reese, T. S. (1975). Structural changes in the membrane of Vero cells infected with a paramyxovirus. *J. Cell Biol.* *67*, 551–565.

CHAPTER 9

The Biologic Role of Host-Dependent Proteolytic Cleavage of a Paramyxovirus Glycoprotein*

PURNELL W. CHOPPIN / ANDREAS SCHEID

INTRODUCTION

For several years our laboratory has been involved in the isolation and purification of the various envelope proteins of paramyxoviruses and the identification of their biologic activities. The glycoproteins of the virion form the projections or spikes on the virus surface. It has been found with three different viruses—simian virus 5 (SV5), Newcastle disease virus, and Sendai virus—that both receptor-binding (hemagglutinating) and neuraminidase activities are associated with one glycoprotein, the largest glycoprotein, now designated HN (8–10, 14). The association of both of these biologic activities with a single paramyxovirus protein is in contrast to the situation with myxoviruses in which hemagglutinating and neuraminidase activities reside on two different glycoproteins.

The finding that the smaller paramyxovirus glycoprotein (F) possessed neither of these activities led us to suggest that this protein might be involved in other important biologic properties associated with the viral envelope, that is, virus-induced hemolysis and cell fusion (8, 14), although no direct evidence was available at the time. Subsequently, such evidence for the involvement of this protein in these activities and also in the initiation of infection was obtained with Sendai virus in our laboratory (9) and independently by Homma and his colleagues (3). In both instances, this demonstration was made possible by the failure of a particular type of host cell to provide the necessary enzyme to accomplish an essential proteolytic cleavage of the precursor of the smaller glycoprotein. We have subsequently obtained mutants of Sendai virus that vary in their susceptibility to proteases, and therefore in their ability to undergo multiple cycle replication in different host systems. These results and some of their biologic implications are summarized briefly. They have been described in detail elsewhere (9–14).

* Research supported by Research Grant Nos. AI-05600 from The National Institute of Allergy and Infectious Diseases, U.S.P.H.S. and BMS 7409873 from The National Science Foundation.

ACTIVATION OF INFECTIVITY, CELL FUSION, AND HEMOLYSIS BY SENDAI VIRUS

Sendai virions grown in the allantoic sac of the chick embryo contain two glycoproteins; the larger (HN) has an estimated molecular weight of 69,000 to 72,000 (depending on the gel system used for estimation) and possesses both hemagglutinating and neuraminidase activities. F has a molecular weight of 48,000 to 53,000. Virions of the same myxovirus strain grown in the bovine kidney (MDBK, Madin Darby bovine kidney) line of bovine kidney cells possess the HN glycoprotein and another glycoprotein with a molecular weight of ~65,000 (designated F_0), but only a small amount of the F glycoprotein (9). This is illustrated in Fig. 9.1. This finding suggested that F was derived from F_0 by proteolytic cleavage, and that the chick embryo provided the necessary protease for this cleavage, whereas MDBK cells did not. That this was the case was demonstrated by cleavage of the F_0 protein of MDBK cell-grown virions *in vitro* with low concentrations of trypsin, for example, 1 to 5 μg/ml, yielding the F protein. The important biologic correlates of the F_0–F cleavage are that the virions grown in the chick embryo, which contain the F protein, are infectious and possess cell-fusing and hemolyzing activities. Those grown in MDBK cells, which contain the biologically inactive F_0 precursor protein, possess none of these activities but are activated upon cleavage of F_0 *in vitro*,

Figure 9.1.
Polypeptides of Sendai virions in MDBK cells (left lane) and the embryonated chicken egg (right lane). The glyco-proteins of the virion are indicated on the left and the nonglycosylated internal virion proteins on the right. The SDS polyacrylamide gel electro-phoresis with the origin at the top. Stained with Coomassie Blue.

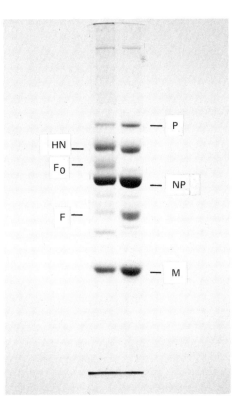

TABLE 9.1 / Correlation between the Glycoprotein Composition and the Biologic Activities of Sendai Virus

		Source of Virions		
		Embryonated Chicken Egg	MDBK Cells	MDBK Cells, Virions Treated with Trypsin
Glycoproteins	HN	+	+	+
present	F_0	−	+	−
in virion	F	+	Small amount	+
Biologic	Infectivity	+	−	+
activity	Hemolysis	+	−	+
of virions	Cell fusion	+	−	+

infectivity, hemolysis, and cell fusion (9). This correlation of biologic activities with the glycoprotein content of Sendai virions is summarized in Table 9.1.

PROTEASE ACTIVATION MUTANTS

Present in Sendai Virus

The production of noninfective Sendai virions by MDBK cells means that the virus cannot undergo multiple cycle replication in these cells and cannot, therefore, form plaques. However, when trypsin, 0.3 μg/ml, is added to the agar overlay, the F_0 protein of the virus produced by the cells is cleaved, and the virus is activated, thus permitting multiple-cycle replication and plaque formation. This is illustrated in Fig. 9.2. The addition of several other proteases, such as chymotrypsin or elastase, will not permit plaque formation. The ability of the virus to undergo multiple-cycle replication when a protease is added to the system has permitted the selection of mutants that are activated by specific proteases (11, 12). Sendai virus was mutagenized with nitrous acid, and MDBK cells were inoculated with the treated virus and incubated in the presence of different proteases, including chymotrypsin, elastase, and plasminogen. Viruses that grew in the presence of these proteases was then plaque-purified, and virus stocks were grown in the presence of the specific protease. The susceptibility to cleavage of the F_0 proteins of these mutants, which were designated protease activation (pa) mutants, and the activation of their biologic properties by specific proteases were then examined. The wild-type (wt) virus is activated by trypsin, but not by chymotrypsin, elastase, or plasmin. One class of mutants isolated in the presence of chymotrypsin is activated by this enzyme and also elastase, but no longer by trypsin. Two classes of mutants were isolated in the presence of elastase, one was activated by elastase alone, and another by both elastase and trypsin. Mutants have also been obtained that were

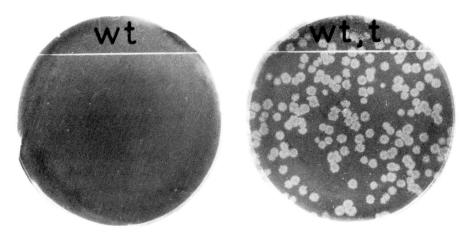

Figure 9.2.
Plaque formation in MDBK monolayers by wt Sendai virus in the presence of trypsin. Confluent monolayers were inoculated with equal concentrations of virus. The agar overlay contained reinforced Eagle's medium alone (left) or medium with N-acetyl-trypsin, 0.3 μg/ml (right). Photographs of unstained dishes after 5 days.

activated by plasmin. Table 9.2 illustrates the spectrum of activation of several pa mutants by proteases. The activation of biologic activities, as tested by assays of infectivity and hemolysis by the mutants, was correlated with cleavage of the F_0 glycoprotein to F.

Altered Host Range

As indicated previously, wt Sendai virus is incapable of multiple-cycle replication in MDBK cells, because it lacks an appropriate protease, but the virus does replicate efficiently in the chick embryo, because this host provides an activating protease. However, as illustrated in Table 9.3, a chymotrypsin-selected mutant, pa-c1, cannot undergo multiple replication in the chick embryo; an appropriate protease is apparently not available in the allantoic sac of the embryo. If chymotrypsin is injected into the allantoic sac at the time of infection, multiple-cycle replication does occur.

TABLE 9.2 / Activation of Wild-Type Sendai Virus and pa Mutants by Proteases in Vivo[a]

	Protease Added			
Virus	None	Trypsin	Chymotrypsin	Elastase
Wild-type	—	+	—	—
Mutant pa-c1	—	—	+	+
pa-e1	—	+	—	+
pa-e2	—	—	—	+

[a] Monolayers of MDBK cells were inoculated with virus and received agar overlays containing proteases as described in Fig. 9.1. Plaque formation was scored after 5 days.

TABLE 9.3 / Requirement for Chymotrypsin for Multiple Cycle Replication of a Sendai Virus pa Mutant in the Embryonated Chicken Egg

	Virus Yield (HAU/ml)	
	---	---
	Protease Injected into the Allantoic Sac	
Inoculum[a]	None	Chymotrypsin (30 μg)
Wild-type virus	2048	2048
Mutant pa-c1	< 4	1024

[a] 10^4 infectious units per egg.

Similarly, an elastase mutant, pa-e1, which requires this enzyme for replication, will not grow in the chick embryo unless elastase is supplied, but another mutant, pa-e2, which can be activated by either trypsin or elastase, can grow in the absence of added enzyme, because it is activated by endogenous protease. It should be recalled here that the wt virus that is also susceptible to trypsin replicates efficiently in the chick embryo.

DISCUSSION

Although the exact chemical mechanism by which paramyxoviruses induce cell fusion and hemolysis remains to be elucidated, the results of studies of cleavage of the F_0 glycoprotein to F have clearly shown that this smaller glycoprotein is involved in these biologic activities, and that the active protein F is derived from a biologically inactive precursor. The finding that hemolyzing and cell-fusing activities are acquired together was not unexpected, since many workers in the field have considered these two activities to be reflections of the same basic alteration in cell membranes, although there has not been unanimous agreement on this point in the past. The finding that infectivity is also acquired on cleavage of F_0 to F required further consideration. The step in infection that is affected by cleavage is clearly beyond adsorption, which is mediated by the HN protein, but prior to the expression of the viral genome. As we suggested previously (9), the most straightforward explanation appears to be that, since the virion acquires infectivity simultaneously with the ability to cause cell membrane fusion, the activation of infectivity is associated with the ability of the viral membrane to fuse with the cell membrane. Thus, these results are compatible with the conclusion that the penetration of the paramyxoviruses involved fusion of viral and cell membranes, an hypothesis suggested by Morgan and Howe (7) on the basis of electron microscopic evidence.

The studies with wt Sendai virus, which indicated that the initiation of biologic activities is dependent on the cleavage of a virion glycoprotein by a protease supplied by the host, have not only established a biologic role for this protein, but also provided a biochemical explanation for host-dependent variation among paramyxoviruses observed previously (1, 2, 4–6, 15).

The isolation of protease activation mutants has provided further evidence that specific proteolytic cleavage of the F_0 protein is required for initiating biologic activity and has emphasized the biologic significance of this phenomenon. The requirement for a specific protease for the production of infective virions, and thus for multiple-cycle replication and spread of the virus, clearly indicates that the tropism and host range of the virus are dependent in part on the presence of an appropriate protease in the tissue, organ, or host. A striking illustration of this is the failure of the pa-cl mutant to undergo multiple-cycle growth in the chick embryo when the F_0 glycoprotein becomes resistant to cleavage by the enzymes available in the allantoic sac. This not only demonstrates the specificity of the requirement of the virus but also indicates the limited variety of proteases available in a host.

The possible implications of host-dependent proteolytic activation of infectivity extend beyond the question of host range and tissue tropism. It is an important question whether, in some persistent infections in which infective virus is not produced, the lack of production of infective virus is due to the absence of a protease required by the virus. In the systems described here with Sendai virus, noninfective particles are produced; however, it is conceivable that in some other virus cell systems, the lack of cleavage could result in failure of efficient virus assembly. Persistent paramyxovirus infections in which few or no infective virions are produced are common in cultured cells but also occur in animals and man, for example, in the disease subacute sclerosing panencephalitis. The possibility should be considered that in at least some of these infections, the defect results from the absence in the tissue of the appropriate protease. Rescue of virus from persistent infections has at times been accomplished by cocultivation with other cells. One function, which now should be added to the list of possible contributions by the "permissive" cell, is the provision of a protease capable of activating the virus.

The finding of protease activation mutants has raised another interesting and perhaps biologically important possibility. The rare infection by a paramyxovirus of a tissue or organ that is not usually affected by that virus, for example, the brain or pancreas, might be due in some instances to the appearance under natural conditions of a mutant susceptible to proteolytic activation by an enzyme present in that tissue. Thus, in addition to the possibility of using proteases to detect the presence of viruses in tissues suspected to be persistently infected with viruses, the question of altered susceptibility to protease of virus isolated under unusual conditions should also be considered.

There is another potentially useful application of paramyxovirus mutants with different protease susceptibilities—mutants that can be selected by the procedure discussed, that is, mutagenizing and infecting in the presence of the desired protease. Such mutants may prove to be very sensitive probes for the presence of specific proteases in various tissues, for example, a plasmin-activated mutant might be useful in the detection of plasminogen activator in normal or transformed cells.

SUMMARY

In order to become infectious and to become active in hemolysis and cell fusion, Sendai virus requires proteolytic activation, which involves the cleavage of a virion glycoprotein precursor F_0 to yield the active protein F. The MDBK cells and certain other lines lack a protease capable of this activation. Treatment of virions grown in these cells with trypsin *in vitro* activates the virus, and the addition of trypsin to such cells infected with wt virus makes possible multiple-cycle replication and plaque formation. The proteolytic activation is specific; several other proteases, including chymotrypsin and elastase, do not activate wt virus. Mutants have been selected that are activated *in vivo* in the presence of enzymes, for example, chymotrypsin and elastase. In addition to being activated by these enzymes, some of these mutants have lost the ability to be activated by trypsin. In contrast to wt virus, such mutants have lost the ability to undergo multiple-cycle replication in the chick embryo unless the appropriate enzyme is added to the allantoic fluid. The findings with these protease activation mutants support the previous conclusion, based on results with wt virus, that a specific host-dependent cleavage of the F_0 protein to F is required for the infectivity and for the cell-fusing and hemolytic activities of Sendai virus. They also indicate that the tissue tropism and host range of the virus are dependent on the presence of a specific activating protease. Other biologic implications of the requirement for a specific proteolytic cleavage for expression of biologic activities, such as a possible role of failure of cleavage in persistent nonproductive infections and the appearance under natural conditions of mutants capable of infecting a tissue not usually affected by the virus, have been discussed.

REFERENCES

1. Homma, M. (1971). Trypsin action on the growth of Sendai virus in tissue culture cells. I. Restoration of the infectivity for L cells by direct action of trypsin on L cell-borne Sendai virus. *J. Virol.* 8, 619–629.
2. Homma, M. (1972). Trypsin action on the growth of Sendai virus in tissue culture cells. II. Restoration of the hemolytic activity of L cell-borne Sendai virus by trypsin. *J. Virol.* 9, 829–835.
3. Homma, M., and Ohuchi, M. (1973). Trypsin action on the growth of Sendai virus in tissue culture cells. III. Structural difference of Sendai viruses grown in eggs and tissue culture cells. *J. Virol.* 12, 1457–1465.
4. Homma, M., and Tamagawa, S. (1973). Restoration of the fusion activity of L cell-borne Sendai virus by trypsin. *J. Gen. Virol.* 19, 423–426.
5. Ishida, N., and Homma, M. (1960). A variant Sendai virus, infectious to egg embryos but not to L cells. *Tohoku J. Exp. Med.* 73, 56–69.
6. Matsumoto, T., and Maeno, J. (1962). A host-induced modification of hemagglutinating virus of Japan (HVJ, Sendai virus) in its hemolytic and cytopathic activity. *Virology* 17, 563–570.
7. Morgan, C., and Howe, C. (1968). Structure and development of viruses as observed in the electron microscope. IX. Entry of parainfluenza I (Sendai) virus. *J. Virol.* 2, 1122–1132.

8. Scheid, A., and Choppin, P. W. (1973). Isolation and purification of the envelope proteins of Newcastle disease virus. *J. Virol. 11,* 263–271.

9. Scheid, A., and Choppin, P. W. (1974). Identification of the biological activities of paramyxovirus glycoproteins. Activation of cell fusion, hemolysis, and infectivity by proteolytic cleavage of an inactive precursor protein of Sendai virus. *Virology 57,* 475–490.

10. Scheid, A., and Choppin, P. W. (1974). The hemagglutinin and neuraminidase protein of a paramyxovirus: Interaction with neuraminic acid in affinity chromatography. *Virology 62,* 125–133.

11. Scheid, A., and Choppin, P. W. (1975). Isolation of paramyxovirus glycoproteins and identification of their biological properties. In *Negative Strand Viruses* (B. W. J. Mahy and R. D. Barry, eds.), pp. 177–192. Academic Press, London.

12. Scheid, A., and Choppin, P. W. (1975). Activation of cell fusion and infectivity by proteolytic cleavage of a Sendai virus glycoprotein. In *Proteases and Biological Control* (E. Reich, D. B. Rifkin, and E. Shaw, eds.), pp. 645–659. Cold Spring Harbor Laboratory, Cold Spring Harbor, New York.

13. Scheid, A., and Choppin, P. W. (1976). Protease activation mutants of Sendai virus: Activation of biological properties by specific proteases. *Virology 69,* 265–277.

14. Scheid, A., Caliguiri, L. A., Compans, R. W., and Choppin, P. W. (1972). Isolation of paramyxovirus glycoproteins. Association of both hemagglutinating and neuraminidase activities with the larger SV5 glycoprotein. *Virology 50,* 640–652.

15. Young, N. P., and Ash, R. J. (1970). Polykaryocyte induction by Newcastle disease virus propagated on different hosts. *J. Gen. Virol. 7,* 81–82.

Discussion/Chapter 9

Dr. Johnson commented on the progressive encephalitis of rubella. It resembles subacute sclerosing panencephalitis (SSPE) in the prolonged "incubation period" of some 12 years and the clinical picture of intellectual and motor deterioration, but it lacks the classic myoclonic jerks and the burst suppression pattern on the electroencephalogram. Pathologically the progressive rubella encephalitis also differs from SSPE in that no inclusion bodies are seen in the affected brain tissue. The key point to bear in mind is that the reported cases had had rubella before the 1964 epidemic, and if 12 years is the approximate length of the incubation period, we might expect to see many such cases soon, as the result of the 1964 epidemic.

Next, the mechanisms that would explain the high circulating antibody titers in SSPE was considered. Dr. Lehmann-Grube drew an analogy to his experiments with mice persistently infected with lymphocytic choriomeningitis (LCM) virus. If these mice are adaptively immunized by injection of syngeneic lymphocytes from immunized donors, they develop exceptionally high antibody titers that exceed those attained under circumstances of ordinary immunization or those following natural infection. He suggested therefore that in SSPE there may be a possibility that late-arising clones of immune lymphocytes may be triggered by the measles antigen to produce high titers of antibodies. The other similarity of SSPE to the experimental LCM in mice is that there are a number of variants of the LCM virus itself. These variants may not be genetically determined, but they do exhibit differences in virulence for tissue culture, ranging from full cytolytic effect to no cytopathic effect at all. The type of cytopathic effect one observes is related to the manner in which LCM, grown in mouse L cells, is harvested. If it is derived from the supernatant and disrupted cells, the virus gives the usual cytolytic effect. However, if infected cells are cocultivated with uninfected cells, in some instances the noncytolytic variants appear, and the virus is transmitted from cell to cell directly. If we now take this noncytolytic variant and inject it into baby mice, the animals become carriers and shed only the noncytolytic variant. Virus harvested from the brains of these animals, however, is cytolytic. Thus there is in one animal a selection for the type of virus within different tissues. It is possible that in the pathogenic process leading to SSPE, virus variants may be selected by the brain.

Dr. Kabat inquired about antigenic determinants of the SSPE virus in comparison with those of the regular measles virus, and Dr. Norrby responded that after serial passage in tissue culture, we cannot detect any differences in the antigenic determinants of the two major envelope components and the internal components of nucleocapsids. In the early stages, however, there seem to be some minor differences. Dr. Kabat stressed that it is the original isolate and its antigenic determinants that are important, rather than those altered by laboratory passage, because almost all microorganisms tend to loose important virulence characteristics or properties in laboratory handling. Dr. Norrby agreed that this would probably also be true of the SSPE virus, which does differ from measles in some of its biologic properties, when it is isolated from the brain, but that this did not necessarily preclude that measles virus was the origin of the SSPE variant. He suggested that the change in what was originally a regular wild measles virus might occur as a result of its residence in the central nervous system. The difficulties with laboratory analysis of this virus were pointed out by Dr. Katz, who commented that the amounts of virus derived directly from the brain were too small to analyze properly in the laboratory and that therefore the process of increasing virus quantity required several passages in tissue culture with the likely consequence that the agent undergoes a change.

Among the available models of virus host interactions, equine infectious anemia was listed by Dr. Kaplan. This disease is characterized by persistent viremia and clinical relapses. Virus isolated from one viremic phase is not susceptible to neutralization by serum obtained during an earlier phase. This suggests an antigenic drift with the result that the serum always neutralizes all the preceding virus isolates, but not the ones that follow. It is likely that the virus variation results from antibody pressure. Dr. Mims stated that he could readily accept the presence of virus in SSPE, or the other infections, in conjunction with a neutralizing antibody, if the virus were cell bound and spread by cell-to-cell passage and that this could continue until the cell became damaged.

In this connection, he wondered whether there was any evidence of antigenic expression of the virus at the cell surface. Dr. ter Meulen responded that there is a suggestion of such antigenic expression, in some tissue cultures, but not in others. The key question of its presence *in vivo* remains unanswered. He agreed that lack of surface expression of the antigen may be a good explanation for the failure of the immune system to contain this infection. Dr. Barbosa claimed that the Doi strain of SSPE causes a nonproductive infection in tissue culture with the cells showing antigen by immunofluorescence and by immunoperoxidase technique on electron microscopy. These cells do show membrane changes, with antigenic expression at the membrane level, at least insofar as the immunoperoxidase test can detect it. However, there is no budding. Addition of immune serum cures this system. This is in contrast to what happens in the brain. The SSPE patients, Dr. Barbosa continued, seem also to have normal cell mediated immunity and yet they do not get rid of their infection.

Dr. Choppin concluded the discussion by supporting one of the explanations for pathogenesis of SSPE listed by Dr. Katz. It is possible, he said, that SSPE results from infection by a variant measles virus that arises in the process of infection itself within the particular host. This would help to explain the rarity of the disease, which would then be dependent on the mutability of the virus.

Comment/Chapter 9

L. H. Barbosa

There are really three questions that must be asked as we view our current knowledge of subacute sclerosing panencephalitis (SSPE). These are: What do we know about the virus? What do we know about the host? and What type of investigations should be planned for the future?

All that can be said about the SSPE virus is that there are a number of examples of a measleslike virus isolated from a variety of patients with SSPE. These isolates cannot really be distinguished from one another by serology, but they do have a variable biologic behavior in experimental animals and tissue cultures. These differences are probably not genetic, and we are glad of the analogy to the lymphocytic choriomeningitis (LCM) infection, elaborated upon by Lehmann-Grube, and of the information about the surface proteins brought forth by Choppin. Both of these comments help us to accept the possibility that the virus isolated from SSPE may be a nongenetic variant of measles.

The initial question about the integrity of the immune system in an SSPE patient remains essentially unanswered. There are, however, interesting experimental suggestions that faulty immunity may play a role in the pathogenesis of this disease. The studies of Rapp, to which Dr. Katz alluded, make us think of an infection of the relatively immature host, perhaps still under the cover of maternal passively transmitted antibodies. It may be well to recall that most SSPE patients seem to have had measles before their second birthday. On the other hand, the suggestion that SSPE may be a manifestation of an autoimmune disease is untenable, in view of two cases of SSPE reported in agammaglobulinemic patients. Failure of cell-mediated immunity is also substantially in doubt, because of the cited studies by our group at the N.I.H. and by Dr. ter Meulen and his associates, which failed to uncover any evidence of a defect in cell-mediated immunity either *in vivo* or *in vitro*. The reports by Sell of a blocking factor in SSPE are intriguing, but must be confirmed by additional studies. Likewise, the hypothesis of plasma membrane modulation by antibodies, brought forth by Kibler at a recent meeting of the N.I.H. awaits more extensive studies.

The obvious question about a genetic predisposition to SSPE remains moot. A preliminary report of a significant increase in the HL-A-W29 gene among SSPE patients awaits elaboration. If there is a genetic predisposition, one wonders how to account for the reported case of identical twins, only one of whom had SSPE.

Quite obviously, we lack answers to many fundamental questions in this disease. Let me conclude by expressing a hope that the immunologic and genetic studies will continue, but that the virologic studies now move into a biochemical phase through which analysis of the basic components of the viruses must be undertaken and the variety of isolates compared in this fashion.

PART III
MULTIPLE SCLEROSIS

CHAPTER 10
Multiple Sclerosis: A Case for Viral Etiology*

V. TER MEULEN

SOME ASPECTS OF THE CLINICAL COURSE

Multiple sclerosis (MS) is currently a leading candidate among human diseases for consideration as a slow virus infection (SVI). Although unequivocal data that would permit us to define MS as a viral disease are still lacking, the available indirect evidence justifies—even mandates—inclusion of MS in these discussions. Whatever the ultimate fate of the concept of infectious etiology for this demyelinating disease will be, the heuristic value of the SVI hypothesis alone will have been immense.

What do we know about the disease itself and what should we emphasize in considering viral etiology of MS? The disease has its onset usually between the ages of 20 and 40 years with a peak incidence at 30 years. The clinical picture is variable. Presenting symptoms may include disturbances of affect, parasthesias, numbness, slurred speech, impaired vision, weak muscles, and poor coordination. Paralysis and myalgia may also occur but are less frequent in the early stages of the disease. Conspicuously, symptoms of a generalized illness, such as fever or malaise, are absent. Whether the symptoms are single or multiple, they usually come on acutely. The first attack tends to subside after a few weeks, but the typical pattern of MS consists of exacerbations or relapses and remissions. There is, however, a progressive development of irreversible changes and eventually permanent disability. According to MacAlpine et al. (13), the complete spectrum of MS ranges from a mild to a rapidly progressive form (Fig. 10.1). He divided the clinical pattern of MS into the seven groups. The clinical course shows severe relapses with increasing disability and early death in Group a. In b, there are many short attacks, which tend to increase in duration and severity. There is in Group c a slow progression from the onset upon which relapses are superimposed with the resulting increasing disability. Group d represents a slow progression from the onset without relapses, and e, an abrupt onset and a remission, followed by a long quiescent phase. f represents relapses of diminishing frequency and severity, and Group g includes an abrupt onset, remission, few or no relapses after

* Supported in part by the Deutsche Forschungsgemeinschaft, Schwerpunkt für Multiple Sklerose und verwandte Erkrankungen.

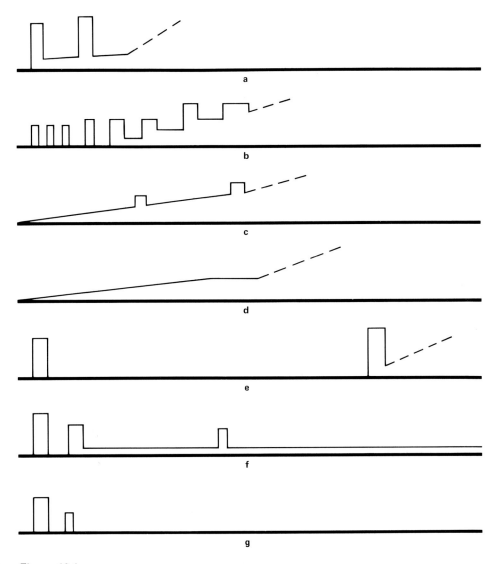

Figure 10.1.
The course of multiple sclerosis: **a.** Severe relapses, increasing disability, and early death; **b.** many short attacks tending to increase in duration and severity; **c.** slow progression from onset, superimposed relapses, and increasing disability; **d.** slow progression from onset without relapses; **e.** abrupt onset with good remission followed by long latent phase; **f.** relapses of diminishing frequency and severity with only slight residual disability; and **g.** abrupt onset with few if any relapses after first year and no residual disability.
[Reprinted with permission from McAlpine *et al.* (14).]

the first year, and no residual disability. Thus there are great differences in the clinical course of MS that are contrary to what has been observed in typical SVI. Such infections characteristically have a progressive course and fatal outcome. Quiescent phases have been observed in subacute sclerosing panencephalitis (SSPE), but they are really arrests, rather than remissions, and the course of deterioration is relentless. In MS, relentless progression is an exception.

EPIDEMIOLOGY

Epidemiologic studies provide a useful approach to MS (2, 14, 17). These studies have revealed certain facts that gave rise to a great deal of speculation. Unquestionably, in the northern hemisphere there is a north to south gradient of the incidence rate of MS. The decreasing incidence of MS from temperate to tropical zones suggests an environmental factor. Studies of immigrants indicate that environment is more important than heredity. Adults migrating from an area of high MS incidence to one of low incidence retain their original risk for the development of the disease. The same holds true for migrants from low risk to high risk areas. On the other hand, individuals migrating as infants or children change their risk factor to approach that present in their new environment. In addition, a certain genetic predisposition, as demonstrated by the HLA-typing, may play a role in the susceptibility to the disease (3, 7). Environmental factors and nativity are not the only determinants, age also plays a role in the susceptibility to MS. The disease is rare in persons under the age of 15 or over 55 years; thus some event in childhood may be an important factor in MS. It may be that some causal event leads to the disease after a latent period of some 20 years. Although the epidemiologic observations do not exclude a nonviral causal factor, they are entirely compatible with the suggestion that exposure to a virus before puberty may be the critical event in the acquisition of MS. The genetic predisposition to MS suggested by the studies of histocompatibility antigens do not preclude viral etiology.

SEROLOGIC AND ULTRASTRUCTURAL FINDINGS

There is substantial evidence in support of viral etiology of MS, such as results of serologic investigations of serum and cerebro-spinal fluid (CSF) (1), electron microscopic observations of nucleocapsidlike structures in MS brain sections (19), and isolation of infectious virus from brain tissues of MS patients (16).

Frequency of antibodies in MS patients against all common viruses has been compared with that of normal individuals and patients with diseases of the central nervous system (CNS) other than MS. Although results vary, they generally indicate that more MS patients tend to have slightly higher antibody titers against measles than do the control groups (4, 18). Increased antibody titers against other common viruses, such as *Herpes simplex*, *Vaccinia* (8), *Varicella zoster*, adeno viruses, influenza C, parainfluenza 3, mumps, and rubella, have also been reported in MS (1). It is of interest that these groups often did not have correspondingly increased measles antibody titers.

However, none of these studies identified a particular candidate causative virus. A candidate virus, especially if it is a common agent, must fit with the established epidemiologic data regarding the differences in incidence of MS in high and low risk areas. It must either itself have a comparable frequency of distribution, or it must act in concert with some triggering event that may determine frequency of MS.

145

More direct evidence of a possible virus involvement in MS derives from electron microscopic studies of fresh plaque areas. Several investigators have seen viral nucleocapsidlike structures resembling those of the paramyxovirus group in the mononuclear cells surrounding the plaques (19, 20, 22, 23). However, these structures cannot be identified unequivocally through morphology alone (5, 10). The ultimate decision as to whether these structures are viral components must await studies by immunologic and biochemical techniques.

VIROLOGIC STUDIES

There have been many attempts directed at isolation of infectious agents from MS brains (1). Recently, Field and co-workers (6) reported an isolation of measles virus in cell cultures derived from brain of an MS patient. The cytopathic effect noted was neutralized with an anti-measles serum. Electron microscopy showed nucleocapsidlike structures in the intra- and extracellular space. However, the investigators themselves cast a doubt on the validity of this observation because they could not rule out the possibility that the virus was a laboratory contaminant.

We have attempted isolation of infectious viruses from MS brain tissue by the method of cell-fusion, which had been successful in SSPE (15). After establishing brain cell cultures, we isolated a parainfluenza type 1 virus named 6/94 virus from two cases of MS (16). As demonstrated in

Origin of cell cultures	MS brain tissue												Indicator cells
	White matter								Gray matter areas				CV-1
	Plaque adjacent area						Plaque distant area						
	1	2	3	4	5	6	I	II	a	b	c	d	
Morphologic changes	–	–	–	NG	+	NG	–	NG	–	–	–	–	–
Nucleocapsids	–	–	–		+		–		–	–	–	–	–
HAD	–	–	–		–		–		–	–	–	–	–
Fusion with CV-1 cells: No. of cultures pooled / Fusion factor	S LL	LL	S	S LL			LL		S			LL	S LL
Morphologic changes after fusion	– –	–	–	–	+①^{x}		–		–			–	– –
HAD	– –	–	–	–	+③^{x}		–		–			–	– –
Nucleocapsid	– –	–	–	–	+③^{x}		–		–			–	– –

Figure 10.2.
History of isolation of virus from brain tissue of EZ, Arrow indicates number of cultures pooled together for fusion experiment; LL = Lysolecithin; S = β-propiolactone inactivated Sendai virus; NG = No Growth; O^{x} Denotes passage number after fusion at which changes were observed; HAD = Hemadsorption of guinea pig RBC. [Reprinted with permission from Koprowski and ter Meulen (9)].

Fig. 10.2, brain tissue cultures were fused with a permanent cell line of African Green Monkey kidney cells in the presence of β-propiolactone inactivated Sendai virus or lysolecithin. Only lysolecithin treated cells yielded infectious virus (6/94). Its characterization was accomplished by hemagglutination inhibition, hemadsorption-neutralization tests and complement fixation cross block titration for the detection of surface antigens. No differences between the 6/94 virus and the Sendai virus strains were identified (9). However, the kinetic hemagglutination inhibition test readily differentiated 6/94 virus from the group of Sendai viruses (11). This finding was further supported by an immunologic characterization of 6/94 and Sendai virus glycoproteins (12). Two glycoproteins GP1 and GP2 were isolated from 6/94 and Sendai virus strain MN according to the method described by Scheid and Choppin (21). Monospecific antisera were prepared in rabbits against these isolated glycoproteins, and in an immunodiffusion test, the specificity of these antisera to the different glycoproteins were determined. As demonstrated in Fig. 10.3, the GP1 fractions of 6/94 and Sendai MN viruses are antigenically different, whereas the GP2 fractions are antigenically identical in both virus strains. The GP1 factor carries hemagglutination and neuraminidase activities in both viruses. This immunologic finding establishes clearly that 6/94 virus is not identical with the common strain of Sendai virus and that isolation of this virus is not laboratory contamination by the Sendai virus used in an inactivated form for cell fusion. We do not doubt that 6/94 virus was derived from the MS brain material. It has neurotropic properties: mice and newborn chimpanzees inoculated with the 6/94 virus developed neuropathologic changes after a long incubation period (11a, 24). However, the role of the 6/94 virus in the etiology of MS is uncertain. Serologic studies of MS patients by standard hemagglutination inhibition or hemadsorption neutralization tests against 6/94 virus have not indicated a hyperimmune reaction to this virus. Antibodies against this virus have been detected in equal frequency in MS patients and controls. It must be emphasized, however, that serologic tests using purified 6/94 glycoproteins as described previously, have not been done yet.

UNANSWERED QUESTIONS OF ETIOLOGY AND PATHOGENESIS

If a virus is a causative agent of MS it must remain latent for many years before expressing itself. This question applies to all SVI whatever the nature of the agent. Therefore, knowledge of the mechanisms of latency in SVI can provide clues to the rescue or identification of such latent viruses in MS. It is useful, therefore, to consider the host–virus relationships in these other diseases.

In SSPE and in the two MS cases studied in our laboratories, isolation of the viruses was accomplished only by cell cocultivation or fusion (15, 16), because the viruses persisted in the brain tissue cultures in a defective form without the spontaneous production of infectious virus. The virus–host relationship that accounts for virus latency in the CNS is not yet under-

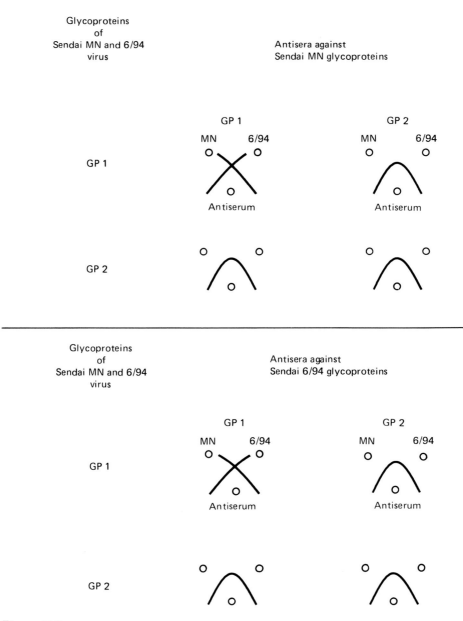

Figure 10.3.
In the immunodiffusion test (Ouchterlony-technique, monospecific antisera against isolated glycoproteins of Sendai MN and 6/94 virus strains are compared. Glyco- protein GP2 from both virus strains are immunologically identical, whereas GP1 differed from 6/94 and MN.

stood even in diseases such as SSPE. For the mechanisms underlying this type of virus persistency, the genetic make-up of the host, the production of subgenomic interfering virus particles and temperature-sensitive mutants, or the integration of viral genomes into host DNA are currently discussed and investigated. However, direct laboratory data to support one of these hypotheses are not yet available.

What might then trigger the disease many years after the original viral infection? Only hypotheses and speculations can be offered. In such slow virus diseases as scrapie, infection of any cell type in the CNS ultimately produces progressive damage accompanied by cell dysfunction and death. Such a process of silent infection takes place in isolation without triggering any immunologic reaction. In contrast, MS is not a smoothly progressing disease but is characterized by exacerbations and remissions. A reasonable hypothesis that would account for the intermittency of MS is an interplay between a slow infection and an immune response of the host. In view of the possibility that the responsible agent could be a budding enveloped virus that causes antigenic changes of the host cell membrane, the infected cell may become susceptible to immune lysis. The immunologic recognition that an infected cell is different may start a chain of events. For example, the destruction of such brain cells may unmask a hidden antigen and trigger an autoimmune process. The resulting combination of a destructive immune process, either cellular or humoral with the underlying infection, can determine the course that the disease takes. The pattern of infection could also be responsible for the intermittency if one assumes that destruction of infected cells is the basis of the formation of an acute lesion. Since infection in the presence of specific antibodies is presumed to spread only by cell-to-cell transfer, the infected cells tend to be clustered in foci. Cell lysis, therefore, would result in multifocal lesions. In view of the slow cycle of replication of the virus, a substantial amount of time must elapse before new infected cell clusters are formed. Additional factors that may also influence the disease process are the restrictions of traffic of lymphocytes into the CNS resulting from its immunologically privileged state or antigenic modulation of infected cells in the presence of extracellular antibodies. The latter prevents immune destruction of the infected cells by antibodies or lymphocytes and permits continuation of virus replication.

CONCLUSION

It is obvious that at present no scheme that would explain the complexity of MS and the many variables that have been observed can be proposed. From a virologic point of view, MS has many features that suggest virus involvement as the first step in the pathogenesis of this disease. The available data do not point to a particular virus as the initiating infectious agent. Indeed, it may well be that the causative agent is one of several or even many viruses. One can expect, however, that such a group of agents would share certain basic characteristics required for the establishment of a latent infection.

REFERENCES

1. Adams, C. W. M., and Leibowitz, S. (1972). In *Research on Multiple Sclerosis*, pp. 135–148. Charles C Thomas, Springfield, Ill.
2. Alter, M., and Kurtzke, J. F. (1968). *The Epidemiology of Multiple Sclerosis.* Charles C Thomas, Springfield, Ill.

3. Bertram, J., and Kuwert, E. (1972). HL-A Antigen frequencies in multiple sclerosis. *Eur. Neurol. 7*, 74–78.

4. Brown, P., Cathala, F., Gajdusek, D. C., and Gibbs, C. J., Jr. (1971). Measles antibodies in C.S.F. of patients with multiple sclerosis. *Proc. Soc. Exp. Biol. Med. 137*, 956–961.

5. Dubois-Dalcq, M., Schumacher, G., and Sever, J. L. (1973). Acute multiple sclerosis: Electron microscopic evidence for and against a viral agent in the plaques. *Lancet ii*, 1408–1411.

6. Field, E. J., Cowshall, S., Narang, H. K., and Bell, T. M. (1972). Viruses in multiple sclerosis? *Lancet ii*, 280–281.

7. Jersild, C., Fog, T., Hansen, G. S., Thomson, M., Svejgaard, A., and Dupont, B. (1973). Histocompatibility determinants in multiple sclerosis with special reference to clinical course. *Lancet ii*, 1221–1225.

8. Kempe, C. H., Takabayashi, K., Miyamoto, H., McIntosh, K., Tourtellote, W. W., and Adams, J. M. (1973). Elevated cerebrospinal fluid vaccinia antibodies in multiple sclerosis. *Arch. Neurol. 28*, 278–279.

9. Koprowski, H., and ter Meulen, V. (1975). Multiple sclerosis and parainfluenza 1 virus: History of the isolation of the virus and expression of phenotypic differences between the isolated virus and Sendai virus. *J. Neurol. 208*, 175–190.

10. Lampert, F., and Lampert, P. (1975). Multiple sclerosis: Morphological evidence of intranuclear paramyxovirus or altered chromatin fibres. *Arch. Neurol. 32*, 425–427.

11. Lief, F. S., Loh, W., ter Meulen, V., and Koprowski, H. (1975). Antigenic variation among parainfluenza type 1 (Sendai) viruses: Analysis of 6/94 virus. *Intervirology 5*, 1–9.

11a. Lief, F. S., Rorke, L. B., Kalter, S. S., Hoffman, S. F., Roosa, R. A., Moore, G. T., Cummins, L. B., McCullough, B., Rodriguez, A. R., and Koprowski, H. (1976). Infection and disease induced in chimpanzees with 6/94, a parainfluenza type-1 virus isolated from human multiple sclerosis brain. *J. Neuropathol. Exp. Neurol.*, in press.

12. Loh, W., and ter Meulen, V. (1976). Comparative antigenic analysis of 2 parainfluenza type I viruses: Sendai MN and 6/94 strain. *J. Gen. Virol.*, submitted.

13. McAlpine, D., Lunsden, C. E., and Acheson, E. D. (1972). In *Multiple Sclerosis, A Reappraisal*, pp. 197–214. Churchill Livingston, Edinburgh and London.

14. McAlpine, D., Lundsen, C. E., and Acheson, E. D. (1972). In *Multiple Sclerosis, A Reappraisal*, pp. 3–80. Churchill Livingston, Edinburgh and London.

15. ter Meulen, V., Katz, M., and Müller, D. (1972). Subacute sclerosing panencephalitis: A review. *Current Topics of Microbiology and Immunology* (Arber *et al.*, eds.). Vol. 57, pp. 1–38. Springer, Berlin, Heidelberg, and New York.

16. ter Meulen, V., Koprowski, H., Iwasaki, Y., Käckell, Y. M., and Müller, D. (1972). Fusion of cultured multiple sclerosis brain cells with indicator cells: Presence of nucleocapsids and virions and isolation of parainfluenza-type virus. *Lancet ii*, 1–5.

17. Millar, J. H. D. (1971). *Multiple Sclerosis, a Disease Acquired in Childhood.* Charles C Thomas, Springfield, Ill.

18. Norrby, E., Link, H., and Olsson, J. E. (1974). Measles virus antibodies in multiple sclerosis. *Arch. Neurol. 30*, 285–292.

19. Prineas, J. W. (1972). Paramyxovirus-like particles associated with acute demyelination in chronic relapsing multiple sclerosis. *Science 178*, 760–762.

20. Raine, C. S., Powers, J. M., and Suzuki, I. (1974). Acute multiple sclerosis: Confirmation of "paramyxovirus-like" intranuclear inclusions. *Arch. Neurol. 30*, 39–46.

21. Scheid, A., and Choppin, P. W. (1974). Identification of biological activities of paramyxovirus glycoproteins. Activation of cell fusion, hemolysis and infectivity by proteolytic cleavage of an inactive precursor protein of Sendai virus. *Virology 57*, 475–490.

22. Tanaka, R., Iwasaki, Y., and Koprowski, H. (1974). Unusual intranuclear filaments in multiple sclerosis brain. *Lancet i,* 1236–1237.
23. Watanabe, I., and Okazaki, H. (1973). Virus-like structure in multiple sclerosis. *Lancet ii,* 569–570.
24. Zgorniak-Nowosielska, I., Iwasaki, Y., Tachovsky, T., Tanaka, R., and Koprowski, H. (1976). Experimental parainfluenza-type-1 virus-induced encephalopathy in adult mice. Pathogenesis of chronic degenerative changes in the CNS. *Arch. Neurol. 33,* 55–63.

CHAPTER 11

In Search of the Abominable Snowman or "deine Viren, meine Viren" in Multiple Sclerosis*

HILARY KOPROWSKI

INTRODUCTION

Some months ago, two fellow workers submitted a paper to *Science* on the ultrastructural observations of a parainfluenza virus in brain tissue of suckling mice (11) that had been infected experimentally with 6/94 virus (7, 16). One of the reviewers, in addition to his factual comments about the contents of the paper, offered the following gratuitous objections: "We remain unconvinced by the studies implicating parainfluenza in multiple sclerosis. The putative isolations of virus have not been confirmed; serological studies do not support an etiologic association and the differences in biological characteristics with 6/94 and Sendai virus are no more than expected of a variant produced by multiplicity reactivation of selection under laboratory conditions. The authors are certainly aware that some authorities are suspicious that the isolation of 6/94 from brain tissue of patients with multiple sclerosis was due to laboratory contamination with Sendai virus and the readers should also be informed of this controversy."

Thurber relates an ironic fable of a man whose wife wishes to see him committed to a lunatic asylum because he claims he sees a unicorn in the garden. When the police and the psychiatrist arrive, the man denies that he ever saw a unicorn in his garden, and his wife is committed instead of himself. The man then joins the unicorn in the garden.[1] To paraphrase the moral of this fable (cited at the end of this paper), it does not pay to make assumptions about what is reasonable or not reasonable until the facts are in.

---

* The experimental work cited here was supported in part by a grant from the National Multiple Sclerosis Society and USPHS grants NS-11036 from the National Institute of Neurological and Communicative Disorders and Stroke and RR-05540 from the Division of Research and Resources.
    [1] James Thurber, *Fables for Our Time*. New York, Harper & Brothers, 1940.

MULTIPLE SCLEROSIS BRAIN TISSUE CULTURE

The reviewer first stated that isolations of virus "have not been confirmed" meaning perhaps that no isolation of parainfluenza virus from human brain tissue has been reported by other laboratories. The truth of the matter is that no other laboratory has studied as extensively as we have brain material obtained from so many multiple sclerosis (MS) patients and maintained for so many passages in tissue culture (3, 18). Since, to the best of my knowledge, no other laboratories have made themselves available to undertake the search for viruses in MS tissue on the same scale as ours, it is unfair to call for "confirmation" of our data when no such confirmations could be immediately forthcoming.

Insofar as our laboratory is concerned, six other MS brains were processed as carefully as the two from which 6/94 virus was isolated, and no virus "either parainfluenza-1" or any other was detected in these specimens over the course of several passages of brain cells *in vitro*. Thus at present, two of eight MS brains have yielded parainfluenza-1 virus; none have yielded any other virus, including measles virus. Such finding are almost self-evident! Compare the results from the isolation of parainfluenza-1 virus with those from the isolation in our laboratory of subacute sclerosing pan encephalitis (SSPE) virus from clinically proved SSPE cases. Again, in only two of eight cases was the SSPE virus isolated, and the failure to isolate the virus in the six other cases "was also consistent in numerous attempts" (6). Despite the fact that SSPE lesions are disseminated throughout the brain (in contrast to MS), and the fact that cells with viral nucleocapsids were observed in three brain specimens from which no infectious virus was isolated, the ratio of brains yielding SSPE virus was identical to the ratio obtained until now in MS. In progressive multifocal encephalopathy (PML), simian virus 40 (SV40) was isolated in only two of the many specimens investigated; in all other cases, another papova virus, JC (a virus clearly distinguishable from SV40), was "incriminated" either through isolation or by immunofluorescence *in situ*. Yet to my mind, there is no doubt that SSPE virus and SV40 are involved in the etiology of SSPE and PML, respectively. On the contrary, I question seriously whether measles virus is involved in the etiology of MS: Neither the virus nor measles antigen has ever been found in any MS tissues, even though (in judging from the frequency of immune reactivity of MS patients allegedly attributed to measles virus) the presence of one or the other in the central nervous system (CNS) tissue of these patients should have been readily ascertainable.

In the course of processing MS brain tissue, we have learned the following: (a) There is no difficulty in establishing cultures from any human brain tissue removed either at biopsy or at autopsy, provided the latter procedure takes place not later than 8 hr after the demise of the patient (3). (b) Though, in general, we have no control over which type of brain cells will adhere either to glass or to plastic, and which grow into a cell line, three morphologically distinguishable cell types were most frequently identified in all brain tissue cultures obtained, regardless of source (10, 18). (c) Like human fibroblasts, brain cells have a finite lifetime in culture, but they can be transformed easily by SV40. After transformation, they display the capacity for infinite growth in culture (12, 13). (d) Several human brain cells maintained in culture express activity similar to that of enzymes involved in the myelination process (1). The fact that only a small number of lesion-containing fragments can be processed from one MS brain because of the limited manpower in a single laboratory, plus the fact that the type of cells growing from each MS brain remains unpredictable, may account both for the paucity of virus isolation from a brain in which the lesions are focal (rather than disseminated) and for the virus (or its "footprints") being confined to a certain type of cell. If cell-sorting procedures succeed in separating easily identifiable types of human brain cells, which can be maintained in culture, and if enough human resources can be mobilized to process *extensively* tissue from an MS brain, the isolation of a viral agent may become more common than it is today.

SEROLOGIC STUDIES

The second argument of the reviewer states that "serological studies do not support an etiologic association." I presume the reference here is to the fact that MS patients do not show an increase in the titer of antibody to parainfluenza-1 virus (9) (or to any other virus) in a serologic assay. Such serologic assay, as routinely performed, provides little information about the host response to a viral infection. With hundreds of antigenic determinants present on a virus particle, there is a heavily heterogeneous antibody population in the serum of the host, some classes of which may not be detectable in a serologic assay. Furthermore, one could hardly expect an increase in antiviral-antibody titer at the time when the MS patient is available for study, if exposure to the virus had occurred decades before the onset of the disease. Moreover, we should remember that in persistent virus infections, the host's immune reactivity may be completely bypassed (as it is in the instances of scrapie, kuru, and other spongioform encephalitides), diminished (as it is with the many viruses that infect lymphocytes (17), or restricted to reacting more strongly with the virus involved in the initial exposure than with the same agent involved in subsequent exposure(s) (2). In the light of all these data, how could one reasonably expect serologic studies to confirm the cause of a chronic disease of possibly viral etiology?

VARIANT VIRUS

The third point made by the reviewer was that 6/94 virus was a "variant [of Sendai virus] produced by multiplicity reactivation of selection under laboratory conditions." I would be quite pleased if 6/94 were simply a variant of a known virus, particularly one of as wide a host range as parainfluenza-1 virus, since it seems to me that there is a good possibility that MS is caused by a variant virus that causes an otherwise banal infection of childhood; from that point of view, 6/94 may be as good a choice as is the putative variant of measles virus.

ISOLATION OF 6/94

The reviewer's last argument is an unwarranted complaint that "the isolation of 6/94 from brain tissue of patients with multiple sclerosis was due to laboratory contamination with Sendai virus." I do not, as a rule, refute such a statement since doing so is an act as futile as the subjective criticism. However, the "laboratory contamination" argument is the more far fetched in the instance of Sendai virus, since after passage in any mammalian cell system, Sendai virus produces a phenotypically deficient variant that is noninfective for other cells. It remains noninfective unless exposed to trypsin or other proteases that may be present [e.g., in the allantoic fluid of the chick embryo (4)]. Hence the virus can be propagated easily in chick embryos, for example, but cannot be maintained after passages in mammalian cells unless it is exposed to trypsin between each passage. As a result, it is hard to visualize a "laboratory contamination" of serially passaged human brain cell cultures by a virus that characteristically loses infectivity after each passage in mammalian cells.

ETIOLOGIC AGENT

The diagnosis of MS is based on an elaborate set of clinical criteria that must be confirmed ultimately by histologic examination. There are no uncontested findings that permit application of chemistry or biology to the characterization of the disease and its lesions. This makes it enormously difficult to furnish proof, even to a reasonably nonopinionated group, that a virus isolated from a MS brain is the etiologic agent of the MS, particularly when the brains of an experimental animal may differ so considerably from human brain in its reactivity to a virus infection which initiates a chronic disease state.

Three approaches to the solution of this problem should be considered: (a) frequent isolation of the same virus from MS patients or their brain tissue, or demonstration of a common viral antigen (b) demonstration of the ability of a virus to become latent in central nervous system (CNS) cells in tissue culture and to initiate, through the infection of the CNS of an animal, a chronic disease state; and (c) vaccination of a newborn human population with a vaccine prepared from a "candidate" virus and relegation to the next generation, or to one thereafter, of the responsibility of finding out if such a vaccine prevented MS. The third approach is in the realm of fantasy; the other two merit further discussion.

It is quite obvious that the frequency of isolating 6/94 virus from brain tissue of MS patients is low; however, attempts to reveal presence of any other virus have failed. Obviously, an increase in the frequency of isolation of a virus from MS tissue requires the examination of a larger number of white matter fragments as discussed previously and the separation of identifiable types of human brain cells for viral assay in tissue culture. Furthermore, structures that may or may not be viral nucleocapsids, observed under an electron microscope in cells surrounding MS plaques (14), are now found in buffy coat cells of MS patients (15); such finding make identification of these structures, and even relating them to a virus infection, more feasible.

Greater progress has been made in the study of 6/94 virus in its ability to induce latent chronic infection. First, human brain cells maintained in culture and infected with 6/94 virus do not show presence of the virus by varied means of hemadsorption, release of hemagglutinins in immunofluorescence, ultrastructural examination, or infectivity. It is necessary to fuse these cells with indicator cells to "free" the virus from its latent state (19). This type of interaction is characteristic for human brain cells since 6/94 virus does cause an overt infection in bovine brain.

Second, a newborn chimpanzee injected intracerebrally (i.c.) with 6/94 virus exhibited convulsions and an abnormal electroencephalogram 14 months afterward. With overt signs of CNS involvement occurring at 23 months of age, the animal was killed (8). Although antibodies reacting specifically with 6/94 virus were detected in serum of the animal shortly after exposure, anti-6/94 antibodies in cerebrospinal fluid were first detected shortly before it was killed. Interestingly enough, no virus was isolated from the animal's brain though the pathologic lesions resembled those observed in mice injected with 6/94 virus as newborns and sacrificed several months later (8).

Furthermore, 6/94 virus injected i.c. into adult mice initiates a series of events leading to chronic, and until now asymptomatic, lesions of white matter (20) that develop in the animal only in the presence of an intact thymus (5). The 6/94 virus can be detected in brain tissue of these animals only during the first week after inoculation. Thus unrelated to the presence of infectious virus, an autoimmune mechanism may be involved in the development of these lesions. The fact that chronic white matter lesions develop after exposure of mice to either inactivated 6/94 virus or to its noninfectious components (5) may indicate further that the autoimmune process may be initiated by antigenic determinants of the virus and not necessarily by its infectivity.

CONCLUSION

The ability of 6/94 virus to induce the latent, chronic infection of the CNS described previously obviously does not constitute proof of its involvement in the etiology of MS. These findings, however, make available for further study a virus that was known until now only for its ability to cause a banal infection (mostly respiratory) in humans and animals, but which has now been shown to cause latent, chronic infection of human CNS in culture and of the CNS of higher primates and of mice *in vivo*. Study of this system limited to interaction between *one* virus and CNS tissue not only will result in improving methods for detecting latent virus infection in CNS, both *in vivo* and *in vitro*, but also will permit development of feasible experimental approaches to link a possible autoimmune mechanism initiated by a viral antigen with chronic CNS disease.

The 6/94 virus presents us with unique features, since no viral agent that may play a role in the etiology of a chronic CNS disease has been found to show the same characteristics as those displayed by 6/94 virus—until now. Thurber's point, therefore, is well taken: "Don't count your boobies until they are hatched."

REFERENCES

1. Duch, D., Mandel, P., and Koprowski, H. (1975). Demonstration of enzymes related to myelinogenesis in established human brain cell cultures. *J. Neurol. Sci.* 26, 99–105.
2. Gerhard, W., and Koprowski, H. (1975). The future in viral immunology and immunopathology. *Viral Immunology and Immunopathology* (A. L. Notkins, ed.), pp. 435–457. Academic Press, New York, San Francisco, and London.
3. Gilden, D. H., Devlin, M., Wroblewska, Z., Friedman, H., Rorke, L. B., Santoli, D., and Koprowski, H. (1975). Human brain in tissue culture: I. Acquisition, initial processing, and establishment of brain cell cultures. *J. Comp. Neurol. 161*, 295–306.
4. Homma, M. (1971). Trypsin action on the growth of Sendai virus in tissue culture cells. Part 1, *J. Virol. 8*, 619–629; Homma, M., and Okuci, M. (1973). Part 3, *J. Virol. 12*, 1457–1465.
5. Iwasaki, Y., Aden, D., and Koprowski, H. (1975). Thymus-dependent sensitizing processing involved in the induction of CNS disease in mice by parainfluenza-type 1 virus. *J. Immunol. 114*, 1846–1847.
6. Katz, M., and Koprowski, H. (1973). The significance of failure to isolate infectious viruses in cases of subacute sclerosing panencephalitis. *Arch. Gesamte Virusforsch. 41*, 390–393.
7. Koprowski, H., and ter Meulen, V. (1975). Multiple sclerosis and parainfluenza-1 virus. History of the isolation of the virus and expression of phenotypic differences between the isolated virus and Sendai virus. *J. Neurol. 208*, 175–190.
8. Lief, F. S., Rorke, L. B., Kalter, S. S., Hoffman, S. F., Roosa, R. A., Moore, G. T., Cummins, L. B., McCullough, B., Rodriguez, A. R., and Koprowski, H. (1976). Infection and disease induced in chimpanzees with 6/94, a parainfluenza type-1 virus isolated from human multiple sclerosis brain. *J. Neuropathol. Exp. Neurol.,* in press.
9. Nemo, G. J., Brody, J. A., and Waters, D. J. (1974). Serological responses of multiple sclerosis patients and controls to a virus isolated from a multiple sclerosis case. *Lancet ii*, 1044–1046.
10. Rorke, L. B., Gilden, D. H., Wroblewska, Z., and Santoli, D. (1975). Human brain in tissue culture: IV. Morphological characteristics. *J. Comp. Neurol. 161*, 329–340.
11. Wolinsky, J. S., and Gilden, D. H. (1975). *In vivo* studies of parainfluenza-1. (6/94) virus: Mononuclear cell interaction. *Arch. Virol. 47*, 25–31.
12. Santoli, D., Wroblewska, Z., Gilden, D. H., and Koprowski, H. (1975). Establishment of continuous multiple sclerosis brain cultures after transformation with PML-SV40 virus. *J. Neurol. Sci. 24*, 385–390.
13. Santoli, D., Wroblewska, Z., Gilden, D. H., Girardi, A., and Koprowski, H. (1975). Human brain in tissue culture: 111. PML-SV40-induced transformation of brain cells and establishment of permanent lines. *J. Comp. Neurol. 161*, 317–328.

14. Tanaka, R., Iwasaki, Y., and Koprowski, H. (1975). Paramyxovirus-like structures in brains of multiple sclerosis cases. *Arch. Neurol. 32*, 80–83.
15. Tanaka, R., Santoli, D., and Koprowski, H. (1976). Unusual intranuclear filaments in the circulating lymphocytes of patients with multiple sclerosis and optic neuritis. *Am. J. Pathol. 83*, 245–254.
16. ter Muelen, V., Iwasaki, Y., Koprowski, H., Käckell, Y. M., and Müller, D. (1972). Fusion of cultured multiple-sclerosis brain cells with indicator cells: Presence of nucleocapsids and virions and isolation of parainfluenza-type virus. *Lancet ii*, 1–5.
17. Wheelock, E. F., and Toy, S. T. (1973). Participation of lymphocytes in viral infections. *Advanced Immunology* (F. J. Dixon and H. G. Kunkel, eds.), Vol. 16, pp. 123–184. Academic Press, New York.
18. Wroblewska, Z., Devlin, M., Gilden, D. H., Santoli, D., Friedman, H., and Koprowski, H. (1975). Human brain in tissue culture: II. Studies of long-term cultures. *J. Comp. Neurol. 161*, 307–316.
19. Wroblewska, Z., Santoli, D., Gilden, D., Lewandowski, L., and Koprowski, H. (1976). Persistent parainfluenza-type-1 (6/94) infection of brain cells in tissue culture. *Arch. Virol. 50*, 287–303.
20. Zgórniak-Nowosielska, I., Iwasaki, Y., Tachovsky, T., Tanaka, R., and Koprowski, H. (1975). Experimental parainfluenza-type-1 virus-induced encephalopathy in adult mice. Pathogenesis of chronic degenerative changes in the CNS. *Arch. Neurol. 33*, 55–62.

CHAPTER 12

Characterization of the Virus Antibody Activity of Oligoclonal IgG Produced in the Central Nervous System of Patients with Multiple Sclerosis

ERLING NORRBY

INTRODUCTION

There is at present no convincing direct evidence of a virus in the central nervous system (CNS) of multiple sclerosis (MS) patients. As mentioned by others, the evidence for such a virus is indirect, that is, serologic. Most of the studies have dealt with antibodies against measles. Adams and Imagawa showed in 1962 (1) that patients with MS had higher titers of measles antibodies than matched controls. Their observation was later confirmed in other studies (2), which demonstrated serum antibodies. We, together with our Finnish colleagues, also carried out such a study (7) in which we compared antibodies to three different components of measles virus, the internal, the nucleocapsid, and the two major envelope components—the hemagglutinin and the hemolysin. In all three serologic tests, one can detect differences in the mean titers between MS patients and the controls, which are carefully matched with regard to age and other characteristics. Furthermore, as shown in other studies (2), mean titers against measles of siblings of MS patients fall between the mean titers of MS patients and controls. Since the increased antibody titers are directed against three different components of the virus, it is highly likely that they represent a true antibody response to measles and not a cross reaction to some other antigen (4).

Other studies (3) have shown that antibodies against measles virus are increased also in the cerebrospinal fluid (CSF). We have made extensive comparative analyses of the serum and CSF antibodies (5, 6, 8). This comparison can give interesting information about the occurrence of locally produced antibody in the CNS and can be illustrated with data from numerous samples of serum and CSF antibodies in a patient with acute measles encephalitis (Table 12.1). For comparison, we have analyzed antibodies against adenovirus and poliovirus as evidence of the integrity of

TABLE 12.1 / Antibody Titers in Serum and CSF Samples from a Patient with Acute Measles Encephalitis[a]

Day of Sampling	Sample	Antibodies to Measles Virus[b,c]			Antibodies to Reference Virus[b,c]	
		HI	HLI	NC–CF	Adeno HE	Polio NE
5	Serum	160 (10)	320 (40)	160 (40)	160 (≥160)	3600 (300)
	CSF	16	8	4	< 2	12
13	Serum	160 (10)	320 (80)	160 (80)	320 (≥320)	5120 (570)
	CSF	16	4	2	< 2	9
37	Serum	80 (40)	80	10	320	2560 (290)
	CSF	2	< 4	< 2	< 2	9
38	Serum	20	32	20	320	
	CSF	< 2	< 4	< 2	< 2	
103	Serum	10	32	20	320	
	CSF	< 2	< 4	< 2	< 2	
145	Serum	10	32	20	320 (≥320)	
	CSF	2	< 4	< 2	< 2	

[a] Onset of Encephalitic Signs on day 1.
[b] Abbreviations: HI, hemagglutination inhibition; HLI, hemolysin inhibition; NC–CF, nucleocapsid complement fixation; adeno HE, adenovirus hemagglutination enhancement; polio NE, poliovirus neutralization enhancement.
[c] The figures to the right of the serum–CSF pairs indicate the ratio of antibody titers in these samples.

the blood-brain barrier. There is no free flow of antibodies into the CNS and only under conditions of damage to the blood-brain barrier can serum and CSF antibodies be freely exchanged. Normally, the proportion between antibodies in serum and CSF is of the order of 300 to 600, as illustrated by adenovirus and poliovirus antibodies. In contrast, antibodies to different measles virus antigens occur in a serum–CSF ratio of the order of 10 to 40 in the early samples. We interpret this to indicate a local production of these antibodies in the CNS.

The data of a patient with acute measles encephalitis are shown not only as an example of the procedure for identification of a local antibody production in CNS but also because this is the first case in which a local production of measles antibodies in the CNS has been demonstrated in connection with acute measles encephalitis. It might be commented that we know remarkably little about the serologic events that occur in connection with acute measles encephalitis. Moreover in this particular case, the fact that there is a local production of measles antibodies in the CNS suggests that measles virus antigen may be present in the brain of this patient. This is of interest since measles encephalitis of the acute type usually is referred to as a type of postinfectious encephalitis with autoimmune characteristics. This acute measles encephalitis may represent different types of reactions sometimes with a direct involvement of the virus. The data in Table 12.1 also indicate that there is a rapid decline of antibody titers in the serum to relatively low levels and that antibodies in the CSF disappear completely. The CNS-associated antibody response is of transient nature.

ANTIBODY PRODUCTION AND IMMUNOGLOBULIN ABNORMALITIES

We have studied a group of 150 MS patients collected in Finland, Norway, and Sweden and compared the CNS and serum antibodies (6). The frequency with which we can find local production of antibodies against different enveloped viruses in these patients is shown in Table 12.2. As in our other studies (8), about 60% of these patients with MS have evidence of local production of measles antibodies in their CNS. Furthermore, there is local production of antibodies against other viruses, for example, rubella in 20% of the cases, mumps in 15% of the cases, and *Herpes simplex* type 1 in 10% of the cases. This means that in some of the MS patients there is a local production of antibodies to more than one virus. In about 7% of the cases, we can find a local production of antibodies against three or more viruses. Thus consideration of the possible etiologic role of viruses must not focus on only one virus.

We then compared the local production of virus-specific antibodies to the immunoglobulin abnormalities in patients with MS. One characteristic feature of this disease is an increase of IgG in the CSF. This IgG is oligoclonal, that is, it consists of homogeneous IgG molecules produced by a restricted number of clones of sensitized cells. Presence of oligoclonal IgG is a very important feature of the MS disease. It occurs in about 95% of all the cases. The major part of this IgG is produced locally.

There is a persistent production of oligoclonal IgG, in contrast to the transient production of such antibodies in the previously mentioned case of measles encephalitis. Other cases of persistent production of CNS-derived IgG are bacterial diseases, such as syphilis, or protozoal diseases, such as trypanosomiasis.

In subacute sclerosing panencephalitis (SSPE), we used two different techniques to study the locally produced antibodies and oligoclonal IgG.

TABLE 12.2 / Percentage of Patients with Significantly Reduced Ratios of Serum–CSF Antibody Titers Against Different Viruses[a,b]

Source of Material	Measles Virus Antibody tests				Mumps Virus HI	Para-Influenza Virus Type 1 HI	Rubella Virus HI[c]	Herples Simplex Virus Type 1 Passive H
	All tests	HI	HLI	NC–CF				
Finland	66(96)[c]	34(72)	62(97)	20(24)	20(30)	6(40)	26(74)	6(84)
Norway	60(98)	48(66)	34(98)	28(30)	12(30)	2(62)	18(60)	16(78)
Sweden	42(80)	16(54)	20(76)	30(34)	14(40)	2(84)	12(68)	12(78)
All countries	57(91)	33(63)	39(90)	26(29)	15(33)	3(62)	19(73)	11(80)

[a] Abbreviations: See legend of Table 12.1.
[b] Values within parenthesis give the percentage of patients with antibodies in CSF plus those with a serum–CSF ratio of >160 in the absence of CSF antibodies.
[c] Ratios were calculated only on patients with a CSF antibody titer of more than 2 or a serum titer >160.

The first made an electrophoretic separation of the various bands of oligo-clonal IgG and determined correlation between different antibody activities and occurrence of the bands. We found that each band of IgG corresponded to antibody activity, and different bands carried different antibody activities (9). The predominant band in all cases contained antibodies against nucleocapsids of the virus. Thus SSPE represents a unique situation in human beings with a local hyperimmunization causing the production of homogeneous antibodies responsible for different antibody activities.

The second was based on absorption–elution experiments. Concentrated CSF or extracts of the CNS were mixed with purified measles virus or with cell extracts of measles virus-infected cells and antigen–antibody complexes were removed by centrifugation. The sediment was dissociated by incubation at pH 4.3 and 2. The usefulness of this technique is exemplified in Table 12.3. Cerebrospinal fluid from a patient with SSPE was found to contain oligoclonal IgG, which was removed by absorption with large amounts of antigen. Considerable amounts of IgG and antibody activities were recovered at the low pH levels. Thus this type of test allows the detection of the specificity of oligoclonal IgG.

Application of preparatory electrophoresis to MS revealed a heterogeneous distribution of antibodies against different structural components. However, we could not correlate these peaks of antibody activities to the occurrence of specific bands of oligoclonal IgG. This is clearly different from the situation that obtains in SSPE. Further differences can be noted in absorption–elution experiments. We found that the major part of all bands remained intact after repeated absorptions with large concentrations of measles virus antigen. However, some oligoclonal IgG was adsorbed to the virus preparation and could be recovered in the low pH eluates (Table 12.4). Therefore, a small fraction of the oligoclonal IgG in MS may represent measles virus-specific antibodies of the type that can be adsorbed to the antigen preparation, the major part cannot be related to measles. This distinguishes MS from SSPE.

TABLE 12.3 / Absorption–Elution of CSF from a Patient with SSPE on Purified Measles Virus Particles[a]

Sample	Electrophoretic Pattern	IgG (mg/ml)	Measles Virus Antibody Titers in[a]			Adenovirus Antibody Titer in HE
			HI	HLI	NC–CF	
Unabsorbed	Oligoclonal IgG	4.2	1280	10240	2560	160
Supernate after absorption	Reduced oligoclonal IgG	1.4	640	5120	80	320
Eluate pH 4.0	Oligoclonal IgG	1.9	20	640	640	10
Eluate pH 3.0	Oligoclonal IgG	0.79	640	10240	320	10
Eluate pH 2.0	Oligoclonal IgG	0.30	320	2560	80	10

[a] HI, hemagglutination inhibition; HLI, hemolysin inhibition; NC–CF, nucleocapsid complement fixation; HE, hemagglutination enhancement.

TABLE 12.4 / Absorption–Elution of Concentrated CSF from an MS Patient with Cell-Associated Measles Virus Antigen[a]

Sample	Electrophoretic Pattern	IgG (mg/ml)	HI	HLI	NC–CF	Antibody Adenovirus Titers in HE
Unabsorbed	Oligoclonal IgG	3.80	80	10240	40	160
Supernate after adsorption	Unchanged	3.45	10	1280	20	160
Eluate pH 4.0	One band of IgG	0.09	10	640	10	10
Eluate pH 3.0	One IgG band different from pH 4.0 eluate	0.11	40	5120	5	10
Eluate pH 2.0	A weaker IgG band corresponding to pH 3.0 eluate	0.05	80	2560	5	10

(Measles Virus Antibody Titers in[a])

[a] HI, hemagglutination inhibition; HLI, hemolysin inhibition; NC–CF, nucleocapsid complement fixation; HE, hemagglutination enhancement.

CONCLUSIONS

What do these findings imply? First, the fact that measles virus-specific antibodies produced locally in the CNS of MS patients have an oligoclonal nature suggests that they result from local hyperimmunization. Thus it is possible, and this is the explanation that we favor, that these antibodies arise in response to measles virus antigen in the brain, most likely as the result of activation of a latent virus infection. However, virus antigen has not yet been identified in the brain. This hypothesis also implies that the activated infection must be present during an early stage of the disease because the oligoclonal IgG is present early and is remarkably persistent throughout the course of the disease, which can be as long as 20 to 30 years.

An alternate explanation for the occurrence of virus specific oligoclonal IgG is some nonspecific activation of clones of cells that produce homogeneous antibodies. This would be analogous to the production of myeloma proteins. Another example of nonspecific activation of the IgG production is chronic hepatitis.

Of considerable interest is the fact that we cannot account for the major part of the oligoclonal IgG produced in the CNS of MS patients. If we could demonstrate specific antibody activity, we would be much closer to a clue of viral etiology of MS. It is possible that the remaining IgG represents antibodies that do not attach efficiently to the antigen used in the absorption studies. This seems less likely because, generally, oligoclonal IgG antibodies have a high avidity. It is also possible that the absorption of oligoclonal IgG is blocked by association with haptens or that they are antibodies against nonstructural virus components or virus antigens that

163

are not present in the preparation we use for absorption. Finally, they may also represent antibodies against viruses other than measles or against non-viral antigens. The oligoclonal IgG is a very important feature of the disease, and major continued efforts should be made to determine its antibody activity.

REFERENCES

1. Adams, J. M., and Imagawa, D. T., (1962). Measles antibodies in multiple sclerosis. *Proc. Soc. Exp. Biol. Med. 111*, 562–566.
2. Brody, J. A., Sever, J. L., Edgar, A., and McNew, J. (1972). Measles antibody titers of multiple sclerosis patients and their siblings. *Neurology 22*, 492–499.
3. Brown, P., Cathala, F., Gajdusek, D. C., and Gibbs, C. J., Jr. (1971). Measles antibodies in the cerebrospinal fluid of patients with multiple sclerosis. *Proc. Soc. Exp. Biol. Med. 137*, 956–961.
4. Field, E. J., Caspary, E. A., and Madgwick, H. (1972). Measles, multiple sclerosis and encephalitogenic factor. *Lancet ii*, 337.
5. Norrby, E., Link, H., and Olsson, J.-E. (1974). Comparison of measles virus antibody titers in cerebrospinal fluid and serum from patients with multiple sclerosis and from controls. *Arch. Neurol. 30*, 285–292.
6. Norrby, E., Link, H., Olsson, J.-E., Panelius, M., Salmi, A., and Vandvik, B. (1974). Comparison of antibodies against different viruses in cerebrospinal fluid and serum from patients with multiple sclerosis. *Infect. Immun. 10*, 688–694.
7. Salmi, A., Gollmar, Y., Norrby, E., and Panelius, M. (1973). Antibodies against three different structural components of measles virus in patients with multiple sclerosis, their siblings and matched controls. *Acta Pathol. Microbiol. Scand. 81b*, 627–634.
8. Salmi, A. A., Norrby, E., and Panelius, M. (1972). Identification of different measles virus-specific antibodies in the serum and cerebrospinal fluid from patients with subacute sclerosing panencephalitis and multiple sclerosis. *Infect. Immun. 6*, 248–254.
9. Vandvik, B., and Norrby, E. (1973). Oligoclonal IgG antibody response in the central nervous system to different measles virus antigens in subacute sclerosing panencephalitis. *Proc. Natl. Acad. Sci. U.S.A. 70*, 1060–1063.

Discussion/Chapters 10-12

Dr. Askonas began by asking Dr. Norrby whether the monoclonal antibodies were directed against certain viral fractions, perhaps the intracellular ones. Dr. Norrby responded that this has not yet been studied, but that in his studies he used virus antigens produced in the cell culture system and absorbed with intracellular and extracellular virus, but not with the cell material itself. The interesting thing, he continued, was the remarkable persistence of the individual clones, which remained relatively constant within each patient, even as there is considerable variation among patients.

This suggested to Dr. Askonas that there is a limited traffic of cells into the central nervous system (CNS), and Dr. Norrby generalized from it that there is a predisposition in the CNS to the development of oligoclonal antibody response, whenever there is hyperimmunization. This would be likely to occur if antibody-producing cells within the CNS had difficulty getting out into the general circulation. Therefore, this would be responsible for the characteristic oligoclonal nature of all antibodies within the CNS.

Dr. Bauer reviewed briefly the reported predominance of the kappa light chains in the CNS oligoclonal antibodies in multiple sclerosis (MS). Dr. Norrby agreed that there was such a shift and wondered whether there was a preference for building up kappa clones. Dr. Kabat offered the explanation that the difference may be statistical only, because there were twice as many kappa chains as lambda chains (and if the antibodies were oligoclonal, there was obviously twice the chance of producing kappa chains as lambda chains). An additional comment about antibodies came from Dr. Harter, who pointed out that there are patients with MS who do not have elevated levels of gamma globulins; therefore, the ones studied by Dr. Norrby and others had been preselected in that respect. Dr. Brody added that it would be useful to examine cerebrospinal fluids of siblings of the patients with MS to see if they had oligoclonal antibodies, but this has not yet been done.

Dr. Dickinson and Dr. Koprowski concluded the discussion by pointing out that it would be far better to study a group of MS patients longitudinally and for a prolonged time period, with respect to many factors, rather than studying large numbers of patients on short term bases. The longitudinal studies would permit, for example, a differentiation of those patients who do have unusual measles antibody titers from those who do not, in terms of their clinical disease pattern and prognosis. Such studies would also obviate the difficulties of selecting proper controls; even siblings may not be the proper controls, since their HLA histocompatibility types may be different.

CHAPTER 13

Demyelination in Experimental Allergic Encephalomyelitis and Multiple Sclerosis

ELLSWORTH C. ALVORD, JR.

INTRODUCTION

Experimental allergic encephalomyelitis (EAE) can be produced by the very simple technique of a single intradermal injection of normal central nervous system (CNS) tissue with Freund's complete adjuvants, killed mycobacteria in water-in-oil emulsion (2). The active component of the CNS is myelin and its "myelin membrane encephalitogenic protein" (17) or, more simply, myelin "basic protein" (BP). Two to three weeks after the injection, the animal becomes paralyzed and usually dies within a few days with a disease that for the past quarter of a century has served as almost the only model for multiple sclerosis (MS).

SPECIES-SPECIFIC DIFFERENCES

Including species-specific differences, EAE has many interesting features, some of which are summarized in Table 13.1. Perivenous inflammatory reactions with lymphocytic infiltrations (Fig. 13.1) are the typical lesion of ordinary acute EAE in all species of experimental animals, specifically

TABLE 13.1 / Comparison of Certain Features of EAE in Different Species of Experimental Animals and in Man

Characteristic Feature of EAE	Guinea Pig	Rat	Monkey	Man
Ordinary, with perivenous lymphocytic inflammation	++	++	++	++
Hyperacute, with fibrinous and polymorphonuclear inflammation	0	++ (with *B. pertussis*)	++	++
Large demyelinating or necrotic lesions	0	0	++	++
Anamnestic acceleration on resensitization	0	0	+	±

the guinea pig, rat, and monkey, which are being compared in Table 13.1, as well as in humans after injections of brain-containing vaccines or certain viral infections. Such lesions may be grossly visible as tiny gray spots scattered through the white matter especially in the monkey (Fig. 13.1a). The hyperacute form of EAE, with hemorrhage, fibrin, and polymorphonuclear leukocytes, is not seen in the guinea pig. In the rat, it can be readily produced if pertussis vaccine is added to the inoculum (29), but in the monkey, it is seen frequently without any specially added procedures (Figs. 13.1b and 13.2a). It is also occasionally seen in humans, more commonly "spontaneously" than after injections of brain-containing vaccines.

One feature worth emphasizing in these species variations is that in the monkey (but not in any other species) one can see an anamnestic acceleration after a second injection of the encephalitogenic emulsion (7). This observation suggests that there is some pathogenetic difference in this species, with perhaps a component of immediate-type immune responsiveness in addition to the classic delayed-type hypersensitivity that is generally considered to underlie EAE. In the human, it is notoriously difficult to document incubation periods except after vaccinia vaccination, where only a very few cases suggesting anamnestic responses have been recorded, and where increased resistance to postvaccinial encephalopathy and encephalomyelitis is the general rule following repeated vaccinations (2).

Large lesions are practically never seen in the guinea pig or rat but are rather frequently seen in the monkey (Fig. 13.2a). These large lesions have fascinated many investigators who have been interested in the possibility that EAE was a good model for MS, and they are well described by the earliest investigators of monkeys, Rivers and Schwentker (41) and Wolf et al. (49) in particular. Recently we have reinvestigated these lesions, which are sometimes hemorrhagic, so that they stand out clearly in photographs as in Fig. 13.2a. There is some gross similarity between such monkey EAE lesions and human MS lesions (Fig. 13.2c), but microscopically, these large EAE lesions in the monkeys are essentially a confluence of small perivenous lesions (Fig. 13.2b). Thus they are not typical of any familiar stage of MS.

One of the main advantages of using monkeys is that they are large enough to permit obtaining repeated blood samples to study other possible correlates of EAE (6, 7, 9). The monkey gives notoriously poor delayed-type skin reactions, so that we did not attempt to measure these. But we did compare animals injected with a nonencephalitogenic BP (lysozyme) as a control on the events temporally related to the use of Freund's adjuvants. Figure 13.3a shows that there are a number of phenomena that are a result of the injection of an antigen in Freund's complete adjuvants in a reasonably regular sequence: "LIF" (leukocyte-inhibiting factor) is released from buffy-coat leukocytes on exposure to the specific antigen (BP or lysozyme, respectively) or to PPD (since Freund's complete adjuvants include killed mycobacteria) so that the migration of the leukocytes (WBC) is inhibited. C-Reactive protein increases in the serum. Both of these changes reach their maxima after 10 days to 2 weeks, at which time there is a

Figure 13.1.
Gross and microscopic features of EAE in rhesus monkeys.

a. Small foci of demyelination in occipital white matter, which becomes confluent on one side (Np 3852, 2-weeks duration).

b. Similar foci in corpus callosum, associated with hemorrhage in confluent lesions in the opposite parietal gyrus (Np 3413, 1-day duration).

c. Perivenous inflammatory exudates in cerebral white matter (Np 3655, 4-days' duration). H & E, ×12

d. Predominantly lymphocytic perivenous exudate in spinal white matter (Np 3849, 4-days' duration). H & E, ×300

e. Perivenous and diffuse exudates of various types of leukocytes (Np 3650, killed 27 days after onset, having had two remissions facilitated by treatments with BP and penicillin). H & E, ×120

f. Predominantly polymorphonuclear (Np 3651, 7-days' duration). H & E, ×300

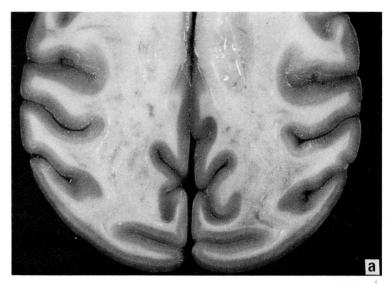

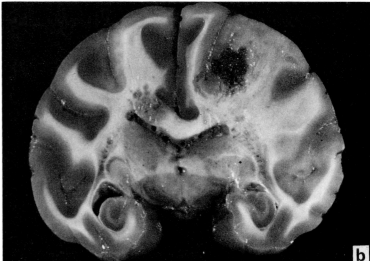

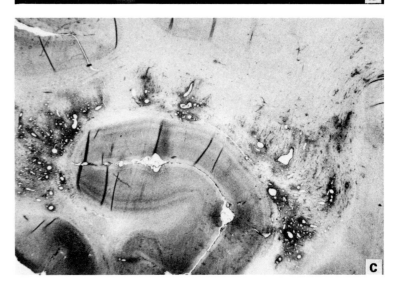

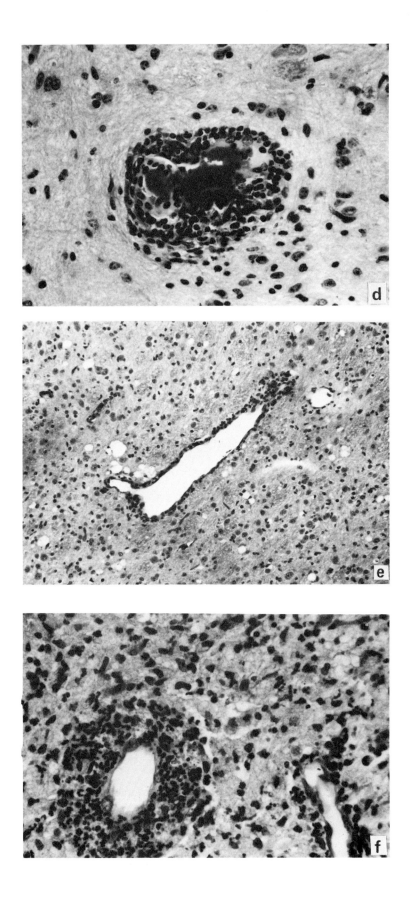

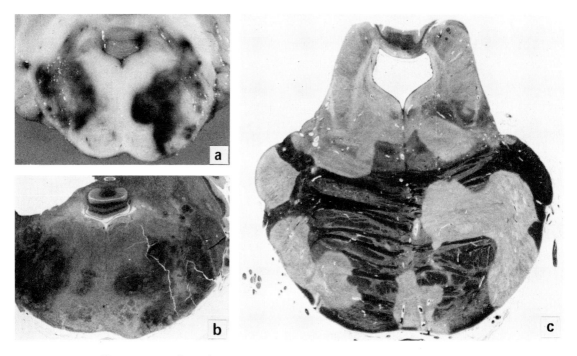

Figure 13.2. **a, b,** and **c.**
Transverse section of the pons from a monkey with EAE (Np 3559). Such lesions need not be grossly hemorrhagic, as seen in other monkeys with similarly large and sharply defined lesions (**b,** H & E, ×2). Although superficially resembling the distribution of MS lesions shown in **c,** the EAE lesions are composed of confluent small perivenous lesions.

precipitous fall in circulating lymphocytes. An increase in total circulating WBC and the clumping of WBC on exposure to the specific antigen (or to PPD) occur after about 3 weeks. When these values are replotted for those monkeys that develop EAE, it becomes apparent (Fig. 13.3b) that practically all of these except LIF, which correlates only with the time of injection!) become synchronized just before EAE becomes clinically apparent. The quantitative degrees of clumping of WBC in BP or PPD differ so greatly that they have been separately plotted, but both reactions increase to maxima as EAE develops. Since most of these tests require only a few hours to do, it should be possible to predict the onset of EAE with remarkable accuracy.

AGE DEPENDENCY

Another feature of EAE that bears emphasizing is age dependency, true in all species, but especially so in humans (44). The similarity in age susceptibility of humans to EAE (44) and MS (39) is so great (Fig. 13.4) that I have been tempted to speculate that the difference in incidences merely represents the 10-fold greater effectiveness of the exogenous BP in the repeatedly injected brain-containing rabies vaccine producing EAE as com-

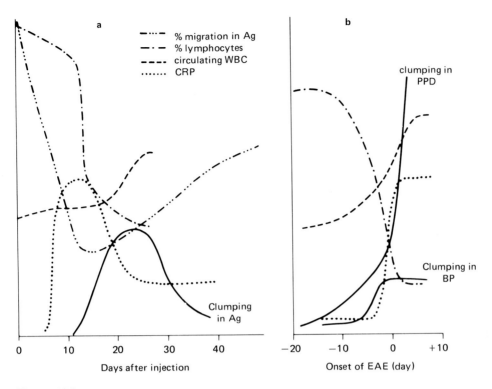

Figure 13.3.
Comparison of various reactions in monkeys sensitized to encephalitogenic myelin BP or to a control nonencephalitogenic antigen (lysozyme) incorporated in Freund's complete adjuvant. The reactions are related to the time of injection at day zero (a) or to the day of onset of EAE (b). Note the synchronization of several of these reactions just before EAE becomes clinically manifest.

pared to the endogenous BP or other brain antigen that could produce MS (2).

Three years ago (3), I plotted the vacillations over the past quarter century of opinions whether EAE and MS were related (Fig. 13.5). When the experimental disease was first produced, even in the 1930s (41) before Freund's adjuvants made the study of EAE so easy in the 1940s (10, 25, 49), many of us were seduced into believing that we had the solution of the MS problem. However, it soon became obvious that the histology of EAE was not quite like that of MS. The fact that there was no adjuvant present in the usual MS patient and the lack of development of new leads in the early 1950s led to increasing disappointment with the possibility that EAE and MS could be related. But no other idea appeared, either. At that time, the concept of a viral etiology of MS was not only discounted but also rather vociferously denounced as inconceivable!

In the late 1950s, the cerebral form of human EAE, which developed in Japan in some individuals inoculated with brain-containing vaccines against rabies and which was characterized by large MS-like lesions (44), provided the impetus for the pendulum's swinging back toward EAE and MS being related. Then, in 1965, when Bornstein and Appel (16) described

171

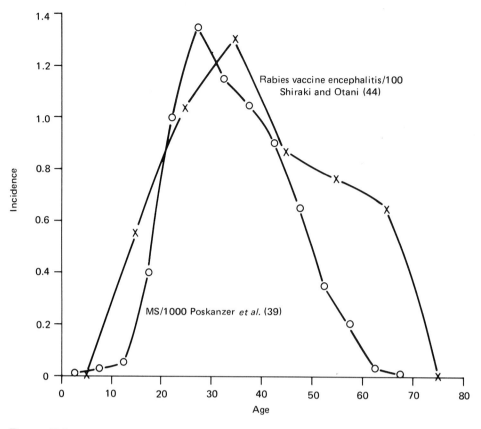

Figure 13.4.
Age specific susceptibility to EAE per 100 persons vaccinated with brain-containing rabies vaccine (9) and to MS per 1,000 population (10). [Reprinted from Alvord (1) by permission of North-Holland Publishing Co., Amsterdam.]

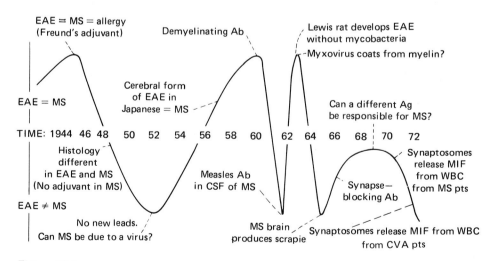

Figure 13.5.
A summary of 25 years of research on EAE and MS, indicating the variations in opinions whether EAE and MS are related (EAE = MS) or not related (EAE ≠ MS). [Reprinted from Alvord (11) by permission of Academic Press, Inc., New York.]

demyelinating antibodies as occurring in both MS and EAE, enthusiasm for EAE as an important and potentially very useful model for MS reached a new high.

However, this enthusiasm was soon tempered by the report of Adams and Imagawa (1) that antibodies against measles could be detected in the cerebrospinal fluid (CSF) of MS patients. Two new hypotheses soon arose: (a) that MS was purely viral or (b) that myxoviruses might become coated with myelin (38), which could act as an antigenic stimulus for the production of autoallergic EAE (and ultimately MS by a process of continued autosensitization). The need for any special adjuvants in particularly susceptible individuals decreased as Levine and Wenk (30) showed that Lewis rats could develop EAE without Freund's adjuvants.

However, although many attempts have been made to demonstrate myelin- or BP-specific antibodies or sensitized lymphocytes in MS patients, the evidence remains unconvincing. A few years ago, we thought we had found evidence of hypersensitivity of MS buffy-coat leukocytes to synaptosomes (4). This observation would have fitted other reports of "synapse-blocking antibodies" in EAE and MS, but we soon found that such cellular hypersensitivity could develop a week or so after a stroke—or any other brain damage—and could, therefore, be secondary to MS. Seil et al. (42) have recently shown that the "synapse-blocking antibodies" are probably not antibodies and are not even characteristics of EAE or MS.

With all these changes in opinions and facts having occurred over the past quarter century, additional changes may be possible with future evidence! But the current situation, coupled with other observations to be presented below, suggests that EAE and MS are not the same, either etiologically or pathogenetically.

PROTEIN COMPOSITION

A remarkable amount of information has become available concerning the particular protein (BP) in CNS myelin that produces EAE. Basic protein consists of a linear sequence of 170 amino acid residues, to which two blank spaces can be added to make each species-specific sequence exactly homologous (17), as schematically shown in Fig. 13.6. The most remarkable thing about BP is that each animal species seems to develop EAE in response to different particular short sequences in the molecule. The guinea pig is especially sensitive to the nonapeptide centered around the single trytophan at residue 118 (8, 48) and to a much lesser degree to other sites (28), and the rabbit to the similarly sized peptide centered around the tyrosine at residue 70 (43) and to a lesser degree to other sites (11, 12). The rat responds to at least two less sharply defined sites (18, 32–35), and the monkey, to several different regions of the BP molecule (7, 20, 26).

In addition to these encephalitogenic sites, there must be at least eight antigenic determinants approximately equally distributed throughout the molecule, as diagrammed in Fig. 13.6. These have been defined by immunoprecipitations in gels (5) by transformation of rabbit lymph node

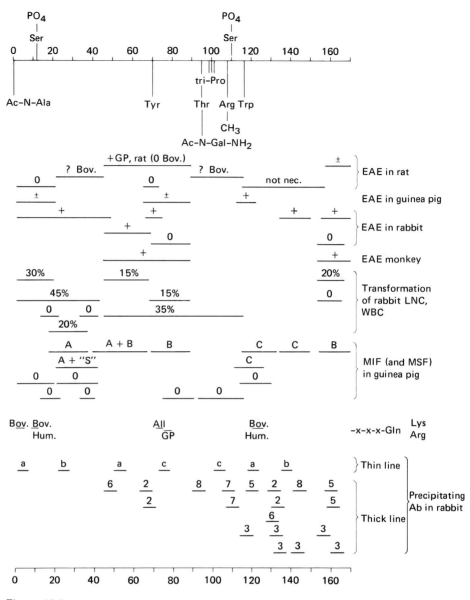

Figure 13.6.
Schematic diagram of the 170 linearly arranged amino acid residues making up the BP molecule, with various interesting features emphasized: regions that are biochemical, regions that are encephalitogenic in various species of experimental animals, and regions that are antigenic by various tests.

cells (LNC) or WBC (14, 15) by tests for MIF (macrophage-inhibiting factor) or MSF (macrophage-stimulating factor) in guinea pigs (13) or by delayed-type skin reactions in guinea pigs where Hashim and Schilling (23) believe that pentapeptides consisting of -x-x-x-Gln-Lys (or Arg) are the antigenic determinant.

Since each species synthesizes BP with substitutions or deletions of a few residues (17), one can begin to appreciate why there may be quantitative differences in encephalitogenic and antigenic activities as assayed in different species. So far, it would appear that only delayed-type hypersensitivity is evoked by the encephalitogenic sites and not circulating antibodies, whereas both are evoked by the antigenic (immunogenic) sites. That is, I know of no evidence that anyone has produced circulating antibodies in one species of animal able to bind to the species-specific encephalitogenic site.

With hyperimmune rabbit antisera prepared against this myelin BP and its several antigenic determinants, one can stain myelin in the normal CNS by the immunoperoxidase reaction shown in Fig. 13.7. This thick immunologic "sandwich" was developed by Mason et al. (36) and Zimmerman et al. (50) for other antigens but was readily adapted for the present experiments. The BP in the tissue is specifically bound by rabbit anti-BP antiserum, the IgG of which has species-specific antigenic sites that bind the next reagent, goat anti-rabbit-IgG antiserum. This, being bivalent, can still react with the species-specific antigenic sites in the IgG of the third reagent, rabbit anti-horseradish-peroxidase antiserum, which then specifically binds peroxidase. The location of the peroxidase is revealed by reaction with diaminobenzidine, and the reaction product is finally fixed and blackened with osmium tetroxide. The serial application of the various specific antisera actually increases both the sensitivity and the specificity of the final reaction. The trick we found necessary with BP, however, was the use of delipidated tissue, as in ordinary paraffin-embedded sections, since BP seems to be masked by lipids and does not stain if the immunoperoxidase reactions are applied to frozen sections of CNS (5). It is fortunate for such studies that BP is stable to formalin fixation, to alcohol–xylol extraction and dehydration, as well as to temperature for embedding in paraffin.

Normal myelin sheaths in MS patients, even at the very edge of MS plaques, also contain BP (Fig. 13.8), confirming immunochemically at the level of the individual myelin sheaths the conclusion that Suzuki et al. (45) came to on biochemical analyses of ultracentrifugally separated myelin. The additional fact that MS macrophages contain myelin debris, which still contains at least some of the antigenic sites in BP (Fig. 13.9), would seem to eliminate two of the more recent hypotheses that have attempted to relate BP to MS: that MS myelin does not contain BP (40) and that in the region of the MS lesion there is increased proteinase activity (19), which either destroys BP or releases it from the myelin and provides it to the body's immunogenic mechanism, thereby setting up the possibility of an EAE-like autosensitization. As in psychology, where dream analysis indicates that one never knows whether one wishes or fears that something be true, so in immunology, one does not know today whether immunogenic determinants should be relatively stable or relatively labile. Perhaps both are true, but at least certain fragments of labile macrophage-digested proteins must be stable enough to complex to RNA to form immunogenic ribonucleopeptides (24). Which of the several antigenic determinants in BP has been revealed by the immunoperoxidase reactions (Figs. 13.7 and 13.8) is not yet clear. It is likely that only part of the BP molecule is still present in MS macrophages (Fig. 13.9). One can imagine that the MS

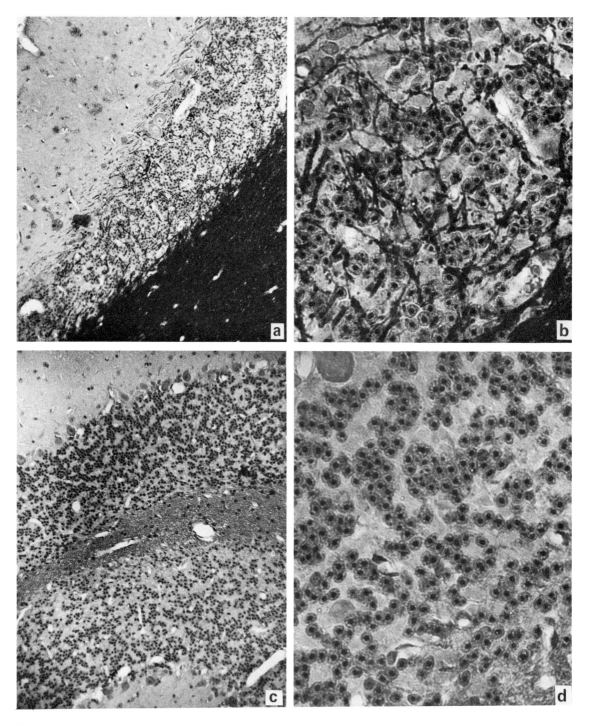

Figure 13.7.
Immunoperoxidase stain of BP in myelin in the cerebellum of a guinea pig, using hyperimmune rabbit anti-bovine-BP serum diluted 1:200 on formalin-fixed paraffin-embedded tissue. Note the heavy staining of the white matter in **a** (× 14) and the individual myelinated fibers coursing through the granule cell layer in **b** (× 490). The nuclei (**c,** × 14) and nucleoli (**d,** × 490) appear black in these photographs but were stained red with nuclear fast red (Kernechtrot) and contrasted sharply with the myelin sheaths, which appeared dark brown to black in the original preparation. All of the control preparations were negative, including the omission or substitution of each reagent.

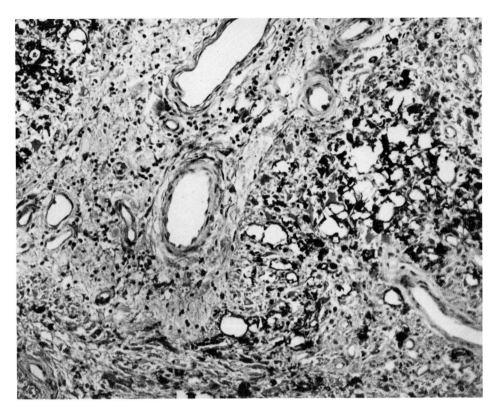

Figure 13.8.
Immunoperoxidase stain of BP in myelin in a section from paraffin-embedded spinal cord from a case of chronic MS (Np 3901), showing the preserved myelin sheaths at the edge of an MS plaque. ×14

patient differs genetically from other people in having macrophages that digest or process BP differently, perhaps uniquely, preserving or destroying one or another peptide component. Since we do not know which region of the BP molecule is encephalitogenic in humans, it may be possible for a particular peptide fragment to produce the EAE-like autosensitization necessary to cause the characteristic MS lesion. Together with the similarity in age susceptibility (Fig. 13.4), this seems to be the only hope of preserving some kind of a relationship between EAE and MS. But, as will become evident soon, even this seems very unlikely.

MULTIPLE SCLEROSIS

Multiple sclerosis is a condition that still has to be defined as a clinico-pathologic syndrome, composed of one or more diseases with multiple demyelinative lesions seen at autopsy. These lesions are multiple both in space and in time (i.e., widely scattered in different sites within the CNS and appearing at different times during the course of the disease in any one MS patient), characteristics that allow MS to be diagnosed clinically with reasonable accuracy. The lesions of MS are still of unknown etiology and pathogenesis.

Figure 13.2c showed typical MS lesions as seen in sections stained for myelin sheaths, which are absent in the plaque. Figure 13.10a shows two sharply defined plaques of demyelination containing lipid-filled macrophages, which were stained bright red in the original preparation stained with oil-red-0 and hematoxylin, contrasting nicely with the normal cylindrical myelin sheaths, which were a rather dull purplish color. Using red or blue filters, I have attempted to increase the contrasting colors in these black-and-white photographs. Figures 13.10b, c, and d show at higher magnifications that in some plaques the edge is really quite sharp: The normal myelin sheaths and the lipid-filled macrophages abut on each other do not overlap. The duration of such a lesion is unfortunately indeterminable. From one point of view, it could be said to be relatively early, before the macrophages disappear, but this process would take several months at least. The lesion probably continues at least a few weeks to months, since the macrophages are well filled with lipids. And one could as accurately estimate that it is relatively late, since there is little evidence of active demyelination at the edge. That is, most of the macrophages appear to be equally well filled with lipids, with few cells at an earlier stage in their progressive enlargement as they ingest and digest the myelin.

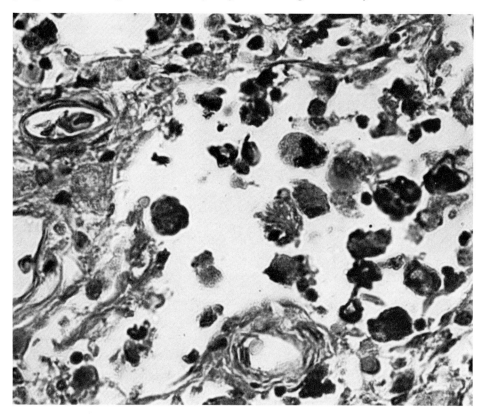

Figure 13.9.
Immunoperoxidase stain showing BP in myelin debris within macrophages within the spinal cord plaque from the same case of MS illustrated in Fig. 13.8. ×490. Again, the nuclei of the cells appeared red in the original preparation in sharp contrast with the dark brown myelin.

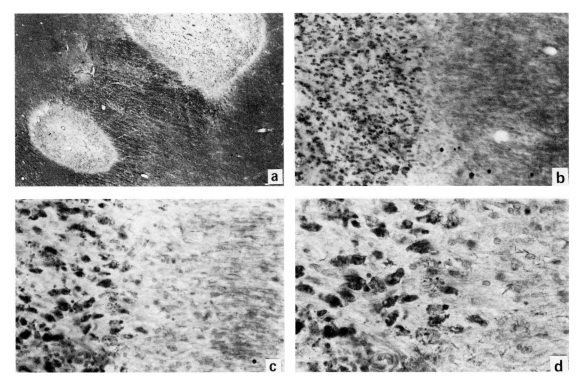

Figure 13.10.
Cerebellar plaques in chronic MS (Np 4249) as seen in a frozen section stained with ORO-H.
a. Low magnification (×8) showing two plaques with lipid-filled macrophages almost completely filling each plaque, most of the normal fibers being cut longitudinally.
b, c, and **d.** Relatively sharp edge of the plaques with few transitional forms of lipid-filled macrophages emphasized by use of a blue filter (**b** ×80, **c** ×200, **d** ×320).

In Figure 13.11, however, one can see part of a large cerebral lesion from the same case of MS with several interesting features. In certain places at the edge of the plaque, under high magnification (Figs. 13.11e and f), one can clearly see that there is a considerable overlap between the normal cylindrical myelin sheaths and the solid lipid-filled macrophages. Furthermore, the sizes and shapes of the macrophages in this edge are quite variable, progressively enlarging as we look deeper toward the center of the plaque. Again, although the duration of this lesion is also indeterminable, from the transitional appearance of many of the macrophages, one would suspect that it is considerably earlier than the one shown in Fig. 13.10, and that some of the myelin is actively breaking down at the edge of the lesion. (A similar transition is illustrated in Fig. 13.12, from the spinal cord, where the normal myelin sheaths are seen in cross section.) It is important to note that there are no other leukocytes at this edge, a distinctive difference from EAE lesions.

However, the center of the large plaque shown in Fig. 13.11 must be very old, since practically all of the macrophages have disappeared, leaving

179

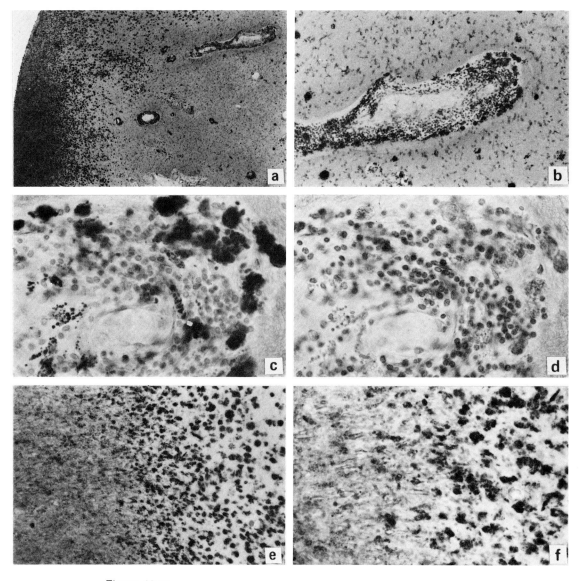

Figure 13.11.
Part of a large cerebral lesion in the same case of MS illustrated in Fig. 13.10 as seen in a frozen section stained with ORO-H.
a. Low magnification (× 20) showing several central venules with leukocytic cuffs, a relatively acellular gliotic center of plaque, and a region at the edge with active demyelination.
b. Central venules with leukocytic cuffs. ×80
c. Central venule with leukocytic cuff, the lipid-filled macrophages emphasized by use of a blue filter. ×320
d. Same field as **c**, the mononuclear leukocytes emphasized by use of a red filter. ×320
e and **f.** Edge of plaque with many transitional forms of lipid-filled macrophages emphasized by use of a blue filter (**e**, ×80; **f**, ×200), most of the normal fibers being cut longitudinally.

a relatively acellular gliotic scar. In addition, in the center, one can see several venules surrounded by cuffs of leukocytes, mostly various types of mononuclear cells (Figs. 13.11b, c, and d). Some of these are lipid-filled macrophages (Fig. 13.11c); others, lymphocytes or a few plasma cells (Fig. 13.11d). Fog (21) has reported that practically all MS plaques surround a venule, and many histopathologists have speculated whether the perivenous leukocytes are primary or secondary. Certainly, the lipid-filled macrophages are secondary carrying the myelin debris away, probably into the venous blood, eventually clearing the whole plaque. But what about the other cells? One can easily imagine that some factor is diffusing slowly and radially through the plaque, either from the blood within the central venule itself or from the mononuclear cells around the veins(s) reaching the edge of the plaque and causing the demyelination there. This factor may be antibodies, immunoglobulins which Lumsden (31) found bound to myelin sheaths at the edge of MS plaques. If there is any rational basis to MS, these should be the demyelinating antibodies which Bornstein and Appel (16) first reported in the serum of EAE animals and MS patients and

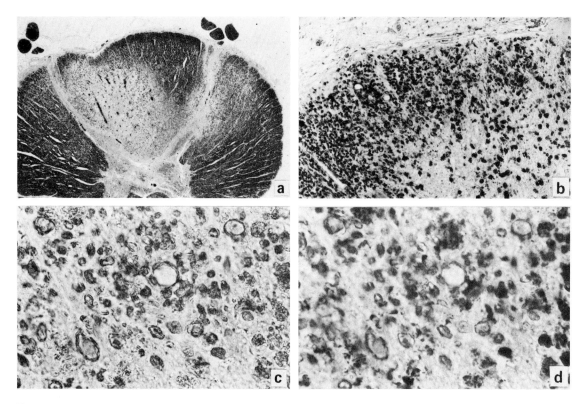

Figure 13.12.
Two plaques in the spinal cord of the same case of MS illustrated in Figs. 13.10 and 13.11 as seen in a frozen section stained with ORO-H. (a) Low magnification (×8) showing plaques in posterior and posterolateral columns. (b) Edge of plaque in posterior column. ×80. (c) Many transitional forms of lipid-filled macrophages emphasized by use of a blue filter. ×320. (d) Same field as c, the normal myelin sheaths in cross section emphasized by use of a red filter. ×320.

which Kim *et al.* (27) have found also in the cerebrospinal fluid (CSF). It would be nice, furthermore, if these were the same relatively cathodic immunoglobulins which Tourtellotte *et al.* (47) first demonstrated to be characteristic of MS CSF and which Toutellotte (46) has repeatedly suggested to be antibodies spilling over from the MS plaque where they are being produced locally, and not systemically.

CONCLUSION

Be that as it may, what are these antibodies directed against? It is clear from the work of Seil *et al.* (42) that demyelinating antibodies are not antibodies to myelin BP. They may be to cerebroside, as Fry *et al.* (22) have reported, but they could perhaps be to viral antigens that have become incorporated into MS myelin. The observations reported by Norrby (37) that 20% of MS CSF oligoclonal IgG can be absorbed by measles antigens suggests a partial solution to the problem.

Are these 20% of the antibodies the important ones, or the other 80%? And what are the other 80% of the MS antibodies directed against? This is the key question in MS: What is the antigen(s) evoking and reacting with these antibodies that are probably being produced by the lymphoid cells around the venule(s) in the center of the MS plaque (Figs. 13.11b, c, and d)? Although the histopathologically visible activity of the demyelinating MS process is at the edge of the plaque (Figs. 13.11e and f), the real action may be at the center of the plaque, where the lymphocytes and plasma cells are, most likely secreting antibodies that cause the characteristic demyelination at the periphery.

REFERENCES

1. Adams, J. M., and Imagawa, D. T. (1962). Measles antibodies in multiple sclerosis. *Proc. Soc. Exp. Biol. Med. 111*, 562–566.
2. Alvord, E. C., Jr. (1970). Acute disseminated encephalomyelitis and "allergic" neuro-encephalopathies. In *Multiple Sclerosis and Other Demyelinating Diseases, Vol. 9, Handbook of Clinical Neurology* (P. J. Vinken and G. W. Bruyn, eds.), Chapter 19, pp. 500–571. North-Holland, Amsterdam.
3. Alvord, E. C., Jr. (1972). Impressions of the conference. In *Multiple Sclerosis, Immunology, Virology and Ultrastructure* (F. Wolfgram, G. W. Ellison, J. G. Stevens, and J. M. Andrews, eds.), Chapter 27, pp. 569–592. Academic, New York.
4. Alvord, E. C., Jr., Hsu, P. C., and Thron, R. (1974). Leucocyte sensitivity to brain fractions in neurological diseases. *Arch. Neurol. 30*, 296–299.
5. Alvord, E. C., Jr., Hruby, S., Petersen, R., and Kies, M. W. (1976). An analysis of antigenic determinants within myelin membrane encephalitogenic protein. Int. Symp. on the Aetiology and Pathogenesis of the Demyelinating Diseases, Kyoto, Japan, September 2–4, 1973. *Acta Neuropathol.*, in press.
6. Alvord, E. C., Jr., Shaw, C. M., Hruby, S., Hsu, P., Thron, R., and Weiser, K. D. (1973). Correlates of acute experimental allergic encephalomyelitis (EAE) in monkeys. *Fed. Proc. 33*, 832.
7. Alvord, E. C., Jr., Shaw, C. M., Hruby, S., and Petersen, A. (1976). Neuro-allergic

reactions in primates. Internat'l. Symp. on the Aetiology and Pathogenesis of the Demyelinating Diseases, Kyoto, Japan, September 2–4, 1973. *Acta Neuropathol.*, in press.

8. Alvord, E. C., Jr., Shaw, C. M., Hruby, S., Petersen, R., and Harvey, F. H. (1976). Correlation of delayed skin hypersensitivity and experimental allergic encephalomyelitis induced by synthetic peptides. In *The Nervous System: 25 Years of Research Progress*, Raven, New York, in press.

9. Alvord, E. C., Jr., Shaw, C. M., Hruby, S., Petersen, R., and Hsu, P. (1974). Diagnosis and treatment of experimental allergic encephalomyelitis in rhesus monkeys. *Trans. Am. Neurol. Assoc. 99*, 63.

10. Alvord, E. C., Jr., and Stevenson, L. D. (1950). Experimental production of encephalomyelitis in guinea pigs. *Res. Publ. Assoc. Res. Nerv. Ment. Dis. 28*, 99–112.

11. Bergstrand, H. (1972). Encephalitogenic activity in rabbits of the C-terminal region of bovine basic myelin protein: Localization to two different regions. *FEBS Lett. 23*, 195–198.

12. Bergstrand, H. (1973). Localization of antigenic determinants on bovine encephalitogenic protein. Disease-inducing activity of fragment 44-68 in rabbits. *Neurobiology 3*, 124–129.

13. Bergstrand, H., and Kallen, B. (1973). Is there a cross-reactivity between different parts of the bovine encephalitogenic protein in the macrophage migration inhibition assay? *Immunochemistry 10*, 471–476.

14. Bergstrand, H., and Kallen, B. (1973). Antigenic determinants on bovine encephalitogenic protein: Studies in rabbits with derivatives of fragments 1-43 and the lymph node cell transformation test. *Neurobiology 3*, 246–255.

15. Bergstrand, H., and Kallen, B. (1973). Antigenic determinants on bovine encephalitogenic protein: Localization of regions that induce transformation of lymphnode cells from immunized rabbits. *Eur. J. Immunol. 3*, 287–292.

16. Bornstein, M. B., and Appel, S. H. (1965). Tissue culture studies of demyelination. *Ann. N.Y. Acad. Sci. 122*, 280–286.

17. Dayhoff, M. O. (1972). *Atlas of Protein Sequence and Structure 1972*. National Biomedical Research Foundation, Washington, D.C.

18. Dunkley, P. R., Coates, A. S., and Carnegie, P. R. (1973). Encephalitogenic activity of peptides from the smaller basic protein of rat myelin. *J. Immunol. 110*, 1699–1701.

19. Einstein, E. R., Csejtey, J., Dalal, K. B., Adams, C. W. M., Bayliss, O. B., and Hallpike, J. F. (1972). Proteolytic activity and basic protein loss in and around multiple sclerosis plaques: Combined biochemical and histochemical observations. *J. Neurochem. 19*, 653–662.

20. Eylar, E. H., Brostoff, S., Jackson, J., and Carter, H. (1973). Allergic encephalomyelitis in monkeys induced by a peptide from the Al protein. *Proc. Nat. Acad. Sci. 69*, 617–619.

21. Fog, T. (1965). The topography of plaques in multiple sclerosis, with special reference to cerebral plaques. *Acta Neurol. Scand. 41* (Suppl. 15), 1–161.

22. Fry, J. M., Weissbarth, S., Lehrer, G. M., and Bornstein, M. B. (1974). Cerebroside antibody inhibits sulfatide synthesis and myelination and demyelinates in cord tissue cultures. *Science 183*, 540–542.

23. Hashim, G. A., and Schilling, F. J. (1973). Allergic encephalomyelitis: Characterization of the determinants for delayed type hypersensitivity. *Biochem. Biophys. Res. Commun. 50*, 589–596.

24. Haurowitz, F. (1973). The role of RNA in antibody formation. Historical perspectives. *Ann. N.Y. Acad. Sci. 207*, 8–15.

25. Kabat, E. A., Wolf, A., and Bezer, A. E. (1947). The rapid production of acute disseminated encephalomyelitis in rhesus monkeys by injection of heterologous and homologous brain tissue with adjuvants. *J. Exp. Med. 85*, 117–129.

26. Kibler, R. F., Re, P. K., McKneally, S., and Shapira, R. (1972). Biological activity of an encephalitogenic fragment in the monkey. *J. Biol. Chem. 247*, 969–972.

27. Kim, S. U., Murray, M. R., Tourtellotte, W. W., and Parker, J. A. (1970). Demonstration in tissue culture of myelinotoxic agents in cerebrospinal fluid and brain extracts from multiple sclerosis patients. *J. Neuropathol. Exp. Neurol. 29*, 420–431.

28. Lennon, V. A., Wilks, A. V., and Carnegie, P. R. (1970). Immunologic properties of the main encephalitogenic peptide from the basic protein of human myelin. *J. Immunol. 105*, 1221–1230.

29. Levine, S., and Wenk, E. J. (1965). A hyperacute form of allergic encephalomyelitis. *Am. J. Pathol. 47*, 61–88.

30. Levine, S., and Wenk, E. J. (1965). Induction of experimental allergic encephalomyelitis in rats without the aid of adjuvant. *Ann. N.Y. Acad. Sci. 122*, 209–226.

31. Lumsden, C. E. (1971). The immunogenesis of the multiple sclerosis plaque. *Brain Res. 28*, 365–390.

32. McFarlin, D. E., Blank, S. E., Kibler, R. F., McKneally, S., and Shapira, R. (1973). Experimental allergic encephalomyelitis in the rat: Response to encephalitogenic proteins and peptides. *Science 179*, 478–480.

33. Martenson, R. E., Diebler, G. E., Kies, M. W., Levine, S., and Alvord, E. C., Jr. (1972). Myelin basic proteins of mammalian and submammalian vertebrates: Encephalitogenic activities in guinea pigs and rats. *J. Immunol. 109*, 262–270.

34. Martenson, R. E., Diebler, G. E., Kramer, A. J., and Levine, S. (1975). Comparative studies of guinea pig and bovine myelin basic proteins: Partial characterization of chemically derived fragments and their encephalitogenic activities in Lewis rats. *J. Neurochem. 24*, 173–182.

35. Martenson, R. E., Levine, S., and Sowinski, R. (1975). The location of regions in guinea pig and bovine myelin basic proteins which induce experimental allergic encephalomyelitis in Lewis rats. *J. Immunol. 114*, 592–596.

36. Mason, T. E., Phifer, R. F., Spicer, S. S., Swallow, R. A., and Dreskin, R. B. (1969). An immunoglobulin-enzyme bridge method for localizing tissue antigens. *J. Histochem. Cytochem. 17*, 563–569.

37. Norrby, E. (1975). Measles virus (in SSPE and MS). This Conference, Würzburg, March 25, 1975.

38. Pette, E., Mannweiler, K., Palacois, O., and Mutze, B. (1965). Phenomena of the cell membrane and their possible significance for the pathogenesis of so-called autoimmune diseases of the nervous system. *Ann. N.Y. Acad. Sci. 122*, 417–428.

39. Poskanzer, D. C., Schapira, K., and Miller, H. (1963). Epidemiology of multiple sclerosis in the counties of Northumberland and Durham. *J. Neurol. Neurosurg. Psychiatry 26*, 368–376.

40. Riekkinen, P. J., Palo, J., Arstila, A. U., Savolainen, H. J., Rinne, U. K., Kivalo, E. K., and Frey, H. (1971). Protein composition of multiple sclerosis myelin. *Arch. Neurol. 24*, 545–549.

41. Rivers, T. M., and Schwentker, F. F. (1935). Encephalomyelitis accompanied by myelin destruction experimentally produced in monkeys. *J. Exp. Med. 61*, 689–702.

42. Seil, F. J., Smith, M. E., Leiman, A. L., and Kelly, J. M., III (1975). Myelination inhibiting and neuroelectric blocking factors in experimental allergic encephalomyelitis. *Science 187*, 951–953.

43. Shapira, R., Chou, F. C. H., McKneally, S., Urban, E., and Kibler, R. F. (1971). Biological activity and synthesis of an encephalitogenic determinant. *Science 173*, 736–738.

44. Shiraki, H., and Otani, S. (1959). Clinical and pathological features of rabies postvaccinal encephalomyelitis in man (Relationship to multiple sclerosis and to experimental "allergic" encephalomyelitis in animals). In *"Allergic" Encephalomyelitis* (M. W. Kies and E. C. Alvord, Jr., eds.), Chapter 2, pp. 58–129. Charles C Thomas, Springfield, Ill.

45. Suzuki, K., Kamoshita, S., Eto, Y., Toutellotte, W. W., and Gonatas, J. O. (1973).

Myelin in multiple sclerosis: Composition of myelin from normal-appearing white matter. *Arch. Neurol. 28*, 293–297.

46. Toutellotte, W. W. (1971). Cerebrospinal fluid immunoglobulins and the central nervous system as an immunological organ particularly in multiple sclerosis and subacute sclerosing panencephalitis. *Res. Publ. Assoc. Res. Nerv. Ment. Dis. 49*, 112–155.

47. Tourtellotte, W. W., Parker, J. A., and Haerer, A. F. (1964). Subfractionation of multiple sclerosis gamma globulin. *Z. Immunol. Allerg. 126*, 85–99.

48. Westall, F. C., Robinson, A. B., Caccam, J., Jackson, J., and Eylar, E. H. (1971). Essential chemical requirements for induction of allergic encephalomyelitis. *Nature 229*, 22–24.

49. Wolf, A., Kabat, E. A., and Bezer, A. E. (1947). The pathology of acute disseminated encephalomyelitis produced experimentally in the rhesus monkey and its resemblance to human demyelinating disease. *J. Neuropathol. Exp. Neurol. 6*, 333–359.

50. Zimmerman, E. A., Hsu, K. C., Robinson, A. G., Carmel, P. W., Frantz, A. G., and Tannenbaum, M. (1973). Studies of neurophysin secreting neurons with immunoperoxidase techniques employing antibody to bovine neurophysin, I. Light microscopic findings in monkey and bovine tissues. *Endocrinology 92*, 931–940.

CHAPTER 14

Genetic Aspects of Multiple Sclerosis*

ERNST K. KUWERT / HANS J. BERTRAMS

INTRODUCTION

The search for the cause of multiple sclerosis (MS) during the past two decades centered primarily on immunologic considerations, and this disease was thought to be a possible expression of allergic encephalomyelitis. Currently, the possibility that viral infection causes MS is being considered. This concept had tended to overshadow the genetic aspects of MS, until some 2 years ago, when three groups of investigators reported that certain histocompatibility determinants of the HLA system were more frequent in the MS patients than in the control populations (1, 3, 15, 21).

Before discussing histocompatibility determinants, the more general aspects of MS genetics, namely its apparent familial incidence, should be reviewed. The increased frequency of MS within families was reported as early as 1896, by Eichhorst (13), and later in 1904 by Reynolds (24) and in 1920 by Curschmann (10). Currently, increased familial incidence of MS is a generally accepted fact (19). In 1933, Curtius (11) conducted the first extensive systematic familial study among 3129 relatives of 106 index cases of MS in Bonn and Heidelberg. On the basis of these observations, Curtius and Speer (12) calculated an incidence rate of MS for siblings of patients of 90/10,000, or 40 to 50 times greater than that observed in the general population. Tables 14.1 and 14.2 summarize these data and others from different locales by different authors. In general, it can be stated that prevalence of MS in siblings and parents of index cases substantially exceeds that in the population at large. It is possible today to criticize these older studies for some imprecisions of design, such as failure to make appropriate adjustments for age and sex and other pertinent variables, but in my opinion, even with such adjustments, these studies would support the concept of familial predisposition to MS.

The next set of important population studies has dealt with twins. As indicated in Table 14.3, 11 different studies had been conducted by different investigators, who scrutinized series of twins, among whom at

* These Studies were supported by the Deutsche Forschungsgemeinschaft (Ku 183/3) and by the Landesamt für Forschung des Landes Nordrhein-Westfalen.

186

TABLE 14.1 / Familial Incidence of MS[a]

Author[a]	Country	Cases of MS	Families with More Than One Case	Familial Incidence (%)
Curtius (1933) Curtius and Speer (1937)	Germany (Bonn and Heidelberg)	106	10	9.4
Pratt et al. (1951)	England (London)	310	20	6.5
Müller (1953)	Sweden (Stockholm)	750	27	3.6
Hadley (1954)	Scotland (Edinburgh)	150	5	3.3
Millar and Allison (1954)	North Ireland	668[b]	44	6.58
Sutherland (1956)	North Scotland	127[b]	14	11
Abb and Schaltenbrand (1956)	Germany (Würzburg)	472	29	6.5
Hyllested (1956)	Denmark	2731	73	2.6
Mackay and Myrianthopoulos (1958)	U.S.A. and Canada	54[b] (twin pairs)	18	22
Alter et al. (1962)	Israel	282[b]	0	—
Fog et al. (1) (1963) (2)	Orkney and Shetland Islands Faroes	60[b] 16[b]	7 2	11.6 12.5
Schapira et al. (1963)	England (Durham and Northumberland)	607[b]	35	5.8

[a] From McAlpine et al. (8). Please see original paper for additional references.
[b] 'Probable' and 'possible' cases.

least one member of each pair had MS. These studies revealed that there was a 27% concordance for monozygotic twins and a 13% concordance for dizygotic twins (8). (We must stress, however, that in some of the older series of reports, proof of zygosity was not always adequate.) Figure 14.1 summarizes these results and those for other family studies.

SINGLE GENE INHERITANCE

Based on these observations and additional data of their own, Myriantho-poulos and Mackay (20) attempted a genetic analysis of the proposed hypothesis that MS is inherited through a single gene. The possibility that the inheritance was through a recessive sex-linked gene was readily ruled out by the observed 1:1 ratio of sexes among MS patients. Autosomal dominance was also untenable, because there were too few affected parents of MS children, unless one postulated the unlikely low penetrance of less

**TABLE 14.2 / The Proportion of Affected Relatives Compared with
Prevalence Rates in the General Population[a]**

Author[a]	Estimated Prevalence Rate per 10,000 in Population	Siblings		Parents		First Cousins	
		Observed	Ratio Observed to Expected[d]	Observed	Ratio Observed to Expected[d]	Observed	Ratio Observed to Expected[d]
Curtius	2.3 Swiss (Ackermann, 1931)	4/414	42 to 1	1/212	21 to 1		
Pratt et al.	5.0 England and Wales (expected prevalence)	6/538	22 to 1	3/620	10 to 1		
Müller et al.	5.8 Simultaneous Survey Northern Ireland	22/2815 34/2939	20 to 1	5/1493 11/1336	14 to 1		
Sutherland	6.7 Simultaneous Survey Northern Scotland	7/547	19 to 1	2/254	12 to 1		
Mackay and Myriantho-poulos	5.0 Estimated rate U.S.A. and Canada (Kurland and Westlund, 1954)	12[b]/204[c]	118 to 1	1/62 (living)	32 to 1	4/663[c]	12 to 1
Schapira et al.	5.0 Simultaneous Survey Northumber-land, Durham	25[b]/2151	23 to 1	7/1206 (47% living)	12 to 1	6/2203	5 to 1

[a] From McAlpine et al. (8). Please see original paper for additional references.
[b] 'Definite' and 'possible' cases.
[c] Over age of 15.
[d] i.e. prevalence expected if the disease is randomly distributed in the population.

than 2%. Thus the only basis for single mode of inheritance that could be proposed was that of an autosomal recessive gene. The authors corrected the data for age and family size and were able to calculate penetrance of this putative recessive "MS gene" of 43%. Therefore, in a population with a 1:2000 prevalence of MS, one out of every 15 people would be heterozygous for the MS gene. This hypothesis has been rejected by most authorities and, as was pointed out by Schapira et al. (25), the presumption of a "genetic factor with incomplete penetrance . . . can be manipulated to explain any disease with a familial occurrence." According to Newcombe (22), who developed a simple scheme for graphic differentiation of a

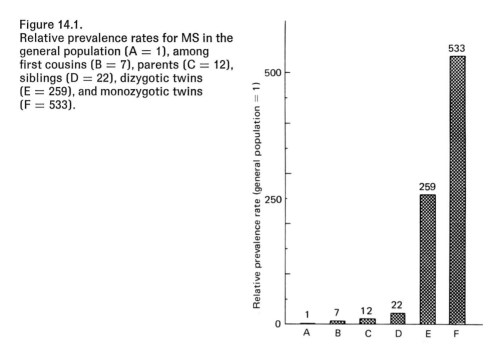

Figure 14.1.
Relative prevalence rates for MS in the general population (A = 1), among first cousins (B = 7), parents (C = 12), siblings (D = 22), dizygotic twins (E = 259), and monozygotic twins (F = 533).

monofactorial inheritance depicted in Fig. 14.2, MS must be a polygenic disease, whose expression depends on exogenous factors. In this sense, it would be analogous to, say, rheumatic fever.

If one accepts the polygenic concept, then one might expect to find certain phenotypic markers that would allow a characterization of an

TABLE 14.3 / Concordance Rates for MS Among Monozygotic and Dizygotic Twins (from Cendrowski (7))

| Authors[a] | Concordance Rate for MS in | |
	Monozygotic Twins	Dizygotic Twins
Koch (1966)	12/28	1/6
Koch and Thums (1952)	1/13	1/30
Schwermann (1955)		1/8
Bammer *et al.* (1960)	1/6	2/7
Schapira, Poskanzer, and Miller (1963)	0/1	0/2+?
Stazio *et al.* (1964)	0/1	
Markov and Leonovich (1964)	1/1	
Mackay and Myrianthopoulos (1966)	9/39	6/29
Cendrowski (1967)		0/3
Holmes, Stubbs, and Larsen (1967)	0/1	
Total	24/90	11/85
= %	26.7	12.9 ($\chi^2 = 5.14$)

[a] From Cendrowski (7). Please see original paper for additional references.

189

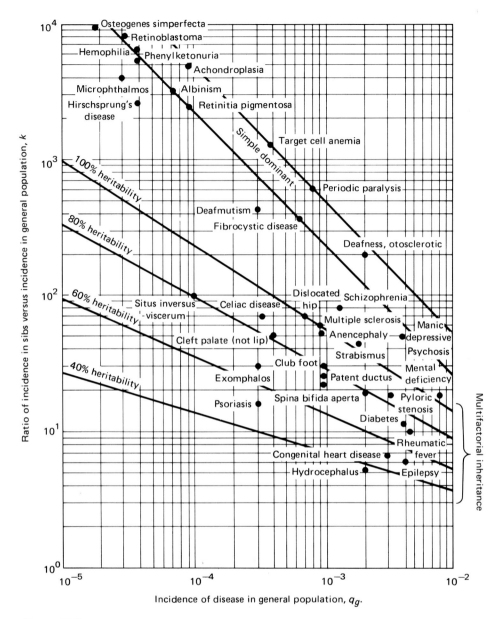

Figure 14.2.
Comparison between the frequency of a disease in siblings of a propositus and the frequency of this disease in the general population. The figure depicts the resulting correlation of single-gene defects and multifactorial inheritance of a disease (21).

individual with a special risk of development of MS under certain environmental conditions that would be safe for others. Such markers might also give clues to the pathogenesis of the disease.

EXPERIMENTATION

In our study of 1,000 German MS patients and a contrast group of 1,000 healthy individuals selected from the same population, we examined such genetic factors as blood groups, enzyme polymorphisms, and histocompatibility antigens, adding up to 73 different phenotypic properties. None of these evaluations was productive, except that of certain HLA antigens, which showed significant deviations in the MS group from the pattern in the contrast group. We, therefore, extended our studies to search for a possible common segregation of the deviant antigens and haplotypes with the disease. Finally, we tested for the lymphocyte defined (LD) MLC (mixed lymphocyte culture)-determinant HLA-DW2 in 39 MS patients and 341 controls (6).

Using 90 highly selected sera for the HLA typing, in accordance with the technique of Kissmeyer-Nielsen and Thorsby (18), we determined that five out of 22 clusters indicated significant differences between the two groups (Table 14.4). The strongest deviation was observed in the HLA-B7, which occurred in 35.3% of the MS patients, but only in 26% of the controls ($p = 0.00008$). The other determinants were also impressively different. HLA-A3 was found in 35.8% of the MS patients and in 28.8%

TABLE 14.4 / HLA-A Phenotype- and Gene-Frequencies in 1,000 MS Patients and 1,000 Controls

Antigen	Phenotype Frequency in MS ($n = 1,000$)	Controls ($n = 1,000$)	p Value	Gene—Frequency in MS ($n = 1,000$)	Controls ($n = 1,000$)
HLA-A1	0.330	0.290	0.05936	0.1815	0.1568
HLA-A2	0.432	0.511	0.00048[a]	0.2463	0.3000
HLA-A3	0.358	0.288	0.00096[a]	0.1988	0.1568
HLA-A9	0.210	0.183	0.14344	0.1112	0.0961
HLA-A10	0.110	0.107	0.88587	0.0566	0.0555
HLA-A11	0.079	0.099	0.13569	0.0403	0.0513
HLA-A28	0.054	0.067	0.26039	0.0274	0.0346
HLA-AW29	n.t.	0.04		—	0.0202
HLA-AW32	0.061	0.033	0.36948	0.0310	0.0165
Blank				0.1069	0.1127
HLA-B5	0.120	0.141	0.18431	0.0619	0.0737
HLA-B7	0.353	0.260	0.00008[a]	0.1956	0.1398
HLA-B8	0.232	0.205	0.15945	0.1236	0.1084
HLA-B12	0.158	0.218	0.00073[a]	0.0824	0.1157
HLA-B13	0.044	0.043	1.00000	0.0222	0.0217
HLA-BW35	0.195	0.172	0.20378	0.1028	0.0901
HLA-BW40	0.112	0.137	0.10406	0.0577	0.0710
HLA-B14	0.068	0.069	1.00000	0.0346	0.0346
HLA-BW15	0.093	0.150	0.00012[a]	0.0475	0.0780
HLA-BW17	0.062	0.080	0.13884	0.0315	0.0403
HLA-B18	0.109	0.100	0.55873	0.0561	0.0513
HLA-BW21	n.t.	0.044		—	0.2222
HLA-BW22	0.033	0.036	0.80650	0.0166	0.0182
HLA-B27	0.074	0.097	0.07853	0.0977	0.0497
Blank				0.1297	0.0853

[a] p corr. $= p \times 21 = 0.05$.
n.t., not tested

of the controls ($p = 0.00096$); HLA-A2 was less frequent in the MS patients (43.2% vs. 51.1%, $p = 0.00048$) as was HLA-B12 (15.8% vs. 21.8%, $p = 0.00073$) and HLA-BW15 (9.3% vs. 15%, $p = 0.00012$) (p values were calculated according to the classic χ^2 test with Yate's correction).

EVALUATION

In order to explore these variations further, we pooled our data of the 1,000 patients with those obtained by Naito et al. (20) in 94 patients and Jersild et al. (14) in 135 patients. These were evaluated by the method of Woolf (27), which takes into account gene frequencies of the populations under study. Table 14.5 and Fig. 14.3 summarize and compare results of these studies. It can be seen that the HLA-B7 determinant has the highest combined estimate for the relative risk value ($\chi = 1.55$, $p = 10^{-7}$; HLA-A3 is the next ($\chi = 1.51$, $p = 10^{-4}$).

On the other hand, HLA antigens -A2, -B12, and -BW15 have the lowest relative risk values ($\chi = 0.7$, 0.69, and 0.68, respectively). With

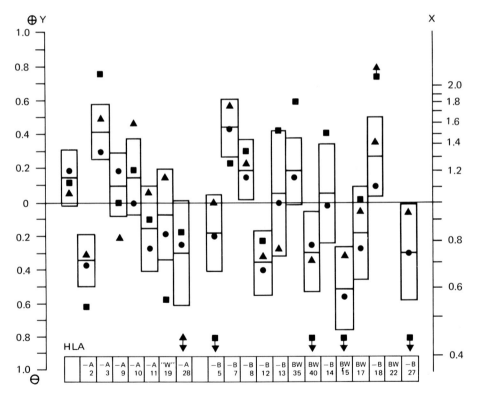

Figure 14.3.
Combined estimate of relative risk for MS in antigen-positive versus antigen-negative individuals. X is the combined relative risk estimate; $Y = 1nX$; the bars indicate the 95% confidence limits of the combined estimate for the relative incidence of MS. Data from this study (●, 1,000 MS patients and 1,000 controls), Naito et al. (20) (■, 94 MS patients and 871 controls), and Jersild et al. (15) (▲, 135 MS patients and 985 controls).

TABLE 14.5 / Calculation of Combined Relative Risk on the Basis of the HL-A Typing Results of Three Groups in Three Different Countries

	Relative Risk[a]			Combined Materials				
Antigen	Own Results ($n = 1,000$)	Naito et al. (20) ($n = 94$)	Jersild et al. (14) ($n = 135$)	Comb. Relative Risk	χ^2 Combined[b]	p Value	χ^2 Heterogeneous[c]	p Value
HLA-A1	1.21	1.13	0.99	1.16	3.15	0.076	0.84	0.657
HLA-A2	0.73	0.54	0.73	0.70	21.29	10^{-5}	1.62	0.445
HLA-A3	1.38	2.20	1.67	1.51	26.50	10^{-6}	3.99	0.136
HLA-A9	1.19	1.03	0.82	1.10	1.03	0.310	1.93	0.381
HLA-A10	1.03	1.21	1.64	1.15	1.48	0.224	2.36	0.307
HLA-A11	0.78	0.91	1.11	0.85	1.50	0.221	1.14	0.566
HLA-AW19	0.84	0.55	1.18	0.93	0.29	0.590	2.16	0.340
HLA-A28	0.79	0.85	0.36	0.73	3.77	0.052	2.66	0.264
HLA-B5	0.83	0.23	1.00	0.83	2.49	0.115	3.61	0.164
HLA-B7	1.55	1.24	1.77	1.55	28.65	10^{-7}	1.32	0.517
HLA-B8	1.17	1.34	1.26	1.21	4.39	0.036	0.28	0.869
HLA-B12	0.67	0.80	0.71	0.69	14.43	0.0001	0.34	0.844
HLA-B13	1.02	1.57	0.76	1.05	0.06	0.806	1.04	0.595
HLA-BW5	1.17	1.80	0.86	1.20	3.38	0.066	3.97	0.137
HLA-BW10	0.79	0.21	0.71	0.74	6.56	0.014	4.75	0.093
HLA-B14	0.98	1.54	0.76	1.05	0.10	0.752	1.73	0.421
HLA-BW15	0.58	0.37	0.74	0.60	17.71	0.0003	1.24	0.538
HLA-B17	0.76	1.03	0.97	0.83	1.69	0.194	0.76	0.684
HLA-BW18	1.10	2.61	1.42	1.30	4.73	0.030	6.36	0.042
HLA-B27	0.74	0.31	0.96	0.74	4.54	0.031	2.60	0.273

[a] Relative risk for an antigen in the ratio of the number of antigen-positive to antigen-negative persons in the disease group divided by analogous values of the control group.
[b] χ^2 combined is the chi square for deviation of the combined estimate of relative risk from 1.0. These χ^2 values have one degree of freedom each.
[c] χ^2 heterogeneous is the chi square for heterogeneity between the relative risks of each study; these χ^2 values have $n - 1$ degrees of freedom, where n is the number of studies.

these five antigens, no significant degree of heterogeneity was found. HLA-BW18, however, did show a significantly increased χ value in Jersild's combined analysis, and a significant degree of heterogeneity could be demonstrated in the combined data. It is possible, therefore, to arrive at the statistical conclusion that an individual carrying the HLA-A3 and -B7 antigens has a 50% higher risk of developing MS than people who lack these antigens.

As might be expected from the increased frequencies of HLA-A3 and -B7 and a decreased frequency of HLA-A2, -B12, and -BW15, the haplotype HLA-A3 -B7 was found significantly more often, and the haplotype HLA-A2 -BW15 less often in the disease group than in the controls (Table 14.6). Both of these haplotypes tend to be quite common in the white populations. Another common haplotype HLA-A2-B2 was decreased in frequency in the MS group but the difference was not statistically significant. There were no significant differences in any other haplotypes.

TABLE 14.6 / Frequency of the Common European Haplotypes (>20‰) in MS-Patients and Controls[a]

| Haplotype | Haplotype-Frequency (‰) | | |
	MS Patients ($n = 1,000$)	Controls ($n = 1,000$)	p Value
HLA-A1-B8	87.9	80.6	n.s.
HLA-A3-B7	92.1	63.4	0.02
HLA-A2-B12	39.4	51.2	n.s.
HLA-A2-BW15	20.5	43.5	0.005
HLA-A2-BW40	25.0	35.0	n.s.
HLA-A3-BW35	32.0	33.6	n.s.
HLA-A2-B5	18.3	26.5	n.s.
HLA-A2-B7	49.5	22.7	n.s.

[a] Haplotype frequencies have been calculated from the phenotypic data.

Haplotype Frequency

The HLA haplotype frequency is influenced by both the antigen frequency and gametic association. Since the general haplotype frequency does not provide useful information about the degree of gametic association between any two antigens of the first and second HLA locus, delta values had to be calculated in order to determine whether the differences in haplotypes of MS patients reflected the nature of gametic association. The following results of 252 haplotype combinations in the two groups under study were obtained. Multiple Sclerosis patients as well as healthy white controls gave evidence of strong gametic association, HLA-A1-B8; HLA-A3-B7; HLA-A2-BW15; HLA-A3-BW35; HLA-A11-BW35; and HLA-A10-B18. The HLA-A7 haplotypes, however, differ significantly between MS patients and controls, with respect to gametic association (Table 14.7).

TABLE 14.7 / Comparison of the Degree of the Gametic Association of all HLA-B7-Haplotypes in MS Patients and Controls

Positively Linked
HLA-A3-B7 in MS ═══════════ in Controls

Weak positive linkage in MS, negatively linked in Controls
HLA-A2-B7 in MS ═══════════ in Controls

Negatively Linked
HLA-A1-B7 in MS ═══════════ in Controls
HLA-A9-B7 in MS ═══════════ in Controls
HLA-10-B7 in MS ═══════════ in Controls
HLA-A11-B7 in MS ═══════════ in Controls
HLA-A28-B7 in MS ═══════════ in Controls
HLA-AW32-B7 in MS ═══════════ in Controls
Blank-B7 in MS ═══════════ in Controls

═══════════ is the symbol for stronger gametic association.

In MS patients, HLA-A3 and -B7 are linked significantly more strongly than in the controls ($p < 0.0005$). The same holds true for HLA-A2 and -B7, which are negatively linked in healthy controls, but show a positive delta value in MS patients. All other HLA-B7 haplotypes of the MS patients and controls are linked by negative gametic associations, which are, however, stronger in the MS patients than in the controls. There is justification, therefore, for concluding that not only single antigens, HLA-A3 and -B7, but also the haplotype, HLA-A3-B7, is associated with MS. Since antigens HLA-A2, -B12, and -BW15 were less frequent in MS patients than in controls, one could predict that the HLA-A2-B12 haplotype would show a significantly weaker delta value in MS patients. This prediction, however, could not be verified. Whereas the gametic linkage between HLA-A2 and HLA-B12 is stronger in MS patients than in controls, the delta values of nearly all other haplotypes, including HLA-A2, -B12, and -BW15 show a weaker gametic association in MS than in the controls. The significant increase of HLA-A3-B7 is not compensated by a decrease of any other haplotype. Apparently the common haplotypes among Caucasians are more strongly gametically linked in MS individuals than in healthy persons. Besides the HLA-A3-B7 and -A2-B12 haplotypes, HLA-A1-B8 shows a trend to a somewhat stronger gametic association in MS.

The fact that 20 out of 1,000 MS patients had the phenotype HLA-A1, -A3, -B7, -B8, but that among the controls only eight out of 1,000 did ($p = 0.036$), may reflect the stronger linkage disequilibrium of these two common haplotypes in MS patients.

Segregation of Haplotypes and Antigens

In order to analyze the segregation of HLA antigens and haplotypes, we tested 36 families, including 72 parents, with 48 MS patients and 65 healthy siblings and derived data summarized in Table 14.8. In backcross families (i.e., where one parent was negative and the other heterozygous positive for the marker under study), we noted a deviation from the expected 1:1 ratio in the offspring of antigen-positive to antigen-negative persons (segregation frequency 0.5). We observed this for the antigens HLA-A3 and HLA-B7 only among MS patients. In 17 families, 18 of 22 MS patients were HLA-A3 positive ($p = 0.003$), whereas 32 healthy siblings showed a 1:1 ratio of HLA-A3 positives to HLA-A3 negative individuals. A similar situation obtains with regard to HLA-B7 antigen in 19 families, in which 17 out of 26 patients were positive, whereas the healthy siblings had a ratio of 21:20 or nearly a 1:1 proportion. Additionally, antigens HLA-B5 and HLA-B8 showed deviations from the 1:1 ratio on backcross situations. HLA-B5 was found in 14 out of 17 MS patients ($p = 0.0076$) and in only 10 out of 29 healthy siblings out of 14 families. HLA-B8 was present in 12 out of 19 MS patients (not significant) and in 21 out of 29 ($p = 0.016$) healthy siblings in 16 families.

The haplotype HLA-A3-B7 was found in 10 out of 12 MS patients in 11 families ($p = 0.021$), whereas the ratio between the positive and

TABLE 14.8 / Segregation Analysis of HL-A Antigens -A3, -B5, -B7, and -B8 and Haplotypes HL-A3-7 and HL-A1-8 in Backcross Families ($+ \times -$)

Antigen	Number of Inform.[a] Families	Number of MS Patients		x^2	Number of Healthy Siblings		x^2
		Positive	Negative		Positive	Negative	
HLA-A3	17	18	4	8.91 ($p = 0.003$)	15	17	n.s.
HLA-B5	14	14	3	7.12 ($p = 0.0075$)	10	19	n.s.
HLA-B7	21	21	10	3.90 ($p = 0.05$)	21	20	n.s.
HLA-B8	16	12	7	n.s.	21	8	5.38 ($p = 0.016$)
Haplotype HLA-A3-B7	11	10	2	5.32 ($p = 0.021$)	10	9	n.s.
HLA-A1-B8	13	11	4	3.27 ($p = 0.07$)	18	7	4.84 ($o = 0.028$)

[a] One parent is negative; the other, heterozygous positive for the marker under examination. The expected segregation frequency in this situation is 0.5.
For Antigens HLA-A1, -A2, -A9, -A10, -A11, -A28, -B12, -B13, -B14, -B18, -B27, -BW15, -BW16, -BW17, -BW21 and -BW22,

$$x^2 = \frac{(\text{Observed} - \text{Expected})^2}{\text{Expected}} \times 2)$$

No significant deviation from the expected 1:1 ratio in both groups was observed.

negative persons among the healthy siblings was nearly 1:1. The haplotype HLA-A1-B8 was present in 11 out of 15 MS patients ($p = 0.07$) in 13 families but was also more frequent among the healthy siblings (18 positive vs. 7 negative, $p = 0.028$) (2).

Additional Correlations

After an analysis of the clinical course of 396 MS patients, we were able to demonstrate a correlation between the frequency of antigen HLA-B7 and the severity of the clinical disease, as measured by its rate of progression (5, 6) (Table 14.9). Although the increase in HLA-B7 was not significant in 128 patients exhibiting either the remittent or the progressive course with exacerbations, this antigen was significantly increased in 152 patients, who only had a progressive course with exacerbations. The highest increase of this antigen was observed in 117 patients, who had the most rapidly progressing form of the disease without exacerbations. Jersild et al. (16) also found a correlation between the rate of progression in 28 MS patients and the histocompatibility determinant HLA-DW2, which is strongly linked to the serologically defined antigen HLA-B7. These data, therefore, may be taken as an indication that certain histocompatibility determinants are not only associated with MS but may also perhaps determine, or at least be associated with, certain clinical patterns of the disease.

TABLE 14.9 / Clinical Course of MS in Relation to HLA-Antigen Frequencies

Clinical Course	Antigen[a]	
	HLA-B7	HLA-BW40
Remittent and progressive with bouts (n = 127)	Increase $p = 0.1612$ n.s.	Normal frequency $p = 0.8930$ n.s.
Progressive with bouts (n = 152)	Increase $p = 0.0429$	Decrease $p = 0.0367$
Progressive without bouts (n = 117)	Increase $p = 0.0299$	Normal frequency $p = 0.6533$ n.s.

[a] Antigen frequencies compared with the corresponding values of 1,000 healthy controls.

Another point of interest may be the increase in the HLA-BW40 antigen in the 152 patients, who had a progressive disease with exacerbations, whereas the other two groups showed a normal -BW40 frequency. Naito *et al.* (21) also observed a very low frequency of this antigen in 94 American MS patients, but they did not correlate these findings with the clinical course of the disease. Although Jersild *et al.* (15) reported in 132 patients an increase in titers of hemagglutination inhibiting antibodies against measles and correlated them with HLA-A3 and -B7 and -B18 antigens, we were unable to demonstrate such a correlation among 941 MS patients tested (5).

Table 14.10 summarizes data relative to the HLA-A, -B, and -D determinants obtained by MLC testing with HLA-DW2, homozygous test cells, and it shows that 12 out of 39 MS patients (30.8%) had this antigen, whereas only 15% of the randomly selected controls were positive. Among patients and controls who had the HLA-A3-B7 haplotype, 66.6% of MS patients and only 41% of the controls were HLA-DW2 positive. Of the MS patients 28.6% compared to 22.4% of the controls with only HLA-B7 antigen were -DW2 positive. Patients and controls who had neither of these two HLA antigens were DW2 positive to the extent of 17.4 and 11.4%,

TABLE 14.10 / HLA-DW2 Frequency in 39 MS Patients and 341 Healthy Controls in Relation to Presence or Absence of HLA-A3 and/or HLA-B7

HLA-A3	HLA-B7	MS Patients (n = 39) -DW2 positive	(%)	Controls (n = 341) -DW2 positive	(%)
+	+	6/9	66.6	44/107	41.1
−	+	2/7	28.6	17/76	22.4
−	−	4/23	17.4	18/158	11.4
Random		12/39	30.8	15/100	15

respectively (6). According to similar data of Jersild *et al.* (17), the relative risk for the development of MS among HLA-DW2 carriers is approximately seven times higher than in the rest of the population.

CONCLUSIONS

The association among the HLA-A3, -B7, and -DW2 is common among Caucasians. Since the delta values among these determinants are relatively high (0.04 to 0.05), there is a strong positive linkage disequilibrium among these entities. The question then arises why this haplotype, common among whites, is even more frequent in patients with MS. One may consider, in this connection, the mechanism for the development of linkage disequilibrium among genetic traits. As pointed out by Bodmer (7), "selection survival advantage" evidently must be linked with those genotypes characterized by extremely high gametic association. Another possible mechanism for the development of linkage disequilibrium, such as inbreeding, random genetic drift, and fusion of populations, cannot reasonably apply exclusively to the widely scattered Caucasian population. The apparent survival advantage of certain gene complexes in a given environment may be associated with certain specific disadvantages, such as hyperreactivity or nonreactivity to certain antigens or infectious agents. Multiple sclerosis patients apparently seem to be unable to develop normal cell-mediated immunity to certain viral antigens, for example paramyxoviruses (9, 26) or antigens in the human white matter (14) and to embryonic mouse fibroblast cells (23). If linkage disequilibrium between SD and LD genes of the human histocompatibility gene complex is a reflection of a "selective survival advantage" for Caucasians in general, then MS might be a concomittant "disadvantage effect" within this population.

In conclusion, let me quote from Eichhorst (13) who stated that "there can be no room for doubt that multiple sclerosis belongs to the inherited, transmissible diseases." It seems to me that in the light of more recent data this remark appears to be valid.

REFERENCES

1. Bertrams, J., and Kuwert, E. (1972). HLA antigen frequencies in multiple sclerosis. *Eur. Neurol. 7*, 74.
2. Bertrams, J., and Kuwert, E. (1976). Distorted segregation of HLA-A3 and -B7 in patients with multiple sclerosis and -B8 in their unaffected sibs. *Immunogenetics,* submitted.
3. Bertrams, J., Kuwert, E., and Liedtke, U. (1972). HLA antigens and multiple sclerosis. *Tissue Antigens 2*, 405.
4. Bertrams, J., Höher, P. G., and Kuwert, E. (1974). HLA antigens in multiple sclerosis. *Lancet i*, 1287.
5. Bertrams, J., von Fisenne, E., Höher, P. G., and Kuwert, E. (1974). Lack of association between HLA antigens and measles antibody in multiple sclerosis. *Lancet ii*, 441.

6. Bertrams, J., Kuwert, E., Grosse-Wilde, H., Metzel, B., and Mempel, W. (1975). Disease-susceptibility genotype for multiple sclerosis: SD-HLA-A3-7-LD-Pi(7a)? *Z. Immunitactsforsch. 148*, 367.

7. Bodmer, W. F. (1972). Population genetics of the HL-A system: Retrospect and prospect in histocompatibility testing. Munksgaard, Copenhagen, p. 611.

8. Cendrowski, W. S. (1968). Multiple sclerosis: Discordance in three pairs of dizygotic twins. *J. Med. Genet. 5*, 266.

9. Ciongolo, A. K., Platz, P., Dupont, B., Svejgaard, A., Fog, T., and Jersild, C. (1973). Lack of antigen response to myxoviruses in multiple sclerosis. *Lancet ii*, 1147.

10. Curschmann, H. (1920). Über familiäre multiple sklerose. *Dtsch. Ztschr. Nervenheilk. 66*, 225.

11. Curtius, F. (1933). Multiple Sklerose und Erbanlage. Thieme, Leipzig.

12. Curtius, F., and Speer, H. (1937). Multiple Sklerose und Erbanlage. *Z. Gesamte Neurol. Psychiat. 160*, 226.

13. Eichhorst, H. (1896). Über infantile und hereditäre multiple sklerose. *Virchows Arch. [Pathol. Anat.] 146*, 173.

14. Finkelstein, S., Walford, R. L., Myers, L. W., and Ellison, G. W. (1974). HLA antigens and hyper-sensitivity to brain tissue in multiple sclerosis. *Lancet i*, 736.

15. Jersild, C., Svejgaard, A., and Fog, T. (1972). HLA antigens associated with multiple sclerosis. *Lancet i*, 1242.

16. Jersild, C., Fog, T., Hansen, G. S., Thomsen, M., Svejgaard, A., and Dupont, B. (1973). Histocompatibility determinants in multiple sclerosis with special reference to the clinical course. *Lancet ii*, 1221.

17. Jersild, C., Dupont, B., Fog, T., Platz, P. J., and Svejgaard, A. (1975). Histocompatibility determinants in multiple sclerosis. *Transplant. Rev. 22*, 148.

18. Kissmeyer-Nielsen, F., and Thorsby, E. (1974). Lymphocytotoxic microtechnique. *Manual of Tissue Typing Techniques.* DHEW Publication No. (NIH) 75-545, p. 50.

19. McAlpine, D., Lumsden, Ch. E., and Acheson, E. D. (1968). *Multiple Sclerosis. A Reappraisal.* Livingstone, Edinburgh and London.

20. Myrianthopoulos, N. C., and MacKay, R. P. (1960). Multiple sclerosis in twins and their relatives: Genetic analysis of family histories. *Acta Genet. (Basel) 10*, 33.

21. Naito, S., Namerow, N., Michey, M. R., and Terasaki, P. I. (1972). Multiple sclerosis: Association with HL-A3. *Tissue Antigens 2*, 1.

22. Newcombe, H. B. (1971). Heritability of threshold characters. In *Genetics of Human Populations*, Cavalli-Sforza, L. L., and Bodmer, W. F. pp. 562–563. W. H. Freeman and Co. San Francisco.

23. Petranyi, G. G.; Ivanyi, P. and Hollan, S. R. (1974). Relations of HL-A and RH System to Immune Reactivity. *Vox Sang. 27*, 420.

24. Reynolds, E. S. (1964). Some cases of fatally disseminated sclerosis. *Brain 27*, 163.

25. Schapira, K., Poskanzer, D. C., and Miller, J. (1963). Familial and conjugal multiple sclerosis. *Brain 86*, 315.

26. Utermohlen, V., and Zabriskie, J. B. (1973). Suppressed cellular immunity to measles antigen in multiple sclerosis patients. *Lancet ii*, 1148.

27. Woolf, B. (1955). On estimating the relation between blood group and disease. *Ann. Hum. Genet. 19*, 251.

CHAPTER 15
Cell-Mediated Immunity in Multiple Sclerosis*

CASPER JERSILD

INTRODUCTION

There is little doubt that immunologic processes play an important role in the pathogenesis of multiple sclerosis (MS). Here we shall review certain aspects of cell-mediated immunity (CMI) in MS, as it may be reflected in various *in vitro* assays.

There are a number of quantitative and qualitative *in vitro* tests of CMI. These tests are important in clinical immunology because evaluation of reactivity toward potentially dangerous antigens may not be carried out readily *in vivo*. *In vitro* tests may correlate with *in vivo* delayed-type hypersensitivity, as has been shown for PPD (14, 43). Differences in sensitivity between the two test procedures may, however, account for certain discrepancies in studies obtained with other antigens (45).

Studies of lymphocytic choriomeningitis virus infections in mice strongly support the concept that T lymphocyte dependent specific CMI against lymphocytic choriomeningitis (LCM) virus is an important immunologic feature of acute infection (1, 11, 38). Immune T cells present early during infection have little effect on virus in chronically infected carriers; however, late occurring immune T cells do have an antiviral effect in these carriers (50). Also of importance in control of virus infections is the effect of macrophages, which limit cell-to-cell spread of herpes virus (33), and participate in the clearance of viral antigen (36).

Other aspects of immunologic control of viral infection are also relevant to the discussion of CMI in MS. The influence of gene(s) within the major histocompatibility system (MHS) of the species on specific immune responsiveness towards viral antigens seems important.

Gorer and Boyse were the first to notice that inbred strains of mice with high incidence of leukemia induced by Gross virus had the same H-2

* Original work from the group at the Tissue Typing Laboratory, Copenhagen University Hospital has been aided by grants from The Danish Multiple Sclerosis Society, Danish Medical Research Council, The Foundation for Research in Copenhagen, Greenland, and Faeroe Islands.

The author acknowledges my colleagues Dr. A. Svejgaard, Dr. P. J. Platz, and Dr. T. Fog for helpful discussion in preparing this manuscript. I am grateful for the excellent secretarial assistance of Mrs. Elly Andersen.

haplotype (30). Experimental evidence for this difference was first provided by Lilly *et al.* in 1964 (31). In 1965, McDevitt and Sela (35) made the original observation that certain genetically determined specific immune responses were controlled by genes closely linked to H-2. Later studies of leukemia induced by Gross virus revealed a more complex genetic control of the disease. The H-2 linked gene for control apparently determines cell-mediated immunity toward virus or virus-infected cells (34). Grumet *et al.* (21) and others have shown that H-2 linked immune response is primarily dependent on thymus-derived T lymphocytes. A selective T cell deficit due to lack of a specific Ir gene can be recognized by the absence of T cell dependent secondary IgG response (20) or absence of production of T effector lymphocytes.

Other experimental models for disease in inbred strains of animals have further indicated histocompatibility-linked genetic control of cellular immunity. Studies of LCM infection in adult mice have shown that certain strains are highly susceptible, whereas other are resistant. Oldstone *et al* (40) demonstrated that susceptibility was linked genetically to the H-2 locus and that the H-2^q haplotype conferring susceptibility was dominant. Since immunosuppression of susceptible mice can induce resistance against infection so that these animals survive infection, it is likely that an H-2 linked Ir determinant, controls cell-mediated immunity against LCM virus or LCM virus-infected cells.

In rats, the ability to develop experimental allergic encephalomyelitis (EAE) is under simple genetic control (17, 37, 51). Here too the mechanism for genetic control seems to involve specific immune response capacity against encephalitogenic factor (EF) of myelin basic protein (BP). The specific Ir gene, named Ir-EAE (51), can be identified by a positive delayed-type cutaneous reaction against EF, *in vitro* lymphocyte transformation, and macrophage migration inhibition with BP as well as EF after challenge of animals with BP (37).

An hypothesis for the biologic role for the MHS has been presented by Doherty and Zinkernagel (13). It applies especially to histocompatibility-linked control of susceptibility to viral infection, since they find that compatibility for H-2 antigens between immune T cells and virus-infected target cells in assays for specific cell-mediated lysis is necessary for the occurrence of lysis (12). They postulate that susceptibility to a particular infectious disease may reflect absence of an immunogenic modification in MHS antigens induced by the infectious agent, rather than operation of controlling immune response genes.

Multiple sclerosis patients have a higher frequency of specific determinants of the MHS and HLA than does the general population (24). There is no explanation for this at present, but it is possible that the MS-associated HLA determinant itself, or some other determinants linked to it, control specific immune response capabilities toward infectious agents, organ specific antigens, or BP. This may be considered analogous to the findings in experimental animals.

IMMUNOLOGICAL STUDIES IN MULTIPLE SCLEROSIS PATIENTS

T and B Lymphocytes in Peripheral Blood

Several methods for characterizing lymphocyte subpopulations in T and B cells have been described (19). Our studies of random MS patients revealed a moderate but significant increase in the percentage of EAC rosette-forming cells (B cells), as well as membrane Ig-bearing cells (23, 41). The percentage of E rosette-forming cells, however, was not decreased significantly. Similar observations have been presented by Oger *et al.* (39), but they noted that fewer T cells in MS patients were able to bind 10 or more red blood cells in the rosettes. There was no pronounced change in patients with active disease. Studies of Lisak *et al.* (32), on the other hand, seem to indicate that there is a decrease in E rosette-forming cells in MS patients during acute exacerbations. It must be stressed that none of these studies followed single patients prospectively. Fluctuations in these measurements have been noted in one of our patients, but decrease in the percentage of E rosette-forming cells could not be related to activity in disease.

In Vitro Lymphocyte Stimulation with Mitogens

Phytohemagglutinin (PHA) stimulation of isolated peripheral blood leukocytes of MS patients was reported impaired (22, 29). It was found later that serum of MS patients contains a factor that reduces the spontaneous transformation of lymphocytes (15, 27) and also influences transformation with PHA (44).

The recent improvements in culture techniques and the use of pooled normal serum in such culture systems have helped to eliminate some of those variables that plagued the earlier studies. With these considerations in mind, there appears to be no evidence of defects in the ability of lymphocytes of MS patients to become transformed by PHA, despite the claims to the contrary (5, 22, 29). Moreover, several other investigators have found normal transformation with PHA (4, 10, 23, 41, 44). Stimulation with pokeweed mitogen has also been reported as normal (2, 23, 41).

In Vitro Lymphocyte Stimulation with Antigens

An increased reactivity of MS leukocytes *in vivo* toward brain extracts or EF was reported (3, 10). These studies reported *in vitro* stimulation of MS patients' leukocytes with measles virus antigen (9, 10, 28). Knowles and Saunders (28) and Cunningham-Rundles *et al.* (9) found no difference between MS patients and normal controls, whereas Dau and Peterson (10) demonstrated a reduced response in MS to measles and respiratory syncytial virus antigens.

It has been difficult in these studies to obtain specific virus antigen preparations capable of lymphocyte transformation *in vitro*. A recent report

202

by Graziano *et al.* (18) showed that a complement-fixing measles virus antigen is able to induce a reasonably good transformation of normal leukocytes *in vitro*. The preparation used contained membrane-bound or membrane-associated viral antigen, which seems necessary for transformation. This observation is consistent with earlier observations of successful stimulation of leukocytes with subacute sclerosing panencephalitis (SSPE) virus infected HeLa cells (47).

Leukocyte Migration Inhibition Tests

Our studies of CMI utilized the leukocyte migration agarose inhibition test (LMAT), originally described by Clausen (18), and various paramyxovirus antigens prepared commercially. Significant differences in inhibition were noted between random MS patients and normal controls (6, 7, 16, 41, 48, 49). Reactivity of MS patients can be restored by the administration of transfer factor to the patients (25, 28, 41) or to the *in vitro* cultures (52).

Lymphocyte-Mediated Cytotoxicity to Virus-Infected Target Cells

Using ^{51}Cr-labeled target cells persistently infected with measles virus, SSPE virus, or rubella virus Rola-Pleszczynski *et al.* (42, 46) demonstrated normal killing effect of MS lymphocytes. They detected a blocking factor for this reaction with specificity for measles and SSPE virus. This factor was associated with the 7 S globulin.

CONCLUSIONS

Study of CMI in MS with *in vitro* methods has revealed a number of abnormalities. There seems to be a slight increase in circulating B cells and perhaps a minor decrease in circulating T cells. Using leukocyte migration inhibition techniques, specific energy toward certain of the paramyxoviruses, especially measles virus, has been demonstrated. Earlier and more recent studies of lymphocyte transformation with virus antigens indicate a normal reactivity among MS patients. Lymphocyte-mediated cytotoxicity indicates the presence of specific K cell activity against measles and SSPE virus-infected cells. Also, a serum factor blocking specifically this reactivity has been demonstrated.

REFERENCES

1. Blanden, R. V. (1974). T cell response to viral and bacterial infections. *Transplant Rev. 19*, 56.
2. Bartfeld, H., and Atoynatan, T. (1970). Lymphocyte transformation in multiple sclerosis. *Br. Med. J. 2*, 91.
3. Bartfeld, H., and Atoynatan, T. (1970). In vitro delayed (cellular) hypersensitivity in multiple sclerosis to central nervous system antigen. *Int. Arch. Allergy Appl. Immunol. 39*, 361.
4. Brody, J. A., Harlem, M. M., Kurtzke, J. F., and White, L. R. (1968). Unsuccessful

attempts to induce transformation by cerebrospinal fluid in cultured lymphocytes from patients with multiple sclerosis. *New Engl. J. Med. 279,* 202.

5. Cendrowski, W., and Niedzielska, K. (1970). Lymphocyte transformation induced *in vitro* by PHA and PPD in multiple sclerosis. *J. Neurol. Neurosurg. Psychiatry 33,* 92.

6. Ciongoli, A. K., Platz, P. J., Dupont, B., Svejgaard, A., Fog, T., and Jersild, C. 1973). Lack of antigen response to myxovirus in multiple sclerosis. *Lancet ii,* 1147.

7. Ciongoli, A. K. (1976). Lack of responsiveness among MS patients to measles virus antigen with leukocyte migration test. Abstract, MS meeting, Copenhagen, September 1975. *Acta Neurol. Scand.,* in press.

8. Clausen, J. E. (1971). Tuberculin-induced migration inhibition of human peripheral leukocytes in agarose medium. *Acta Allergy 26,* 56.

9. Cunningham-Rundles, S., and Dupont, B. (1976). Lymphocyte stimulation with measles virus in multiple sclerosis. MS meeting, Copenhagen, September 1975. *Acta Neurol. Scand.,* in press.

10. Dau, P. C., and Peterson, R. D. A. (1970). Transformation of lymphocytes from patients with multiple sclerosis. *Arch. Neurol. 23,* 32.

11. Doherty, P. C., and Zinkernagel, R. M. (1974). T-cell-mediated immunopathology in viral infections. *Transplant Rev. 19,* 89.

12. Doherty, P. C., and Zinkernagel, R. M. (1975). H-2 compatibility is required for T-cell-mediated lysis of target cells infected with lymphocytic choriomeningitis virus. *J. Exp. Med. 141,* 502.

13. Doherty, P. C., and Zinkernagel, R. M. (1975). A biological role for the major histocompatibility antigens. *Lancet ii,* 1406.

14. Federlin, K., Maini, R. N., Russel, A. S., and Dumonde, D. C. (1971). A micromethod for peripheral leukocyte migration in tuberculin sensitivity. *J. Clin. Pathol. 24,* 533.

15. Field, J., and Caspary, E. A. (1971). Lymphocyte response depressive factor in multiple sclerosis. *Brit. Med. J. 4,* 529.

16. Fuccillo, D. A., Abela, J. E., Traub, R. G., Gillespie, M. M., Beadle, E. L., and Sever, J. L. (1975). Cellular immunity in multiple sclerosis. *Lancet i,* 980.

17. Gasser, D. L., Newlin, C. M., Palm, J., and Gonatas, N. K. (1973). Genetic control of susceptibility to experimental allergic encephalomyelitis in rats. *Science 181,* 872.

18. Graziano, K. D., Ruckdeschel, J. C., and Mardiney, M. R. (1975). Cell-associated immunity to measles (rubeola). *Cell. Immunol. 15,* 347.

19. Greaves, M. F., Owen, J. J. T., and Raff, M. C. (1974). *T and B Lymphocytes. Origins, Properties and Roles in Immune Responses.* Excerpta Medica, Amsterdam and American Elsevier, New York.

20. Grumet, F. C. (1972). Genetic control of the immune response. A selective defect in immunologic (IgG) memory in non-responder mice. *J. Exp. Med. 135,* 110.

21. Grumet, F. C., Mitchell, G. F., and McDevitt, H. O. (1971). Genetic control of specific immune responses in inbred mice. *Ann. N.Y. Acad. Sci. 190,* 170.

22. Jensen, M. K. (1968). Lymphocyte transformation in multiple sclerosis. *Acta Neurol. Scand. 44,* 200.

23. Jersild, C., Ciongoli, A. K., Fog, T., Good, R. A., Platz, P. J., Svejgaard, A., Thomsen, M., and Dupont, B. (1976). Histocompatibility linked immune responsiveness in autoimmune diseases and possible implications for immunostimulatory therapy with special reference to multiple sclerosis. In *Infection and Immunity in Rheumatic Diseases* (D. C. Dumonde, ed.). Blackwells, Oxford, in press.

24. Jersild, C., Dupont, B., Fog, T., Platz, P. J., and Svejgaard, A. (1975). Histocompatibility determinants in multiple sclerosis. *Transplant Rev. 22,* 148.

25. Jersild, C., Platz, P., Thomsen, M., Hansen, G. S., Svejgaard, A., Dupont, B., Fog, T., Ciongoli, A. K., and Grob, P. (1973). Transfer-factor therapy in multiple sclerosis. *Lancet ii,* 1381.

26. Jersild, C., Platz, P., Thomsen, M., Dupont, B., Svejgaard, A., Ciongoli, A. K., Fog,

T., and Grob, P. (1976). Transfer factor treatment of patients with multiple sclerosis. I. Changes in immunological parameters. *Scand. J. Immunol.*, in press.

27. Knowles, M., Hughes, D., Caspary, E. A., and Field, E. J. (1968). Lymphocyte transformation in multiple sclerosis. *Lancet ii*, 1207.

28. Knowles, M., and Saunders, M. (1970). Lymphocyte stimulation with measles antigen in multiple sclerosis. *Neurology 20*, 700.

29. Koulischer, L., Stenuit, J., and Ketelaer, P. (1966). La croissance 'in vitro' de leucocytes de malades atteints de sclérose en plaques. *Acta Neurol. Belg. 66*, 274.

30. Lilly, F. (1971). The influence of H-2 type on gross-virus leukemogenesis in mice. *Transplant Proc. 3*, 1239.

31. Lilly, F., Boyse, E. A., and Old, L. J. (1964). Genetic basis on susceptibility to viral leukemogenesis. *Lancet ii*, 1207.

32. Lisak, R. P., Levinson, A. I., Zweiman, B., and Abdou, N. I. (1975). T and B lymphocytes in multiple sclerosis. *Clin. Exp. Immunol. 22*, 30.

33. Lodmell, D. L., Niwa, A., Hayashi, K., and Notkins, A. L. (1973). Prevention of cell-to-cell spread of herpes simplex virus by leukocytes. *J. Exp. Med. 137*, 706.

34. McDevitt, H. O., Oldstone, M. B. A., and Pincus, T. (1974). Histocompatibility-linked genetic control of specific immune responses to viral infection. *Transplant Rev. 19*, 209.

35. McDevitt, H. O., and Sela, M. (1965). Genetic control of the antibody response. I. Demonstration of determinant specific differences in response to synthetic polypeptide antigens in two strains of inbred mice. *J. Exp. Med. 112*, 517.

36. McFarland, H. F. (1974). In vitro studies of cell-mediated immunity in an acute viral infection. *J. Immunol. 113*, 173.

37. McFarlin, D. E., Hsu, S. C.-L., Slemenda, S. B., Chou, F. C.-H., and Kibler, R. F. (1975). The immune response against myelin basic protein in two strains of rat with different genetic capacity to develop experimental allergic encephalomyelitis. *J. Exp. Med. 141*, 72.

38. Marker, O., and Volkert, M. (1973). Studies on cell-mediated immunity to lymphocytic choriomeningitis virus in mice. *J. Exp. Med. 137*, 1511.

39. Oger, J. F., Arnason, B. G. W., Wray, S. H., and Kistler, J. P. (1975). A study of B and T cells in multiple sclerosis. *Neurology 25*, 444.

40. Oldstone, M. B. A., Dixon, F. J., Mitchell, G. F., and McDevitt, H. O. (1973). Histocompatibility-linked genetic control of disease susceptibility. Murine lymphocytic choriomeningitis virus infection. *J. Exp. Med. 137*, 1201.

41. Platz, P., Jersild, C., Thomsen, M., Svejgaard, A., Fog, T., Midholm, S., Raun, N., Hansen, S. K., and Grob, P. (1976). Transfer factor treatment of patients with multiple sclerosis. II. Immunological parameters in a long-term clinical trial. In *Proc. II Int. Congr. on Transfer Factor*, in press.

42. Rola-Pleszczynski, M. (1975). Lymphocyte-mediated cytotoxicity to viruses in patients with multiple sclerosis: Presence of a blocking factor. *Neurology 25*, 491.

43. Rosenberg, S. A., and David, J. R. (1970). Inhibition of leukocyte migration: An evaluation of this *in vitro* assay for delayed hypersensitivity in man to a soluble antigens. *J. Immunol. 105*, 1447.

44. Saunders, M., Knowles, M., and Field, E. J. (1969). Lymphocyte stimulation with phytohæmagglutinin in multiple sclerosis. *Lancet i*, 674.

45. Senyk, G., Hadley, W. K. (1973). *In vitro* correlates of delayed hypersensitivity in man: Ambiguity of polymorphonuclear neutrophils as indicator cells in leukocyte migration test. *Infect. Immun. 8*, 370.

46. Steele, R. W., Hensen, S. A., Vincent, M. A., Fuccillo, D. A., and Bellanti, J. A. (1973). A ^{51}Cr microassay technique for cell-mediated immunity to viruses. *J. Immunol. 110*, 1502.

47. Thurman, G. B., Ahmed, A., Strong, D. M., Knudsen, R. C., Grace, W. R., and Sell, K. W. (1973). Lymphocyte activation in subacute sclerosing panencephalitis virus and cytomegalovirus infections. *J. Exp. Med. 138*, 839.

48. Utermohlen, V., and Zabriskie, J. B. (1973). Suppressed cellular immunity to measles antigen in multiple sclerosis patients. *Lancet ii*, 1147.

49. Utermohlen, V., and Zabriskie, J. B. (1973). A suppression of cellular immunity in patients with multiple sclerosis. *J. Exp. Med. 138*, 1591.

50. Volkert, M., Marker, O., and Bro-Jørgensen, K. (1974). Two populations of T lymphocytes immune to the lymphocyte choriomeningitis virus. *J. Exp. Med. 139*, 1329.

51. Williams, R. M., and Moore, M. J. (1973). Linkage of susceptibility to experimental allergic encephalomyelitis to the major histocompatibility locus in the rat. *J. Exp. Med. 138*, 775.

52. Zabriskie, J. B., Espinoza, L. R., Plank, C. R., and Collins, R. C. (1976). Cell mediated immunity to rival antigens in multiple sclerosis. MS meeting, Copenhagen, September 1975. *Acta Neurol. Scand.*, in press.

Discussion / Chapters 13-15

Dr. Dickinson expressed an uneasiness about the genetic interpretation of multiple sclerosis (MS) by recalling the history of scrapie and the early explanation of the disease on an exclusively genetic basis. Yet the concentration of this disease among relatives was ultimately explained on the basis of a transmissable agent and not on a heritable basis. The correlations among relatives, therefore, do not necessarily imply a genetic correlation. Both Dr. Kuwert and Dr. Jersild agreed that the background of MS depended on many factors and that it was not possible at present to identify all of them and to assign appropriate weights to them.

Some additional problems of the analysis of MS cases were discussed by Dr. Kurland who cited his studies in Winnipeg, Canada. There was a substantial rate of error of diagnosis in a quarter of the patients, because MS is a disease for which there is no specific test and therefore clinical diagnosis is subject to interpretation. If we allow for "dilution" of the true MS patients by some, who do not have MS, then the increased frequency of the LD7A type becomes somewhat more convincing, because it is possible that the individuals who lack it are the ones in whom the diagnosis of MS had been made in error.

Regarding the study of twins, Dr. Kurland pointed out that selection of the subjects through radio and newspaper advertisements was such that one could expect a higher degree of reporting if the twins were concordant for the disease than if they were discordant. Therefore, the apparent degree of association or concordance of twins may be subject to serious question. Finally, erroneous classification of non-MS patients as MS patients in even a very small number of cases— for example, hereditary ataxia—may have a tremendous effect on the data and suggest an apparent familial aggregation in the entire series.

Dr. Kabat also expressed substantial concern about the genetic data. He said that it is a fundamental principle of statistics that a difference is a difference only if it makes a difference. In the relationship between blood groups and disease, for example, it has been well established that there is a slightly higher incidence of carcinoma of the stomach in blood group A and a slightly higher incidence of gastric ulcer in blood group O, but this does not explain anything about the diseases themselves. There is no question that the association is statistically significant, but it is of no interpretive value.

How much does the HLA association tell us in prognostic terms about the outcome of a specific case of MS? Dr. Kuwert responded that there were quite striking differences between the studies of blood groups and their relationship to diseases and the HLA studies in MS. First, there was an *a priori* reason to think that the differences in HLA had more to do with the disease and at a much higher level of correlation than the blood groups. For example in the case of ankylosing spondylitis, there is a difference between 90% correlation in patients and 8% in the population at large. In MS, of course, the HLA 7 association is not as high as it is with ankylosing spondylitis, but all the data are not as yet at hand. Dr. Jersild contributed additional information that among patients with MS those who were LD7A exhibited both the fast and the slowly progressing course of the disease, whereas those who were LD7A-negative followed only the slowly progressing course.

Finally, the significance of the differences in T lymphocytes between MS patients and normal individuals was questioned by Dr. Kabat, who stated that the improvement in techniques of enumeration has led to the gradual increase in identifiable T cells, to the point that now some 90% of the lymphocytes are so classified. Therefore, by reciprocity, the B cells constitute only some 10% of the lymphocytes, and the various studies of enumeration of these cells in MS patients may have to be reevaluated.

Comment/Chapters 13–15
David Porter

The virologic and genetic concepts may actually obscure the principal issue, i.e., the identification of the cause or causes of multiple sclerosis (MS). Epidemiologic data strongly suggest that some environmental factor(s), that operates during the first 15 years of life, eventually leads to MS. The epidemiologic studies do not indicate whether there is a single factor, perhaps 20 factors, or a requirement for several factors operating together or sequentially. Although the epidemiologic studies clearly state the geographic regions where the factor(s) was present some years ago, they cannot identify the nature of the factor(s).

Multiple sclerosis is a heterogeneous disease that could have multiple causes. Several well-studied examples of a clinical viral disease caused by different agents are known. Infectious mononucleosis can be caused by EB virus or cytomegalovirus, and subacute sclerosing panencephalitis can be caused by either measles or rubella virus. Acute hepatitis can be caused by hepatitis A virus, hepatitis B virus, and probably one or more additional viruses. On the other hand, a single agent such as *Treponema pallidum* may present protean manifestations. Experiences with well-defined infectious diseases should make us wary of taking a narrow approach to the problem of multiple sclerosis.

We should clearly distinguish between studies of the etiology of MS and studies of the pathogenesis of MS. Although there is considerable variation in the size and location of the lesions of MS, the basic lesion is stereotyped with only some variation in the apparent age. It is likely that the brain responds to injury in a limited number of ways, and the apparent similarity of lesions in MS may delude us into believing that we are dealing with a single disease. Investigators of liver disease have long been aware that different insults to that organ often result in lesions that are similar or even identical.

Isolation of a viral or other infectious agent from or demonstration of an antigen in MS brain should be interpreted with considerable caution. Gajdusek and his co-workers have isolated over 150 viruses of 11 main groups from the brains of chimpanzees used in experiments with kuru and Creutzfeldt–Jakob disease, none of which have any relevance to the diseases being studied. Although virologists working with human brain have not had similar experiences, there is no reason why man should differ completely from the chimpanzee, and the 6/94 agent could even be analogous to some of Gajdusek's isolates. It is clear that we will have to apply some version of Koch's postulates to agents that are isolated from MS patients. Huebner's[1] restatement of Koch's postulates offers guidance for agents that cannot be returned to their natural host.

A large prospective study involving the families of perhaps 500 MS patients might give useful clues about an etiologic agent(s) of MS. Such a study would require participation of epidemiologists, virologists, geneticists, immunologists, and neurologists. The nature of a proper control population is a real problem for such a study. Although such a study would be expensive and may require a commitment of 20 years, it may represent the only approach to the etiology of MS that will yield meaningful data if the present, somewhat fragmented, approaches fail.

The remarks about the present lack of evidence for a viral etiology of MS are not meant to be negative, but are meant to encourage definitive experimentation on this difficult medical problem. Everyone with an interest in MS should be encouraged to demand rigid experimental evidence concerning the etiologic agent(s) of this disease and to remain open-minded about the interpretation of experimental results.

REFERENCE

1. Heubner, R. J. (1957). The virologists dilemma. *Ann. N.Y. Acad. Sci. 67*, 430–438.

PART IV
CRITIQUE ON THE INVESTIGATIONAL APPROACHES TO ETIOLOGY AND PATHOGENESIS

CHAPTER 16
The Virologist*

LUDVIK PREVEC

In considering the virologic aspects of slow virus diseases by an outsider to the field, it is probable that answers to some of the questions or approaches suggested may already be experimental fact. Conversely, other suggestions may well have been considered and rejected, either because of their obvious naivete or because of the strong existing negative evidence. By approaching the area from the view point of a molecular virologist, I may restate ideas that have been and are being considered by those in the field.

One of the first necessities from the virologic point of view is the identification and characterization of the virion—that physical entity that may be capable of transferring the disease from individual to individual by either horizontal or vertical transmission. Although the direct implication of the isolated virus as the primary cause of the neurologic lesion from which it was obtained remains to be confirmed in many instances, it is probably safe to say that the viruses of subacute sclerosing panencephalitis (SSPE) and progressive multifocal leukoencephalopathy (PML) possess physical and structural characteristics that place them in known virus groups.

Presently, only the agents of scrapie and kuru suggest the possible existence of a novel structural group having some conventional viruslike properties. With the use of the assay procedures described by Dickinson and Fraser, it may be possible to sort out the biologic diversity of these agents and begin to examine their biochemical nature. In the case of the scrapie and scrapielike agents, I can only suggest that inactivation studies employing specific enzymes—that is, proteinases, nucleases, lipases, and glycosidases—either separately or in selected combination, may provide more biochemical information concerning the nature of the infectious agent than the use of physical or more nonselective chemical treatments.

The relationship of the more conventional viruses of SSPE and PML to other members of their respective groups is, of course, of primary concern. This is especially true in the case of SSPE virus, which is anti-

* This investigation was supported by Public Health Service research grant AI-06264 from the National Institute of Allergy and Infectious Diseases; it was conducted under the sponsorship of the Commission on Influenza, Armed Forces Epidemiological Board, as well as being supported by the U. S. Army Medical Research and Development Command, Department of the Army, under research contract DADA 17-67-C7046.

The author expresses his sincere gratitude to Dr. C. P. Stanners and Dr. John J. Holland for their assistance and access to data prior to publication.

213

genically similar to measles virus. Since this difference is apparently central to the function of SSPE as a slow infection, it deserves considerable attention.

Comparisons of the antigenic and structural relationships of the virus proteins and of the nucleic acid genomes need to be made. This latter feature may be compared by sizing in polyacrylamide gels and by oligonucleotide comparisons. The extent of nucleic acid homology (as measured by nuclease resistance after annealing with complementary RNA) can be determined using virus complementary RNA obtained either by *in vitro* transcription or by extraction from infected cells. This technique is sufficiently sensitive to indicate virus relatedness but not so sensitive that it responds to minor base substitutions or mutations.

In a somewhat analogous manner, a comparison of the PML viruses with known simian virus 40 (SV40) viruses and with each other can be obtained by restriction endonuclease mapping and by DNA–DNA hybridization analysis.

The thorough characterization of these viruses should provide unequivocal proof for or against the possible derivation of these viruses from the conventional ones and hence suggest the probable etiology of the disease.

Although the term "neurotropic" tends to suggest that the virus has a predilection for neural tissue, this need not be so. For the purpose of slow virus diseases, it is a necessary and sufficient condition that the virus be capable of infecting and persisting in neural tissues, not necessarily to the exclusion of similar behavior in nonneural tissue. In those circumstances in which the neurologic disease may be only a delayed sequela of infection by a normal cytopathic virus, the state of the virus during the latent phase requires some examination.

One basic feature of slow virus disease is the latent period between exposure to the agent or virus and the clinical manifestation of the disease. It is this problem of persistence that is of particular interest from the molecular point of view. At the cellular level, it would seem that there are two fundamental methods by which the latency can be maintained. The virus may attain a nonreplicative or dormant state within a cell or group of cells, or there may be progressive, but attenuated, virus replication in cells. In this latter circumstance, the fact that the disease remains subclinical may be due either to the relatively nonessential nature of the infected cells, the absence of a cytolytic response during virus growth, or extremely slow virus growth approaching the condition of total dormancy.

If the virus is dormant, then we must consider the biochemical state of the viral genome during the dormant phase. The DNA genome of the human SV40 may exist in either an integrated or proviral state within the cell. Since virus particles can be obtained, this problem is open to direct analysis utilizing the procedures employed for cells transformed by the comparable simian virus.

The most obvious dormant state, a paramyxo-like RNA virus within the cell, would seem to be in the form of ribonucleic protein moiety within either the cytoplasm or nucleus of the infected cell. Whereas the possibility of visna virus and similar reverse transcriptase-containing entities existing as latent DNA integrated within the cell seems likely, the possibility of a similar situation for the RNA paramyxo-like viruses did not seem tenable until the recent transfection experiments of Simpson (8). It is not difficult to conceive, at a superficial level, of mutations in a viral replicase or transcriptase that enable the enzyme to accept deoxy substrates, but the possibility that this simple effect is sufficient to produce a DNA transcript with full biologic activity must be evaluated further. In this regard, the observation that a persistent Newcastle disease virus (NDV) strain may catalyze DNA synthesis is of some interest (2).

Although the nature of the block on virus replication during latency is not clear, it is not difficult to conceive of such a situation when we consider that even as unfastidious an organism as vesicular stomatitis virus (VSV) may be under cellular regulation as shown by the host range mutants obtained by Szilagyi and Pringle (11). Thacore and Youngner have also shown that rabbit corneal epithelium cells are highly restrictive for this virus (12). When we consider the more demanding growth requirements of most other mammalian viruses, it is possible that some neural cells may be deficient in the growth requirements of a particular virus mutant. Accepting this line of reasoning will necessitate the later consideration of a compensating mechanism for virus activation.

The possibility that virus growth continues throughout the latent period at a very low level must be considered and evaluated by examining mechanisms for the attenuation of virus replication. Apart from unspecified cell-related regulation, the easiest possibilities are the occurrence of missense mutants, which replicate at a greatly reduced growth rate. The frequency of spontaneous temperature sensitive (ts) mutants in negative-stranded RNA viruses can be of the order of 1% suggesting that the number of possible missense mutants that restrict but do not completely block virus synthesis in a mammalian host may be quite large.

Studies of the kinetic analysis of virus protein synthesis suggest that the membrane associated proteins, the external glycoproteins and the internal matrix or membrane protein, are the rate limiting proteins of virus synthesis. Mutations in these proteins would most readily lead to a reduction in virus yield and could result in a situation in which considerable quantities of viral ribonucleic protein accumulate within infected cells. Alternations in the glycoproteins would have the possible selective advantage of conferring an altered antigenicity to the virus particle, thus protecting the virus produced from neutralization by antibody raised to the initial viral infection. Similarly, mutant infected cells may not be susceptible to a cell mediated immune response elicited by the original infection.

Yet another mechanism by which virus replication may be altered is the activation of defective particles as proposed by Huang and Baltimore (6). Coreplication of defective and infectious virions can greatly reduce the yield of infectious particles produced by that cell. The ability of defective virions to regulate the growth of virus in tissue culture has been amply demonstrated by Huang (5) for the cytopathic VSV and by

Lehman-Grubbe (7) for the relatively noncytocidal virus of Lymphocytic choriomeningitis (LCM). The cyclic rise and fall of infectious virions seen after continuous passage of defective-producing virus provide a possible analogy to the *in vivo* situation.

Finally, some combination of defective particle production and partially attenuated infectious particles may provide yet another fine tuning level on the attenuation of virus growth.

Regardless of the mechanism by which the virus remains in a relatively dormant or clinically unrecognized state, it seems necessary to postulate some form of induction or reactivation mechanism to explain the relatively rapid progressive disease that ensues. Whether the neural destruction is an immunologic or viral cytopathic function, the reactivation may cause the expression of viral antigen and perhaps the more rapid dissemination of infectious virus.

By analogy with RNA tumor viruses, the induction of dormant viruses may be effected by chemical changes that temporarily disrupt cellular protein synthesis. The possibility of hormonal induction might also be considered. Once activated, the virus may now have access to another cell type—one in which normal cytolytic replication is possible—leading to expanded virus synthesis and possible neuron involvement. The role of tissue macrophages in the replication and amplification of virus might be considered.

The observation by Youngner that VSV virus can be "rescued" from rabbit corneal cells or from some interferon-treated cells by superinfection with a poxvirus suggests an interesting mechanism for virus reactivation. Rescue of a latent or mutant virus from relatively nonpermissive neural cells may be due to coinfection of these cells by another virus. In analogy with Youngner's experiments, the superinfecting virus need not be closely related to the latent virus but must be capable of providing some function to overcome the block. Alternatively, particularly if we consider the case that the "latent" virus has a defective glycoprotein function, the superinfecting virus may now allow the formation of phenotypically mixed "pseudotypes." As before, the induced virus may now have access to cells in which replication can occur. It is possible to envisage on the basis of the data presented by Choppin regulation due to the presence or absence of specific cleavage proteases in the cellular plasma membrane. Rescue of virus by pseudotype formation from the nonpermissive cell line might then begin the infective process.

Superinfection by a related viral genome may effect rescue through recombination as well as complementation. In this case, it might be expected that recombination may generate a particle capable of progressive, if attenuated, replication in neural tissue. If this mechanism does indeed exist, then one may postulate that the latent period between initial infection and subsequent reactivation of the virus is a direct measure of the immunologic resistance to the superinfecting virus present in the host animal as a result of the first infection.

Biochemical approaches to some of the postulates already presented are currently possible. In particular, in those instances in which viruses can be isolated in quantity, it should be possible using DNA–DNA hybrid Cot analysis in the case of the DNA viruses to gain some information on the possible cell type or intracellular location of viral DNA. In the case of RNA viruses, the technique employed will be determined by the ability to synthesize virus-complementary RNA or DNA. In the case of SSPE virus it may be possible that the ribonucleic protein complexes in infected cells contain sufficient plus as well as minus strand viral RNA to allow the isolation of complementary pairs of labeled RNA, which could then be used with the nucleic acids from donor cells in a manner analogous to the DNA–DNA Cot procedure. The search for infectious nucleic acid by extraction from test cells and transfection of potentially permissive cells may provide yet another useful technique in searching for the latent viral genome.

Expression of the latent genome may also be examined by nucleic acid hybridization procedures using unlabeled RNA extracted from test cells and highly labeled minimal quantities of viral DNA or RNA. The use of I^{25}-labeled nucleic acids may be particularly useful in this procedure. Attempts to detect specific viral induced antigens in the cytoplasm and on the surface of the cells in a manner analogous to the antigens of cells infected with tumor viruses should continue to be actively pursued.

Attempts to activate latent virus from potential carrier cells should be extended to include not only cell fusion to possible permissive cells but also attempts at chemical induction or induction by superinfection with both related and unrelated viruses. This procedure may require the selective use of appropriate mutant viruses in order to create a situation in which induced and inducing viruses can be differentiated, but it should be feasible in many instances.

Yet another approach to the understanding of slow virus infection, which is distinct from the relatively straightforward attack described previously, is the use of a well-characterized virus that possesses many of the possible attributes of the agents producing slow virus infections, but which is not yet known itself to be responsible for any slow virus diseases. If such a virus can, through manipulation, be brought to such a state that it now gives rise to a slow virus disease, it may be possible to reconstruct the features of natural slow virus infections. One such virus used by a number of virologists interested in the field of neurologic disease is the virus of VSV. In particular, I would like to describe briefly some experiments of John J. Holland in California and C. P. Stanners in Toronto that utilize this virus and this approach.

Holland and Villarreal (3) showed that coinfection of cells in culture with a ts mutant of VSV together with interfering defective particles could result in the establishment of a noncytocidal infection. An interesting feature of this persistent infection is the fact that though the original defectives were standard "short T" particles; cocultivation of the carrier culture with normal cells led to the production of a longer "long T" defective particle. The "long T" defective allowed the establishment of a carrier culture upon coinfection with normal wild-type (wt) virus. Since the defective particle appeared to affect the transcriptase activity of purified infectious virions, it was felt that reduced virus yield and hence reduced cytopathology derived from this fact.

Doyle and Holland (1) have gone on to show that preinoculation of high-purified defective particles into the brain of young mice can ameliorate the course of disease after subsequent injection of wt virus. Instead of dying within 2 to 3 days, the animals either survived indefinitely or died after protracted periods of time with a neurologic disease. There seems to be little doubt from these results that defective viruses have the capability of attenuating virus replication in a manner appropriate to the development of a slow virus infection. More recently, Holland's group found that defective particles of VSV can be generated in brains of newborn animals but not of adults (4). Whether this particular observation bears any relationship to a possible mechanism of induction of latent virus in older animals remains to be determined. This observation has, at least in part, helped to overcome the conceptual difficulty of transposing experiments performed in tissue culture into *in vivo* situations. A number of problems concerning the frequency of defective particle production and the spread of these particles *in vivo* remain to be worked out before the model can be strictly applied to slow virus infection.

In yet another approach using this model system, Stanners and his co-workers screened existing ts mutants of VSV for reversion frequency, cytopathic effect in tissue culture, and animal pathogenicity (9). A representative picture of the survival times of newborn hamsters injected subcutaneously (s.c.) with wt or mutant virus is shown in Fig. 16.1. Virus Its$^+$ is wt VSV and kills the hamsters within 2 days, whether it is injected at 10 or 10^4 p.f.u./animal. The result observed for mutant T1025 is characteristic of a number of ts mutants, all of which give rise to revertant virus when grown at 37°C. In this case, the hamsters died at approximately the same time as observed with wt virus. At the other extreme, mutant G114 is representative of a number of ts mutants with an extremely low reversion frequency. In these cases, the virus presumably does not replicate to any significant extent in the hamster, and the animals survive indefinitely. Between these two situations was the mutant of greatest interest from the point of view of slow virus infections. Mutant 1026 was shown to be extremely "leaky" and to produce very high virus yields at 37°C. The virus produced at this temperature were all ts in nature and did not give rise to plaques at 39.5°C showing that "leakiness" and not reversion to wt was involved. As seen in Fig. 16.1, this particular mutant allowed 50% survival of the hamsters for approximately 7 days; the animals dying had neurologic symptoms.

Another particularly relevant aspect of the study by Stanners and Goldberg is their analysis of the distribution of virus between brain and kidney as a function of the time elapsing between s.c. injection and death (10). A large number of different virus stocks, both wt (HR and Its$^+$) and ts mutant (prefixed by the letters T, G, W, or O) were employed.

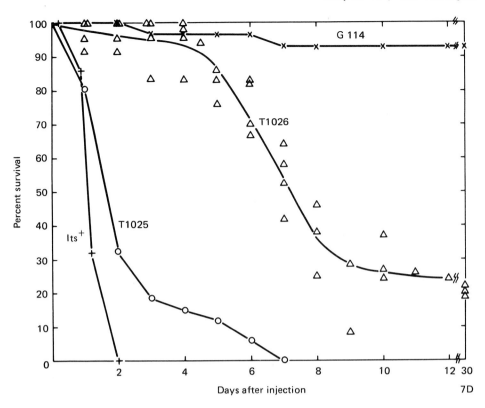

Figure 16.1.
Survival of newborn hamsters injected s.c. with wt and three ts VSV mutants. For lts+, 30 animals were injected with 10 to 10^4 p.f.u./animal; for T1025, 30 animals were injected with 10^3 to 10^5 p.f.u./animal; and for G114, 30 animals were injected with 10^3 to 10^6 p.f.u./animal. For T1026, the results of four independent experiments, three of which employed single but different doses ranging from 10^3 to 10^6 p.f.u./animal and involving approximately 20 animals each, are shown.

As seen in Fig. 16.2, the ratio of virus in brain to virus in kidney increased to a plateau level as the survival time of the animal reached 4 days or longer. It would appear that if a virus, regardless of its genotype, allows survival of the animal for approximately 4 days, it now shows apparent neurotropism. As seen in Fig. 16.2 in many of the long-lived animals, no virus was recovered from the kidney, whereas high titers were observed in the brain. This result suggested that s.c.-injected virus, after replication at the injection site, spread quickly to peripheral organs such as the kidney, as well as to the brain, and that in those animals surviving for 3 days a resistance mechanism was stimulated which cleared virus from the peripheral organs but not from the brain.

As a test of this hypothesis, newborn hamsters injected s.c. with T1026 at birth were reinoculated after 3 to 4 days s.c. with wt virus. Instead of dying within 2 days, the hamsters showed the survival characteristics of T1026, and although virtually no wt virus was recovered from either brain or kidney, the expected titer of T1026 was recovered from the brain. In a complementary experiment, animals injected with T1026 at birth were given

219

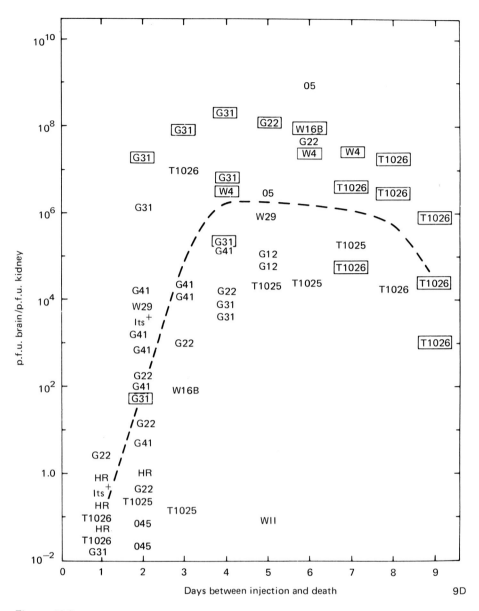

Figure 16.2.
Neurotropism in newborn hamsters versus VSV mutant and time of death. Hamsters were injected s.c. with doses of different mutants of VSV ranging from 10^3 to 10^6 p.f.u./animal within 24 hours after birth (a few animals were injected 3 days after birth). The ratio of p.f.u. in the brain to p.f.u. in the kidneys is presented for individual dead or dying animals. The dashed line represents the approximate logarithmic average. Where no virus could be recovered from the kidney, the point is surrounded with a box and represents the actual brain titer.

intracerebral (i.c.) injections of wt virus after 3 or 4 days. Inoculation i.c. of wt virus into nonpreinjected animals led to the pressence of virus in both brain and kidney at death; the inoculation into preinjected animals yielded wt virus principally from the brain. Thus, an inducible mechanism capable of clearing virus from peripheral organs but not from the brain appears to be a real possibility. This mechanism coupled with an attenuated virus may explain the neurotropic behavior of slow virus diseases.

While the analogies from the animal model systems to the known slow virus diseases observed in man may, in many ways, appear more superficial than real, the results being obtained may introduce concepts and direction that could not be observed or tested in the natural disease.

REFERENCES

1. Doyle, M., and Holland, J. J. (1973). Prophylaxis and immunization in mice by use of virus-free defective T particles to protect against intracerebral infection by vesicular stomatitis virus. *Proc. Natl. Acad. Sci. U.S.A. 70*, 2105–2108.
2. Furman, P. A., and Hallum, J. V. (1973). RNA-dependent DNA polymerase activity in preparations of a mutant of Newcastle disease virus arising from persistently infected L cells. *J. Virol. 12*, 548–555.
3. Holland, J. J., and Villarreal, L. P. (1974). Persistent noncytocidal vesicular stomatitis virus infections mediated by defective T particles that suppress virion transcriptase. *Proc. Natl. Acad. Sci. U.S.A. 71*, 2956–2960.
4. Holland, J. J., and Villarreal, L. P. (1975). Defective interfering T particles of VSV and rabies virus *in vivo*. In *Third International Congress for Virology Abstracts*, Madrid, p. 155.
5. Huang, A. S. (1973). Defective interfering viruses. *Ann. Rev. Microbiol. 27*, 101–117.
6. Huang, A. S., and Baltimore, D. (1970). Defective viral particles and viral disease processes. *Nature 226*, 325–327.
7. Lehmann-Grubbe, F. (1971). *Virol. Monogr. 10*, 1–173.
8. Simpson, R. W., and Iimuna, M. (1975). Recovery of infectious proviral DNA from mammalian cells infected with respiratory syncytial virus. *Proc. Natl. Acad. Sci. U.S.A. 72*, 3230–3234.
9. Stanners, C. P., Farmilo, A. J., and Goldberg, V. J. (1975). Effects *in vitro* and *in vivo* of a mutant of vesicular stomatitis virus with attenuated cytopathogenicity. In *Negative Strand Viruses*, pp. 785–798. Academic Press, New York.
10. Stanners, C. P., and Goldberg, V. J. (1975). On the mechanism of neurotropism of vesicular stomatitis virus in newborn hamsters. Studies with temperature-sensitive mutants. *J. Gen. Virol. 29*, 281–296.
11. Szilagyi, J. S., and Pringle, C. R. (1975). Virion transcriptase activity differences in host range mutants of vesicular stomatitis virus. *J. Virol. 16*, 927–936.
12. Thacore, H. R., and Youngner, J. S. (1973). Rescue of vesicular stomatitis virus from interferon-induced resistance by superinfection with vaccinia virus I and II. *Virology 56*, 505–522.

CHAPTER 17
Temperature-Sensitive Viruses: Possible Role in Chronic and Inapparent Infections

JULIUS S. YOUNGNER

INTRODUCTION

For the last 5 years my colleagues and I have been working on cell culture models of persistent viral infections. Currently, our hypothesis concerns the establishment and maintenance of certain persistent infections. We believe that in the process of infection with wild-type (wt) virulent viruses that later lead to persistent infection there is frequently a selection of temperature-sensitive (ts) virus mutants uniquely suited to maintain the persistent infection.

Our original observations were initiated studying the abortive infection of mouse L cells by Newcastle disease virus (NDV). We soon found that the abortive infection quickly led to a persistent infection of L cells (15, 16). The persistently infected cells were morphologically similar to the parental wt L cells and could be passaged at the same intervals as the uninfected ones. Although their growth characteristics were not remarkably different, other alterations were noted. Culture fluid from the persistently infected L cells (L_{NDV}) always contained infectious virus and 10 to 20 units of interferon; these activities were absent from control L cell cultures. The L_{NDV} cells were completely resistant to challenge with vesicular stomatitis virus (VSV), whereas L cells were completely susceptible.

PROPERTIES OF TEMPERATURE-SENSITIVE VIRUSES

The L_{NDV} cells have now been maintained in continuous culture for over 6 years. Table 17.1 compares some properties of the virus (NDV_{pi}) recovered from the persistently infected cells to the properties of the wt Herts strain (NDV_0) used to initiate the infection. Less virulent for embryonated eggs, NDV_{pi} produced small plaques in primary chick embryo cell cultures. There were also indications of structural differences between the two viruses: The inactivation rates of infectivity and hemagglutinin activity of the two viruses were significantly different. Most important to the present discussion was the difference in replication of the two viruses in permissive CE cells incubated at 37° and 42°–43°C. Whereas NDV_0 replicated with almost equal efficiency at both temperatures, the replication of NDV_{pi} was

TABLE 17.1 / Comparison of Properties of wt Herts NDV (NDV$_0$) and Virus (NDV$_{pi}$) Recovered from Persistently Infected L Cells

Property	NDV$_0$	NDV$_{pi}$
Lethality for embryonated eggs (10^4 P.F.U.)	100% at 48 hr	65–70% at 48 hr
Plaque size in chick embryo cells (3 days, 37°C)	Large (2–3 mm)	Small (< 1 mm)
Stability of infectivity at 50°C	Stable	Unstable
Stability of hemagglutinin at 50°C	Unstable	Stable
Interferon production in L cells	Yes	Yes
Replication in L cells at 37°C	Covert infection	Productive infection
Replication in chick embryo cells at 42–43°C	Yes	No

effectively inhibited at the higher temperature. Details of the isolation of stable ts mutants of NDV$_{pi}$ and their characterization have been published elsewhere (8, 9). Biochemical characterization of NDV$_{pi}$ ts mutants showed that all NDV$_{pi}$ clones isolated did not synthesize virus-specific RNA (RNA$^-$) at the nonpermissive temperature and appeared to have defects associated with RNA polymerase activity (9). Other alterations in the virion-associated polymerase of virus mutants isolated from L$_{NDV}$ cells have been reported (1).

SELECTION OF TEMPERATURE-SENSITIVE MUTANTS IN PERSISTENT INFECTIONS

We found that the selection of ts mutants by persistent infection of L cells was not a peculiarity of the Herts strain of NDV, but was also true for two other strains, the Texas GB and the Kansas-Man. When L cells were infected with low multiplicities of these two strains, the infection became persistent (10). The infected cells had the characteristics of L$_{NDV}$ cells. The virus present was ts, and isolated mutants exhibited RNA$^-$ phenotypes.

When cell lines from other species were used to initiate persistent infections with Herts NDV$_0$, evidence was obtained that confirmed that ts mutants with an RNA$^-$ phenotype are spontaneously selected (18). A persistently infected hamster cell line (BHK-21), maintained since 1973, produces no interferon and is completely susceptible to VSV. This is in marked contrast to L$_{NDV}$ cells, which constantly produce interferon and are resistant to superinfection with VSV. Twenty-six virus plaques isolated from BHK$_{NDV}$ culture fluid were tested for efficiency of plating at 37° and 43°C; all were found to have 43°/37°C ratios ranging from 7.7×10^{-3} to $< 7.0 \times 10^{-7}$, in contrast to ratios of ≤ 0.5 for six wt NDV$_0$ clones. Clearly, BHK$_{NDV}$ had spontaneously selected a population of ts viruses, similar to the selection previously recorded with L$_{NDV}$ cells. Seventeen stable ts clones tested proved to be defective in RNA synthesis (RNA$^-$) at the nonpermissive temperature.

Permissiveness

Persistent infection of a canine kidney cell line (MDCK) terminated with the destruction of all cells at about 100 days due to the permissiveness of this cell line for NDV. Even with this degree of permissiveness, 33% of the virus clones isolated at 60 to 70 days were ts mutants. Table 17.2 summarizes our findings to date with several cell lines and several strains of NDV. The findings illustrate several important points regarding persistent infection of cell lines with NDV. First, selection of ts mutants occurs in mouse (L), hamster (BHK-21), and canine (MDCK) cell lines infected at low multiplicities of infection with several strains of NDV. In the case of L$_{NDV}$ and BHK$_{NDV}$ cell lines, a long-term persistent infection was established in which ts mutants completely replaced the wt population. Despite the permissiveness of MDCK cells for NDV and the loss of the persistently infected cell lines about 100 days after initiation of the infection, a large proportion of the viruses present (33%) was ts mutants. Second, all the ts mutants isolated from persistently infected L, BHK-21, and MDCK cells were defective in RNA synthesis at the nonpermissive temperature. This evidence points to the possible importance of a viral transcriptional defect in establishing persistent infection (10). Third, in complete contrast to L$_{NDV}$ cells, BHK$_{NDV}$ and MDCK$_{NDV}$ cells made no interferon and were completely susceptible to VSV, suggesting that interferon mediation is not essential for establishing or maintaining the persistently infected state.

TABLE 17.2 / Summary of Persistent Infections Established with Various Strains of NDV and Selection of ts Mutants

NDV Strain	Cell Line Persistently Infected	Interferon Production	Susceptibility to VSV	NDV$_{pi}$ Mutants Isolated and ts Defect
Herts	L cells	Yes	No	RNA$^-$ phenotype polymerase (?) defect
Texas-GB	L cells	Yes	No	RNA$^-$ phenotype polymerase (?) defect
Kansas-Man	L cells	Yes	No	RNA$^-$ phenotype polymerase defect
Herts	BHK-21	No	Yes	RNA$^-$ phenotype polymerase defect
Herts	MDCK (7 passages only)	No	Yes	RNA$^-$ phenotype polymerase defect

Low Multiplicity of Infectious Virions

More recently, we have succeeded in establishing a line of mouse L cells persistently infected with VSV. This was accomplished by initiating the infection with a low multiplicity of infectious virions in the presence of large numbers of defective-interfering particles, as described by Holland and Villarreal for BHK cells (3). In the months that this persistent infection has been maintained, there has been a gradual selection of ts mutants with an RNA$^-$ phenotype. The details of these experiments will be published elsewhere.

Additional Work

The literature on persistent viral infections deals mostly with qualitative and quantitative changes in the cells harboring the virus. Comparatively little has been done to analyze properties other than the virulence of the carried virus. An increasing number of reports indicates that virus recovered from many different types of persistent infections in cell cultures has an impaired ability to replicate at higher temperatures. A sampling of these reports is given in Table 17.3. A plaque-type mutant was isolated from a line of Fructo mouse sarcoma cells persistently infected with Western equine encephalitis virus (WEE) (12). This mutant was attenuated in virulence for mice and was also ts at 42°C (13). In contrast to the results from our laboratory with NDV, temperature-shift experiments suggested that the ts mutants of WEE virus might be defective in a late stage of virus maturation at the nonpermissive temperature.

Several other reports have associated ts virus mutants with establishing persistent infections. As shown in Table 17.3, in BHK-21 cell cultures persistently infected with Sendai virus, virus maturation was normal at 31°C but was ts at 37°C (6). Two reports also link persistent measles virus infections in cell cultures with ts mutants (2, 4).

Selection of ts mutants in persistent infections can also occur in prokaryotic cells. Valentine *et al.* (17) described a commonly occurring spon-

TABLE 17.3 / Persistent Infections in Cell Cultures that Select ts Viruses

Virus	*Cell Line*	*ts Defect*	*References*
Western equine encephalitis	Fructo mouse sarcoma	Late step (42°C)	13, 14
Sendai	BHK-21	Maturation defect—37°C	6
Measles	Hamster embryo	Maturation defect 37 and 39°C	2, 4
Qβ bacteriophage	*Escherichia coli*	RNA$^-$ mutants replicase defective 41°C	7

TABLE 17.4 / Persistent Infections in Vivo **that Select ts Viruses**

Virus	Animal	Virus Defect	References
Foot-and-mouth disease (picornavirus)	Cattle (12 month carriers)	Reduced yield and plaque size 41°C (BHK cells)	15
Aleutian disease (parvovirus)	Mink	Immunofluorescent foci at 31.8°C; not at 37°C (feline renal kidney cells)	8
6/94 (paramyxovirus)	Human (? MS)	Reduced yield 37°C Normal yield 33°C	5

taneous mutant of bacteriophage Qβ, which caused a persistent infection of its host *Escherichia coli*. Virus isolated from the turbid plaques produced by this mutant was strongly ts at 41°C due to defective RNA polymerase production at the higher temperature. Valentine concluded that the non-virulent state of the phage was important for virus development under certain environmental conditions.

Selection of ts mutants also occurs during persistent infection *in vivo*, and some examples of this are given in Table 17.4. The observations with such diverse agents as the viruses of foot-and-mouth disease and Aleutian mink disease suggest that a certain degree of caution be exercised in the use of any ts viruses in humans. To date, there is no evidence of long-term adverse reactions in humans to live virus vaccines that consist of ts viruses, that is, polioviruses and measles. However, increasing evidence of the possible role of measles virus in subacute sclerosing panencephalitis and multiple sclerosis warrant continuing follow-up studies in those who have been vaccinated.

CONCLUSIONS

The observations that have been summarized, together with other information, have led us to make a practical suggestion to investigators seeking to isolate viruses from tissue explants from patients in which latent or persistent virus infections are suspected (11). Since some of these viruses could be ts mutants, the parental strain of which has long been lost, the routine practice of incubating such cell cultures at temperatures below 37°C should be adopted. In addition to the conventional 37°C incubation, by culturing cells from tissues suspected of harboring latent or persistent viruses at 31 or 33°C viruses that have heretofore gone undetected may be isolated.

REFERENCES

1. Furman, P. A., and Hallum, J. V. (1973). RNA-dependent DNA polymerase activity in preparations of a mutant of Newcastle disease virus arising from persistently infected L cells. *J. Virol. 12*, 564–569.

2. Haspel, M. V., Knight, P. R., Duff, R. G., and Rapp, F. (1973). Activation of a latent measles virus infection in hamster cells. *J. Virol. 12*, 690–695.

3. Holland, J. J., and Villarreal, L. P. (1974). Persistent noncytocidal vesicular stomatitis virus infections mediated by defective T particles that suppress virion transcriptase. *Proc. Natl. Acad. Sci. U.S.A. 71*, 2956–2960.

4. Knight, P., Duff, R., and Rapp. F. (1972). Latency of human measles virus in hamster cells. *J. Virol. 10*, 995–1001.

5. Lewandowski, L. J., Lief, F. S., Verini, M. A., Pienkowski, M. M., ter Meulen, V., and Koprowski, H. (1974). Analysis of a viral agent isolated from multiple sclerosis brain tissue: Characterization as a parainfluenza virus type 1. *J. Virol. 13*, 1037–1045.

6. Nagata, I., Kimura, Y., Yasuhiko, I., and Tanaka, T. (1972). Temperature-sensitive phenomenon of viral maturation observed in BHK cells persistently infected with HVJ. *Virology 49*, 453–461.

7. Porter, D., Larsen, A. E., Cox, N. A., Porter, H. G., and Suffin, S. C. (1975). Isolation of Aleutian disease virus of mink in cell culture. *Fed. Proc. 34*, 947.

8. Preble, O. T., and Youngner, J. S. (1972). Temperature-sensitive mutants isolated from L cells persistently infected with Newcastle disease virus. *J. Virol. 9*, 200–206.

9. Preble, O. T., and Youngner, J. S. (1973). Temperature-sensitive defect of mutants isolated from L cells persistently infected with Newcastle disease virus. *J. Virol. 12*, 473–480.

10. Preble, O. T., and Youngner, J. S. (1973). Selection of temperature-sensitive mutants during persistent infection: Role in maintenance of persistent Newcastle disease virus infections of L cells. *J. Virol. 12*, 481–491.

11. Preble, O. T., and Youngner, J. S. (1975). Temperature-sensitive viruses and the etiology of chronic and inapparent infections. *J. Infect. Dis. 131*, 467–473.

12. Simizu, B., and Takayama, N. (1969). Isolation of two plaque mutants of Western equine encephalitis virus differing in virulence for mice. *J. Virol. 4*, 799–800.

13. Simizu, B., and Takayama, N. (1971). Relationship between neurovirulence and temperature sensitivity of an attenuated Western equine encephalitis virus. *Arch. Gesamte Virusforsch. 34*, 242–250.

14. Straver, P. J., and van Bekkum, J. G. (1972). Plaque production by carrier strains of foot-and-mouth disease virus in BHK-monolayers incubated at different temperatures. *Arch. Gesamte Virusforsch. 37*, 12–18.

15. Thacore, H. R., and Youngner, J. S. (1969). Cells persistently infected with Newcastle disease virus. I. Properties of mutants isolated from persistently infected L cells. *J. Virol. 4*, 244–251.

16. Thacore, H. R., and Youngner, J. S. (1970). Cells persistently infected with Newcastle disease virus. II. Ribonucleic acid and protein synthesis in cells infected with mutants isolated from persistently infected L cells. *J. Virol. 6*, 42–48.

17. Valenti, R. C., Ward, R., Strand, M. (1969). The replicative cycle of RNA bacteriophages. *Adv. Virus Res. 15*, 1–59.

18. Youngner, J. S., and Quagliana, D. (1975). Temperature-sensitive mutants isolated from hamster and canine cell lines persistently infected with Newcastle disease virus. *J. Virol. 16*, 1332–1336.

Discussion / Chapters 16-17

Dr. Koprowski expressed concern that so much work on the defective viruses has been carried out in vesicular stomatitis virus, which is so highly virulent. He voiced doubts that defective, interfering particles played a significant role in multiple sclerosis (MS). He felt, however, that the question of temperature-sensitive mutants and the types of mutants described by Dr. Choppin may play a larger role in the development of chronic neurologic diseases. Dr. Gajdusek added that a search for temperature-sensitive mutants in spongiform encephalopathies, conducted in his and Dr. Gibbs' laboratories, has been unsuccessful.

Dr. Lehmann-Grube raised the subject of the persistent infection of mice with the lymphocytic choriomeningitis (LCM) virus. He asked, rhetorically, why the virus was not eliminated in such animals and yet why it did not kill them. In his view, this situation obtains because of the animal's immunologic tolerance. Yet the virus does not increase in the animal to an unlimited extent. The virus growth is not inhibited by interferon, or by defective interfering particles, but because a variant arises, which is less virulent than the wild-type virus. This variant does not damage the cell; it spreads to other cells directly and protects them against infection with the more virulent, cytolytic virus. Yet, it apparently is not a mutant in the genetic sense, because it reverts rather quickly into the more virulent form under certain laboratory conditions.

Dr. Youngner commented that the temperature-sensitive mutants allow a theoretical situation to exist wherein the viruses do not kill the cells, but form a vegetative cycle, which produces virus and viral products. Under such circumstances viral proteins of these mutants can be inserted into cell membranes, forming neo-antigens. This can lead to immunologic diseases.

Dr. Porter described studies with temperature-sensitive mutants of the Aleutian mink disease virus. Using five different sources of the virus it was possible to reach higher titers at 37°C than at 31.8°C. However, after growing the virus at the lower temperature for four to six passages, the temperature sensitivity becomes lost. Upon inoculation into animals, the temperature-sensitive mutant causes persistent infection, and when it is reisolated at 10 or 30 days after infection, the agent does not have temperature sensitivity, whereas if it is reisolated at 180 days it is again temperature sensitive.

Dr. Youngner stated that this type of *in vivo* experiment mimics what his laboratory accomplished in cell culture. The temperature-sensitive mutants can establish a persistent infection and revertants, which are virulent, may appear. He advised that caution be exercised in the widespread use of temperature-sensitive virus mutants.

CHAPTER 18
The Geneticist

A. D. BLOOM

My information regarding slow virus infections has grown logarithmically. I want to share a few of my "genetic" reactions to a fascinating and important area of investigation. Whatever biases I may have were acquired here. Furthermore, since my work is in the area of gene expression in Epstein–Barr (EB) virus-infected human lymphocytes, my focus has to be on the somatic cell genetics rather than on the population genetics of, for example, kuru and multiple sclerosis (MS). In order to indicate some of the most interesting aspects of slow virus infections from a genetic point of view, I shall cover the so-called conventional virus infections of MS and subacute sclerosing panencephalitis (SSPE) first, and then look at the genetically more complex, unconventional scrapie and kuru agents.

Two questions of a genetic nature come to mind. First, are large numbers of individuals being infected with these agents? If the answer proves to be yes, then the question is: Why do so few come down with the overt disease? This is the question of genetic susceptibility. Second, if large numbers of individuals of the species that develops disease are *not* infected and yet the virus or agent is relatively widespread in other species, then we must ask why are the few individuals singled out? At the cellular level, the question becomes still more intriguing, namely, What specific tissues are infected? There have been several references to specific tissues beside the central nervous system (CNS) that may harbor these agents or viruses. The specificity of the virus for particular cell types seems important. Last, how does the virus infect and survive within the cell for so long and how is it transmitted from cell to cell? These are fundamental questions of population genetics and somatic cell genetics.

In the case of progressive multifocal leukoencephalopathy (PML), the common denominators apparently are immunosuppression and consistent recovery of papovaviruses from individuals with this subacute demyelinating disease, which is seen in a small proportion of immunosuppressed patients. The high mortality of the primary diseases probably does not allow a sufficient time interval to elapse between infection and the onset of demyelination in all of those who might be infected. With time, however, and more prolonged survival of immunosuppressed patients, such as those having renal transplantation, it will become clearer what percentage of patients have the infection with these papovaviruses, especially the BK type, which has been isolated in some 90% of them. Furthermore, if immunosuppression is really the key issue here (and I am not absolutely sure that it is), then patients with genetically determined immunologic deficiency disorders, whether B cell variety, specific immuno-globulin deficiency, or T cell diseases, or patients with combined T and B cell disease ought also to harbor these papovaviruses. Immunodeficient patients would then be a reasonable group in which to look for these viruses. In SSPE, we have a situation in which the high measles antibody titers imply that measles virus or a variant thereof is involved in the etiology of that disease. If this is so, then we must determine why we get so few patients with SSPE while so many are infected with measles virus. Apparently, there is no underlying genetic predisposition to SSPE, since familial SSPE has not been reported. If, as seems likely, the SSPE inducing agent is either a variant or mutant of the measles virus, then we have to explain the origins of that mutant or variant, how it is transferred from person to person and from cell to cell. The most likely genetic explanation is that in SSPE we are dealing with a genetic mutant of measles virus (perhaps encouraged to mutate in vaccine preparation), a mutant that is probably antigenically the same as measles virus but with an enhanced specificity for the CNS. If this mutant virus had arisen by vaccine modification, it would be more widespread than it apparently is. If, on the other hand, it arises *in vivo* by a specific mutation after infection, then the neurotropism of the mutant may preclude intrafamilial transmission. From a genetic point of view, repeated *in vivo* mutation at a specific site in the paramyxovirus genome is certainly possible, given the large number of virus particles replicating and the presumably limited number of codons. We must distinguish variant virus from mutant virus. A mutant virus is one that has a permanent heritable change in its nucleic acid. The variant, on the other hand, may be far less permanent and may be merely an adaptation of the virus to its milieu without any fundamental genetic alteration. For some of these para-myxoviruses the likelihood of mutation to neurotropism may be consider-able under certain environmental conditions since there may exist a rela-tively small number of mutable sites within the virus. Under these condi-tions, we might expect no primary immunologic abnormalities in SSPE, but abnormalities that are only secondary to the basic disease. Support for this notion comes from studies that have been presented here. Variants of lymphocytic choriomeningitis virus (LCM) that have an enhanced affinity for cells *in vitro* were also described; and variants of paramyxovirus muta-genized by nitric acid, which altered tropism of the virus. The wild-type virus failed in that instance to plaque in the presence of trypsin, whereas the mutant did plaque. This occurrence suggests that multiplication and spreading of that virus are altered in the mutant. This approach to the genetic analysis of slow virus infections is likely to be extremely rewarding. As Choppin noted, the mutation frequency is very high (10^{-4}), and it should therefore be possible using mutagens to isolate a whole range of mutants among agents of slow virus infections and to carry out sequential analysis of the entry replication and release steps. This is all the more possible, since these viruses seem to replicate (sometimes well, sometimes badly, but they more or less all replicate) in tissue culture. One has, therefore, means at hand for mutagenizing the cells and viruses in the cells containing them. Thus, to a geneticist, a major tool is available for study of viral mutants, which should enable us to determine precisely what the nature of some of these viruses is, their pathogenic range, cell-type specificity, and so on.

The biohazards that may be associated with mutagenized virus will obviously be a major problem and one to which considerable attention will have to be paid. There are certain mutagens that might lend themselves to the induction of mutant virus better than others. Among those that have been used extensively in mammalian cells *in vitro* are the alkylating agents, such as MMNG EMS, and frameship mutagens, such as some acridine dyes. One could then extend these observations to the induction of mutant virus in cell cultures.

There are basically two important levels at which genetics of MS must be considered: the population level and the cellular level. There seems to be considerable evidence in the literature that first-degree relatives of patients with MS have an incidence of this disease some 10- to 20-fold greater than the population at large. On the basis of this suggestive evidence, geneticists can estimate such factors as heritability and frequency of sibling/ sibling and parent/child associations. What is the nature of the genetic defect? At most it is a genetic predisposition rather than a clear-cut gene control etiology to the disease.

The HL-A data of Kuwert and others are interesting but of themselves not especially informative. There are, however, a number of interesting aspects of this approach that may lend themselves to future studies. First, the finding of the association of A7 with MS really does need confirmation. Furthermore, the HL-A haplotypes 1-8 and 3-7 are among the most common, so it is sometimes difficult to interpret data based on frequencies of these haplotypes. The same approach has basically been used in systemic lupus erythematosus (SLE) and Hodgkin's disease. These findings are also suggestive of an association between specific HL-A antigens and susceptibility to the diseases. The question remains what the association means, even if we accept it as truth. The linkage of HLA-A to chromosome 6 in the human karyotype is well established, and if the HL-A is proved to be linked to the I-R gene, we may have an important clue relating HL-A specificity, the immunologic response, and MS. This is, then, an area that may be fruitful for future investigation. The effect of the HL-A gene, whether antigen 7 or 3, on the I-R region is of major interest, and the problem appears to be how to test for it. The relationship of SLE and Hodgkin's disease and the HL-A specificities is important. Some investigators have inferred that the HL-A specificity confers sensitivity to specific viral infections in some way —an idea that may or may not be valid.

The reports of localized homogeneous antibodies in MS, presumably measles antibody, at the site of specific lesions are intriguing. One wonders whether the lymphocytes of these lesions could be isolated to determine whether they are clonally derived. Banding the chromosomes of these cells, if the cells can be stimulated to divide *in vitro* and if they have specific markers, as they well might, would permit a definitive statement about the clonal origin of the infiltrating mononuclear cells. It was suggested that these are localized monoclonal, immunoglobulin-producing cells, and it is possible that these lymphocytes are triggered to divide by virus infected brain cells in some way. The description of macrophage activation *in vitro* by 6/94 is interesting and suggests that macrophages *in vivo* might carry or activate the virus. Macrophage studies in these lesions would certainly be rewarding.

In PML and possibly also in MS, it might reasonably be asked whether the virus infects specific subpopulations of brain cells; whether integration into the host genome occurs early or, alternatively, late because of the slow cell turnover time; and whether a specific stimulus is required to trigger proliferation of the clonal cells that are infected with the virus. In the EB virus, it is becoming increasingly clear that the EB virus does infect a specific subpopulation (the B cells). One wonders whether there are other systems in which this type of cellular specificity is demonstrable. There is little evidence that these disorders are primarily caused by defects in cell-mediated immunity.

The problems of scrapie and kuru are really the most difficult for a geneticist to analyze. The early replication of scrapie agent was said to take place in the reticuloendothelial system (RES) with later manifestations in the CNS. If the evidence for this selective replication in the RES is firm, then we would have to view the RES as a passenger tissue for the virus, perhaps with migratory cells, presumably lymphocytes, acting to transmit the virus to the CNS or acting as sites of virus release into the blood stream. Again the idea of mutant virus returns, the 22A scrapie of Dickinson has virologic properties that are different from those of the ME7 scrapie agent. Dickinson has designated the *sinc* gene as the factor responsible for the control of the incubation period and the rate of replication. Thus, his idea that two loci, S7 and P7, of the *sinc* gene act together in ME7 to encourage more rapid replication seems to be a good one. I have not been able to review his evidence regarding the multiple-host site concept, but the principle of viral agents that differ at specific loci is important. The S7 allele encourages shorter incubation in ME7, the P7 prolonging that incubation time in ME7. Alternatively, in 22A the S7 effect is reversed, resulting in prolonged incubation and P7 shortens it. The host, C57 inbred mice, obviously presents additional variables. The derivation of these different strains of agents was from serial passages in the different mouse strains. The genetic analysis allowed initially for genotype determination, that is, S7S7 as the homozygote, S7P7 as the heterozygote, and so on, and for demonstration of the effects of these various genotypes. This type of genetic variant of an original scrapie agent is informative and the kind of study than can be done profitably, even though the specific agent is not yet defined. The mere demonstration of the genetic properties of the agents, as long as they are consistent, inheritable, and mutable, will tell us something about the nature of the virus itself: the number of viral genes, which may be a measure of size, for example; the nonnucleic acid proteins present; and so on.

The collection of families in which Creutzfeldt–Jakob disease (CJD) is seen in two or more members is much needed. It is likely, on the basis of what we know about slow virus diseases generally, including MS, that we will again be dealing in CJD with an infectious disease involving possibly, but not necessarily, a genetic predisposition on the part of the host. That seems to be a common denominator that runs through a number of these conditions. To determine the nature of that genetic predisposition will not be easy. Present evidence is not overwhelmingly impressive, but there appears to be an underlying immunologic problem. The T and B cell function, I have been told, is normal in kuru and CJD, and the transmitted virus does not transform lymphocytes, so it is difficult to decide how one could evaluate the defects if there are specific immunologic or genetic predisposing factors. There is a great need for an assay system for both scrapie and kuru. This issue is not an easy one to resolve, but there is no biologic assay for the agent except in terms of the passage *in vivo*, which does not qualify as a proper assay. At this time, one can establish clearly the passage number and the response of the cells at different passages; but it would be informative to have some way of measuring the biologic end-point, the number of cells destroyed, the transformed cell membrane alterations, and so on. From what we have heard about these atypical, unconventional viruses, they seem to be intracellular with no grossly apparent cell surface effects, inflammatory responses, or localized immunologic reactions, with a few minor exceptions. If the virus attaches to the cell membrane, we can reasonably ask Why is there no apparent response? Is there an alternative pathway that does not elicit a systemic response? Perhaps there is cell-to-cell transmission without release of viruses.

In many ways, the study of gene function in EB virus-infected lymphocyte is similar to the conventional virus infections. The EB virus infection *per se* is almost always inapparent, but antibodies do develop. In acute disease, such as infectious mononucleosis, a rising antibody titer is diagnostic. If lymphocytes from EB virus-infected persons are incubated in culture these cells will transform spontaneously. One can, under cell culture conditions, get replication of the virus with hundreds of copies of the EB virus genome per cell. *In vitro*, however, when one establishes these cells, one tends not to get EB virus release, except under certain conditions that have now been defined. Those conditions are the ones that lead to cell senescence. When the cells reach senescence, then free virus is released as the cells begin to die. Maintenance of EB virus infection in culture requires establishment of the metabolic and nutritional requirements of the virus. It has been shown conclusively that the arginine concentration in the medium is critical to the proper survival of EB virus *in vitro*. In some ways, it might prove useful to explore as fully as possible the optimal *in vitro* nutritional conditions for cell growth and for virus survival in tissue culture. With respect to EB virus, there was initially a question of genetic susceptibility to the virus. The epidemiologic evidence clearly pointed to an infectious etiology. Nonetheless, one still has in that story the same kind of residual genetic-type question that one has with the slow virus infections: If 90% of individuals in the population are serologically EB virus positive, why then do so few get Burkitt lymphoma or infectious mononucleosis. The question whether there is a genetic predisposition recurs, and this is one of the things that bind the EB virus story to the slow virus disease story.

Discussion/Chapter 18

Dr. Koprowski commented that antigenic changes on the surface of the virus in, for example, influenza viruses occur in the presence of antibodies and that perhaps the original infection produces such an enormous variety of antibodies that some of them can take care of mutants that may develop *in vivo.* If we have an infection that produces only oligoclonal antibodies against the parent virus, the mutants can escape neutralization and cause damage, despite the presence of antibodies. The already cited example of equine infectious anemia is a case in point.

Dr. Brody asked how we can manage the concept of polygenic somatic influences in multiple sclerosis (MS) and subacute sclerosing panencephalitis (SSPE), both of which have unequal sexual distribution. (In SSPE a male to female ratio is at least 3:1, and in MS there is predominance of females.) Dr. Bloom stated that no genetic explanation could be put forth, but that there are nongenetic differences in susceptibility to infection. Some examples of this may be the greater susceptibility of the male to lethal or severe infection in the first year of life.

Dr. Lehmann-Grube concluded the discussion by recalling that in regard to any infectious agent a very small proportion of the infected hosts develop clinical disease. The ratios may be 1:1000, or 1:100 in case of, say, poliomyelitis. In some instances, this may be determined by the virus; in other instances, by the host, either genetically or on some other basis.

CHAPTER 19
Critique: Afterthoughts of an Immunologist

EBERHARD WECKER

Any discussion regarding pathogenesis of virus diseases must consider the immune system. This is an intricate system in which various cells interact with each other either by collaboration that brings about an immune reaction or by suppression of one another, which results in the abolition of positive reactions of some cells. In principle then, the pathogenic involvement of the immune system can result either from failure of the collaboration or through institution of the suppression, either of which can lead to reactions that are not beneficial to the host.

All of the diseases discussed in this volume affect the central nervous system (CNS). Therefore it is important to consider the function of the immune system in two phases of the disease. The first is at the time when the host is infected by the specific viral agent, but before this agent has reached the CNS and the second phase which begins when the agent enters the CNS.

It is obvious that a certain lack of reactivity must prevail on the part of the host if the virus is to escape destruction before it makes its way into the CNS. On the other hand, once the virus does reach the CNS, failure of immune response, as well as an exaggerated, or modified immune response may bring about expression of the disease. It seems appropriate to discuss some of the major aspects of these various possibilities from the point of view of an immunologist. Even if one cannot establish which of these phases is more important, or even assign to them specific pathogenic values, it is possible, at least, to consider them as basis for future research.

Whenever a virus infects a host the evoked immune response attempts to block the infection in various ways. One may be through the production of specific antiviral antibodies, which neutralize the infectious agent and render it susceptible to removal by phagocytic cells. Alternatively antiviral antibodies may bind to viral antigens associated with the infected host cell membrane and may destroy the cell, provided that complement is present. It is possible, however, as has been shown in a number of viral infections, for the agent to affect cellular antigens themselves, in particular those coded for the major histocompatibility complex.

The other major type of immune defense mechanism is the cellular immune response. Either T lymphocytes (1), so-called K cells (12),

236

"activated macrophages" (5), or "natural killer cells" (3, 10) may be the effector cells. These cells can attack other cells, e.g., virus-infected cells, and destroy them. Again, viral antigens in the cellular membrane or altered normal membrane constituents can be the immunogens and the antigens recognized by these effector cells.

The first intriguing problem for our consideration therefore is the mechanisms by which the putative infectious agent responsible for a particular slow virus disease can escape immune defense mechanisms as it makes its way from the tissues into the central nervous system. There are unfortunately no precise answers to some of the questions that must be posed in this regard:

1. What is the nature of the viruses involved?
2. How and where does the virus enter the body?
3. What is the type of cells in which the virus initially multiplies?
4. How does the virus reach the CNS?

Regarding 1, some viruses are known to be poor immunogens. Dr. Dickinson mentions that in scrapie one cannot detect any evidence of an immune response. The fact, however, that amyloid is present suggests that there must be some immunologic response.

Considering 2, if a virus enters a site that is anatomically and functionally close to the CNS, e.g., the olfactory epithelium, it may proceed swiftly along olfactory nerves and thus reach the CNS, without causing any significant peripheral immune response.

As for 3, if a virus multiplies within the cells of the immune system themselves, e.g., T or B lymphocytes and macrophages, the agent may severely suppress the immune response. Indeed, when T cells are activated they can become much more susceptible to infection with certain lipid-containing viruses (9). The activation may result from the presence of a viral antigen itself and thus the virus might infect and harm only the T clones that are immunologically responding to it.

Regarding 4, if a virus reaches the CNS along the nerve axons, it escapes the immune mechanisms. If a virus chronically infects cells of the lymphoid system, even without causing any direct harm to them, it may use these cells as means for rapid transport throughout the body. Under certain pathologic circumstances lymphoid cells can pass through the endothelial cell lining of blood vessels of the CNS and thus virus carrying lymphoid cells may bring the infection into the CNS.

In addition there are some complications of a strictly immunologic nature that may lead to the general failure of the immune defense of the body. The killing of virus infected targets by effector cells can be blocked in those instances when antibodies have covered the recognizable cell surface antigens (4). It has been shown that antibodies binding to antigens within the cell membrane may lead to "modulation" of the membrane (11). In the case of viral components within the cell, the antigenic modulation may remove them from the surface and also may lead to inhibition of resynthesis of the virus. In some sites the suppression exerted by suppressor T cells upon either the humoral (6) or the cellular immune response may prevail. The immune responsiveness is primarily controlled genetically (2) and there are animal models that clearly show presence of high and low responders to a given antigen and that this differential has a genetic basis. It may be worthwhile to investigate low and high responder animal strains to a study of a pathogenesis of diseases following infection with specific viruses derived from slow infections.

One thing that can be stated with certainty is that a virus disease manifesting itself in the CNS results from an infection by a virus that has escaped the defense mechanisms of the host. This escape, however, alone is not enough to explain a viral disease. Lymphocytic choriomeningitis virus infection is an example of an agent that does escape the immune mechanisms and is able to enter the CNS, but its presence there does not necessarily result in disease. The prevailing evidence indicates that pathogenesis of this infection depends on the participation of the immune system.

The second puzzle before us is the possible role of untoward, non-beneficial positive immune responses in the development of slow virus diseases. For failure of the immune system within CNS to be responsible for disease we must have an agent that is directly pathogenic to the neural tissue. The same reasons that may be responsible for general immune failure may also apply to the immune reactions within the CNS. Since CNS has been considered a privileged site for immune reactions, mere presence of lymphoid cells within this compartment can be taken as evidence of a pathologic state. The emphasis of any hypothesis regarding the contribution of the immunologic reactions to disease of the CNS must be directed toward false positive immune reactions, rather than to any lack of a normal immune reaction. It is possible to envision a direct immune response by the host to his own nervous tissues, which under ordinary circumstances are protected from direct contact with the cells of the immune system. If for some reason lymphoid cells get into the privileged compartment they may become the aggressors. It appears, however, that this is not the case. There are a number of conditions in which lymphocytes are found within the CNS, e.g., trauma and bacterial and viral infections. Autoimmune disease is not the usual consequence of these events. Perhaps it is simply a matter of chance whether particular clones of lymphoid cells happen to enter the CNS. This is a possible explanation and is supported, in part, by the data presented by Dr. Norrby who gives evidence that the antiviral antibodies within the cerebrospinal fluid were of oligoclonal nature. Quite clearly much more research is required to determine the circumstances under which experimentally transferred lymphoid cells can react against the components of the normal CNS.

A humoral immune response directed against infectious, primarily cytopathic, viruses in the CNS would be expected generally to be beneficial. Agents causing slow virus infections are not likely to be neutralized by such antibodies. It seems obvious that these agents tend to create a prolonged infection of the host cell. In such a case the infected cell itself will be the prime target of the immune reactions.

As indicated earlier, components within the cell membrane, or altered membrane constituents can be immunogenic and they can be recognized by either cytotoxic antibodies or cytotoxic cells (7). Such mechanisms are clearly involved in the pathogenesis of lymphocytic choriomeningitis in which the virus itself does not cause any functional disorder. The actual destruction of infected cells is due solely to a cell mediated immune response and the consequences are particularly bad if there is no regenerative power to the affected tissue, as is the case in the CNS.

It is important to consider also the intensity of immune reaction that takes place in the CNS. From the extraordinarily high titers of oligoclonal antibodies to several viruses sometimes found in the CNS in the several diseases mentioned, one can infer that there is a lack of a controlling cerebral mechanism. This may be the result of the restricted clones of lymphoid cells and thus only a small number of the suppressor cells that enter the compartment. Moreover, the antigen, e.g., any one of the viruses, may not be removed and in fact may accumulate in large concentrations and continue to stimulate the immune cells for an unusually long time.

There is very little information about the flow, if any, of lymphoid cells and macrophages, antigens and antigen–antibody complexes in and out of the CNS. (For example, what is the significance of immune complexes in the CNS?) It may be quite interesting to study the consequence of immune responses to antigens experimentally brought into the CNS together with limiting numbers of lymphoid cells.

Thus far I have discussed the obvious damaging effects on the central nervous system through direct or indirect immune responses, based on the assumption that the agent itself does not cause harm to the neural tissues. If, in fact, the agent were cytopathic, then the immune response can be expected to be predominantly beneficial.

There exists, however, one other intriguing possibility to be considered. In most cases viral populations consist not only of infectious particles, but rather of a mixture of infectious and noninfectious ones, existing in various ratios. Usually the noninfectious particles tend to outnumber the infectious ones. Noninfectious defective particles have been shown to interfere with the replication of the infectious viruses and hence are called "defective interfering particles." They share most surface antigens with the infectious viruses and their interference can be neutralized by antisera that also neutralize infectious viruses.

A properly maintained balance between infectious virus and interfering particles can result in a persistent infection of cells. The interference can be sufficiently strong to prevent actual virus replication and damage in most of these cells. If one speculates that some of the agents causing slow infections, in fact, produce such a type of persistent infection of the CNS, an immune reaction would have disastrous consequences. Neutralization of the extracellular interfering viral material by specific antibodies would cause a severe imbalance of the otherwise self-limited system. Some experimental evidence does support such a notion (8).

This explanation differs from all the other proposed pathogenic mechanisms in that it is based on the presence of a normal humoral immune response to a viral antigen that is not of itself unusual.

There remain additional possibilities that would explain the means by which the immune system, usually the indispensable defense mechanism of higher organisms against infectious agents, can be the basis for bringing about disease. There are many such explanations, but none of them seems to be very likely. It is my intention to focus on those hypotheses that have a more immediate relevance.

It appears clear that virology must provide additional data for the immunologists to be able to offer an educated guess about the next steps in investigation of slow virus diseases. It seems also clear that this battle should be fought—and perhaps even won—not in the CNS but in the extraneural parts of the host. Once the agents penetrate the CNS it is much more difficult to conceive of any effective therapeutic measures. Nevertheless considerations of the immune responses within the CNS are likely to provide a useful insight into the immunopathology of this long neglected compartment of the body.

REFERENCES

1. Brunner, K. T., and Cerottini, J. C. (1971). Cytotoxic lymphocytes as effector cells of cell-mediated immunity. In *Progress in Immunology* (B. Amos, ed.), p. 985. Academic Press, New York.
2. Gershon, R. K. (1974). T cell control of antibody production. *Contemporary Topics in Immunobiology 3*, 1–40.
3. Glaser, M., Bonnard, G. D., and Herbermann, R. B. (1976). *In vitro* generation of secondary cell-mediated cytotoxic response against a syngeneic gross virus-induced lymphoma in rats. *J. Immunol. 116*, 430–436.
4. Hellström, K. E., and Hellström, J. (1974). Lymphocyte-mediated cytotoxicity and blocking serum activity to tumor antigens. *Adv. Immunol. 18*, 209–277.
5. Lohmann-Matthes, M. L., and Fischer, H. (1973). T-cell cytotoxicity and amplification of the cytotoxic reaction by macrophages. *Transplant. Rev. 17*, 150–171.
6. McDevitt, H. O., and Benacerraf, B. (1969). Genetic control of specific immune responses. *Adv. Immunol. 11*, 31–74.
7. McFarland, H. F., and Johnson, R. T. (1975). The role of the inflammatory response in viral infection. In *Viral Immunology and Immunopathology*, p. 137–148. Academic Press, New York.
8. Martin, S., and ter Meulen, V. Personal communication.
9. Nowakowski, M., Feldman, J. D., Kano, S., and Bloom, B. R. (1973). The production of vesicular stomatitis virus by antigen-or mitogen-stimulated lymphocytes and continuous lymphoblastoid lines. *J. Exp. Med. 137*, 1042–1059.
10. Nunn, M., Djeu, J. Y., Lavrin, P. H., and Herbermann, R. B. (1973). Natural cytotoxic reactivity of rat lymphocytes against syngeneic Gross' leukemia. *Proc. Am. Assoc. Cancer Res. 14*, 87.
11. Old, L. J., Stockert, E., Boyse, E. A., and Kim, J. H. (1968). Antigenic modulation. Loss of TL antigen from cells exposed to TL antibody. Study of the phenomenon *in vitro*. *J. Exp. Med. 127*, 523–539.
12. Perlmann, P., Perlmann, H., and Wigzell, H. (1972). Lymphocyte-mediated cytotoxicity *in vitro*. Induction and inhibition by humoral antibody and nature of effector cells. *Transplant. Rev. 13*, 91–114.

Discussion / Chapter 19

Dr. Wecker reemphasized the point made earlier that by the time the viral agent has reached the central nervous system (CNS), the immunologic response was unlikely to cope with the infection. In line with this, he asked what the time interval might be between infection of the organism and the arrival of the virus in the brain. Dr. Lennette began the response by commenting that in viremia, the viruses can enter CNS quite rapidly. Therefore, in this respect, the time interval would be determined by the interval between infection and viremia.

Dr. Wecker then extended his question to include also those infections without viremia—for example the ones in which the virus travels along the nerve trunk. Dr. Mims stated that, in fact, there could be no general answer to this question, because essentially every route has been taken by some virus or other. The time interval is likely to be quite variable.

Regarding the immunologic response within CNS, Dr. Mims stated that our knowledge of the immunological defense mechanism within CNS was quite limited. There is still much ignorance about the turnover of the immune cells. We do not know, for example, how the lymphocytes arrive in the normal cerebrospinal fluid. Once the cells do reach the brain, added Dr. Askonas, there seems to be a shut-off mechanism that prevents the immune response from continuing. This may be caused by restriction on circulation of the cells, since none of them seem to leave the system, but perhaps also through some shutting down of the cells already there and possibly this is responsible for viral persistence.

Dr. Johnson requested a clarification about this hyperreactivity or lack of shut off, and Dr. Askonas put the case of Dr. Norrby's reports of oligoclonal antibodies. She indicated that in a single clone reproducing very large amounts of protein, perhaps on the order of that seen in multiple myeloma, we might expect 500,000 cells to produce this particular immunoglobulin. Some discussion then followed about the quantity of this globulin and whether it represented a relatively large amount, but it was apparently resolved by the statement from Dr. Kabat that the amounts in the spinal fluid are quite significant, because only a very small portion of that gammaglobulin was necessary for its biologic, protective effect.

At this point, the discussion returned once again to classification and definition of slow virus infections. Dr. Askonas stressed that the slowness did not refer to the replication of the virus in a particular compartment, but rather to the slowness of the disease that develops. For example, in the scrapie situation, did the *sinc* gene affect the incubation period or rather the length of time required for the escape from the immune system? If there is a long incubation period, this might indicate that the organism is combating the pathogen.

Dr. ter Meulen raised the question about the K cells. He wondered if these cells were able to eliminate other cells with foreign antigens and whether a blocking antibody, such as has been described in tumor virology, might play a role here. Dr. Askonas responded that, in her opinion, the K cell works very well *in vitro*, but *in vivo*, it has not yet been demonstrated and its role is uncertain, perhaps because there are only very few such cells. Dr. Askonas then also commented about the suppressor T cells, which may have some function in tolerance, or induction of tolerance. There could be two types of tolerance: one a central tolerance perhaps resulting from neonatal or prenatal exposure, and another tolerance mediated by the suppressor cells.

CHAPTER 20
Critique: The Epidemiologist

BRIAN MACMAHON

Epidemiologic methods may be applied to elucidation of slow virus infections. In the aims of the Workshop, the organizers have written "it seems to us that a considered effort, perhaps more prosaic than that which characterizes studies in the recent past, must now be made." I cannot suggest any *new* ways in which epidemiologic methods can be applied in this field, but it does seem to me that epidemiology is one of the fields that deserve increased attention here, perhaps in a more prosaic but also in a more systematic way than in the past.

Before indicating some possible lines of enquiry, I should point out that one of the difficulties of discussing the application of epidemiology to the slow virus infections is the definition of the area of discourse. Epidemiology is often more useful in determining to what category a disease belongs, e.g., whether it is infectious or noninfectious, than in elucidating the specific etiologic agent within that category. Thus, epidemiology has often been useful in suggesting that one should look for a microbial agent as cause of a disease—and sometimes even in suggesting where to look for what kind of agent—but the actual identification of agents does not come from epidemiologic studies. Epidemiologic methods may be more likely to be useful in suggesting diseases that may be considered slow virus infections than in investigating the known slow virus diseases themselves. I take my area to be, therefore, not epidemiology and the slow virus diseases, but epidemiology and the search for evidence of slow virus infection.

There are four main kinds of epidemiologic study: (a) descriptive, i.e., the compilation of readily available data on incidence and/or mortality to ascertain whether patterns emerge that stimulate new directions of thought about possible mechanisms of etiology—the classical questions asked are Who (what kind of person) is affected? When? and Where? (b) Case-control studies are studies in which information on the past histories of affected individuals and comparable unaffected persons is assembled (either from the individuals themselves or from records) and compared. Differences in the histories of the cases and control groups may suggest areas that should be explored for etiologic clues. (c) Cohort studies are studies in which a group of persons known to have been exposed to a particular agent is followed over time to ascertain its disease experience; that experi-

242

ence is compared with the experience of a similar group of individuals not exposed to the particular agent. (d) A special type of cohort study may be conducted in which exposure to the agent is not permitted to occur haphazardly, as it does under natural circumstances, but is manipulated by the investigator. Thus in this experimental study, assignment to exposure or nonexposure is determined by the investigator, or some random procedure established by him. Experimental studies, at least in epidemiology, as distinguished from clinical experimental studies, are nearly always conducted to evaluate the effects of an agent thought to be protective against disease (e.g., a vaccine) rather than one thought to cause a disease.

With respect to the objectives of epidemiologic studies, these can be categorized into three groups: (a) hypothesis initiation—in the present context, for example, this might be accomplished if epidemiologic data suggested that a disease of unknown etiology might in fact be a slow virus infection; (b) hypothesis specification—for example, if suspicion is aroused that a disease is a slow virus infection (confirmation of this hypothesis will be facilitated if we can specify the age at probable infection, the incubation period, the source of infection, and other such characteristics); and (c) hypothesis testing—the epidemiologic component of this procedure is basically one of determining whether the distribution of a disease with regard to specific variables follows that which would be predicted on the basis of the hypothesis under test. Other aspects of the testing of causal hypotheses, such as the identification of specific agents or of plausible cellular mechanisms, fall more within the province of the experimentalist in the laboratory and are seldom contributed to in a major way by epidemiologic methods.

The cross classification of these three objectives with the four general methodologies listed earlier produces a matrix containing 12 cells. The remarkable breadth of the epidemiologic work that has been done or is needed on the suspected slow virus diseases is suggested by the fact that one could identify an actual or potential contribution corresponding to nearly all of these cells—the exception being those involving experimental procedures on humans. Since no protective agents have yet been identified, there has been little opportunity for experimental epidemiologic studies. Otherwise, I think all the cells of the matrix can be filled.

Take, for example, the use of descriptive data. With respect to hypothesis initiation, there is no more fascinating story in medical history than the way in which the peculiarities in the distributon of kuru by age, sex, and other variables finally led to suspicion of the role of cannibalism and, hence, of a transmissible agent present in the central nervous system (CNS). There is another story, which has not yet been mentioned at this meeting, but which to me is equally fascinating, even though its final outcome remains undetermined. This concerns the 85% or so cases of Parkinson's syndrome that are still referred to as "idiopathic." In studying time trends in patients with this disease at the Massachusetts General Hospital, Poskanzer and Schwab (2) noted two things: (a) There were very few cases before 1915 but a gradual and consistent increase in numbers since that time, and (b) there had been a change in the age distribution of cases over time, with consistent increase in the mean age at diagnosis. In fact, the increase in mean age was so great as to suggest that Parkinson's syndrome was occurring predominantly in the cohort of people who were alive in 1925 and were at that time in the age range in which most cases of von Economo's encephalitis occurred, even though these "idiopathic" cases gave no history of clinical infection at the time. A great many persons were infected and showed no clinical disease at the time but developed the characteristic symptoms decades later. This hypothesis, if confirmed by other data, would seem to be capable of explaining the majority of cases of idiopathic Parkinson's syndrome.

With respect to hypothesis specification, the descriptive studies of multiple sclerosis (MS) in migrants illustrate how such studies can be used to define the age at which persons are probably infected, if indeed a virus is responsible.

As for hypothesis testing, a very clear example of the use of descriptive data is in testing the prediction that if cannibalism is the method whereby the virus is transmitted, there should be no new cases after the termination of the ritual. As we have heard, this prediction appears to be borne out. Similarly, the cohort of individuals exposed to von Economo's disease in 1925 is dying out rapidly. If Parkinson's syndrome is occurring only (or predominantly) in this cohort, we should now be seeing a rapid decline in prevalence of this syndrome. To my knowledge, such a decline has not been looked for.

Case-control studies are used mainly to test hypotheses, but in the field of concern to this conference, there are a few instances of use of information of this type to initiate, or at least strengthen, a hypothesis. For example, it was shown that persons who had tonsillectomies were at higher risk of bulbar poliomyelitis, particularly in the 2 to 3 months after the tonsillectomy, but also on a long-term basis. Noting certain similarities in the epidemiologic features of poliomyelitis and MS, Poskanzer, Schapira, and Miller (1) enquired whether there was also a higher frequency of tonsillectomy among patients with MS than among comparable unaffected individuals. Such an increase was found. The observation has not been confirmed by all subsequent investigators, but it is the kind of question that needs further evaluation, on other neurologic disorders, as well as MS. For example, I am not aware that the possibility of a relationship between tonsillectomy and idiopathic Parkinson's syndrome has been investigated.

Some of the known viral diseases of infancy and childhood have immediate effects, in some cases, on the CNS. It is possible that, in other cases, as in von Economo's disease, the effects may be delayed and that some diseases that are now of unknown origin, such as childhood autism and other psychiatric abnormalities with organic components, may result from subclinical infections with these same viruses. Case-control studies of the frequency of exposure to specific viral infections would seem to be worthwhile. The appearance of encephalitis in cohorts of children over the age of 12 years with congenital rubella is evidence of the need to watch for other late manifestations of early viral infections. It also illustrates the utility of the cohort approach when groups of seriously exposed individuals can be identified.

Until recently, few cohort studies of infants exposed to viruses *in utero* included observations of neurologic damage appearing late in childhood. The collaborative perinatal study of the National Institute for Neurologic Diseases and Blindness (now National Institute of Neurological and Communicative Diseases and Stroke) is a notable exception; detailed follow-up has been continued in children up to 7 years of age. The experience with rubella suggests the importance of such long-term follow-up of cohorts of exposed infants.

Groups of people with immunodeficiency diseases, whether congenital or acquired, have been shown to have increased risk of a number of diseases, as well as the progressive multifocal leukoencephalopathy (PML) discussed at this meeting. These increased risks have all been observed empirically, there being no theoretical reasons to suspect that the particular diseases involved would show the observed increases. Cohort studies of such groups should certainly be continued. They might identify new, unexpected associations as well as elucidate the specifics of known associations; for example, they may provide data on the incubation period of PML.

The greatest gap between potential utility and current epidemiologic resources appears to me to lie in the area of descriptive data. Knowledge of the frequency of a neurologic disease in a population (or a population similar to the one of immediate interest) nearly always requires a special study. This is in marked contrast to the situation in regard to cancer, for which over 50 registries across the world routinely collect information on incidence in geographically defined populations. I realize that in the establishment of registries or other forms of surveillance for neurologic disorders there would be substantial problems of diagnosis, as in MS, or recording, as in Parkinson's disease. However, the same problems exist in cancer, albeit to a less degree, and, moreover, since mortality is a better index of frequency in most forms of cancer than in most neurologic diseases, the application of resources to registries of incidence is more readily justifiable for neurologic disorders than for cancer. I do not believe that we need 50 registries, but the development of half a dozen, strategically located throughout the world, would do a great deal to accomplish all three of the objectives that I have indicated might be approached by epidemiologic research.

REFERENCES

1. Poskanzer, D. C., Shapira, K., and Miller, H. (1963). Multiple sclerosis and poliomyelitis. *Lancet ii*, 917–921.
2. Poskanzer, D. C., and Schwab, R. S. (1963). Cohort analysis of Parkinson's syndrome. *J. Chronic Dis. 16*, 961–973.

Discussion/Chapter 20

Dr. zur Hausen began by asking whether there were any epidemiologic criteria by which multiple sclerosis (MS), or any other disease, could be considered either an infectious disease or not. Dr. MacMahon responded that there was no evidence that one could accept as proof, but that there may be factors tending to point a little in one or another direction. For example, the allegation that tonsillectomy predisposes to MS, if true, would tend to be an argument in favor of the infectious etiology. All such considerations are necessarily indirect.

One problem with correlations was emphasized by Dr. Gajdusek who recalled that arrival of Australian and European missionaries in New Guinea produced an epidemic of goiterous cretinism in the valleys of New Guinea. This might have been interpreted as evidence of infectious etiology, if the real etiology were not known. What actually happened was that the missionaries brought with them noniodized salt to a people who were pregoitrous, but who used the native salt sources that contained a small amount of iodine.

Comment / Chapter 20
D. D. Reid

I agree with Dr. Porter on the importance of historical analogies. Infectious mononucleosis is a case in point where investigators sought a single agent, but they did learn that two or three agents were involved. With respect to multiple sclerosis (MS), it may be the ultimate heresy to suggest that it could turn out to be quite unrelated to a viral infection. But it is important to keep an open mind in the initial stages of all etiologic inquiries. A perfect candidate for an infectious disease of the nervous system may be found, in the end, to be caused by something else. This misunderstanding happened in the case of pellagra where some very simple epidemiologic observation indicated that, although its distribution in families and seasonal peak suggested a viral origin, it was in fact a vitamin deficiency found in poor families before harvest time.

History does teach us that history teaches us nothing; but one of the important things it ought to teach us is the need for scientific humility. In other words, it warns us to look at the broader distribution of disease along the lines that MacMahon has made clear, to initiate etiologic theories and not to start with a preconceived notion. We need the broad picture of the distribution of mortality in different groups of the population that can be derived from vital statistics. These statistics are a much despised kind of clinical or scientific information, but they may nevertheless prove useful. Despite their limitations, this source of data could be used much more widely. For example, the Registrar-General for England and Wales has studied the social class distribution of mortality from MS among married women around 1951. The rates were relatively high among women married to men in professional classes, but lower in those married to men in the laboring and semi-skilled occupations. When we look at hospital admission statistics in relation to multiple sclerosis, we face the problem that one individual with this disease is responsible over his lifetime for many hospital admissions. But we must use all such sources of information to the best of our ability. The experience of military service populations is of particular interest. Acheson's studies of American veterans showed very clearly that there is a north–south latitude effect in relation to the prevalence of severe MS. It would be interesting to do something similar in Europe where national military service is much more usual.

To decide whether these findings really represent differences in disease distribution and not mere artifacts due to differences in diagnostic standards, we need special field surveys in the population. In our own work in the field of chronic respiratory disorders, we have come to appreciate the need for precise definitions of the clinical syndrome involved. This is especially important in international studies. When people from different countries use what seems to be the same diagnostic label, they may mean something quite different. Standardization of approach must be accomplished among clinical epidemiologists working in different areas. An important contribution made by epidemiology has been the emphasis on human variation, both in the character of a specific disease and between the clinical observers in their description and classification of it. There is thus the need for the development of standard methods for the diagnosis and classification of MS and the training of observers in their application.

Migrant studies are examples of large-scale "human experiments" where people moving from one country to another provide an excellent basis for epidemiologic data gathering. They are usually from the same genetic stock changing from one environment to another, thus providing their own control group. Members of such populations can be analyzed even more precisely by observing individuals who have moved and comparing them with their siblings who stayed in the original environment. Studies of migrants to Israel have shown, for example, that MS is commoner among those who came from Europe than those from North Africa. Moreover, the age at which they left their original environment was also important. This suggests that exposure to infection in early life rather than after the age of 15 affects the immune response and thus the emergence of clinically obvious disease.

A study of the experience of successive generations or cohorts may be as helpful in MS as it has been in pinpointing the role of early infection in the study of carcinoma of the cervix. Valerie Beral has recently pointed out peaks in mortality from this disease in cohorts of women who lived in the United Kingdom during three important periods. These were World War I, World War II, and a period of several years after World War II, when there was a relaxation in sexual morals with a great deal of promiscuity. Since promiscuity increased the risk of the opportunity for herpes virus infection, the increased incidence of cervical carcinoma in this group of women may be a manifestation of a late effect of that infection.

As MacMahon pointed out, there are many variants of the epidemiological approach to the problems of MS. They may not offer a final solution but at least they can indicate the areas in which all methods of investigation might most usefully be concentrated.

CHAPTER 21
Conclusions: Outlook on Future Research

C. A. MIMS

A great variety of slow or persistent virus infections have been discussed, and each of these infections has its own fascination for us. We must, however, come to grips with the central problems that we face. It is in front of us on the landscape with its stern forbidding slopes, a mountain whose name is multiple sclerosis (MS). A few useful preliminary observations have been made, and some promising approaches have been seen, but the problem is still there. The great new hope that may help us scale this MS mountain is the possibility that it is caused by an infectious agent.

What can be learned from the known slow or persistent infections of the central nervous system (CNS) that will help us to understand MS? First, we are learning something in a very general sense about the immunology of these infections. However, it has been suspected that immunologic factors play only a secondary role in MS. It is very difficult to identify the earliest histologic lesion in MS, but should it consist of a decrease in oligodendroglial cells and some demyelination before there is a detectable cell infiltration, then this would suggest that immunologic factors were secondary. Whatever the case, we need to know about the immunology of the CNS in general if we are to understand MS. There are many important areas of ignorance. For instance, we know nothing about the small lymphoid cells present in normal cerebrospinal fluid (CSF)—how these cells get there, their turnover rates, and so on. We also need to find out more about neurons and glial cells. Are there any specific neuronal or glial cell membrane antigen markers that would assist immunologic studies and also help us to identify these cells? Antigens on neuronal and glial cells have been described, but some of these have been shown to be present in other types of cell in the normal embryo. In any case, most of the studies have been done with tumor cells from oligodendrogliomas or astrocytomas rather than with normal cells.

The second general area that deserves more study is genetics. The genetic studies point to a predisposition to MS, in that people with certain histocompatibility antigens on their cells are more likely to get MS. The parts of chromosome 6 that determine the histocompatibility types are closely associated with the immune response genes. Conceivably, genetically determined weak responses to a theoretic infectious agent causing

MS make one more susceptible to the development of MS. On the other hand, it might be that this genotype confers susceptibility to the infection by coding for virus receptors on cell surfaces. But these are no more than possibilities, and it is really only our current bias that makes us think in terms of immune responses or receptors at all. It is possible that these genotypes are closely linked with factors that control quite separate things, such as the ability of a circulating microorganism to localize in the CNS or the susceptibility of certain enzymes to viral damage or even the presence of enzymes controlling cell susceptibility. The question of the basis of genetic predisposition is still open.

What about the infectious hypothesis of MS? What things should we be thinking of? What lessons should we have learned from the known slow virus infections? First, we cannot count on any infectious agent responsible for MS being a conventional virus. There is one human representative of the scrapie group, and we have to accept the possibility that there are other representatives in man of this same group of infectious agents. Moreover, additional agents of an unconventional type may be found that do not cause spongiform encephalopathies, and, of course, they might be very hard to detect if, like scrapie, they induce no trace of an immune response in the host.

Second, if we are thinking about a conventional virus, we will have to keep an open mind about it and not get bogged down, thinking only, for instance, about measles. In fact, we should perhaps remind ourselves that past cancer virus research has been described as a graveyard with the names of prominent virologists inscribed upon the tombstones. We have to recognize that we are in the same danger with MS. Nor can we expect that MS will necessarily operate just like any of the known slow virus infections of the CNS. The importance of these slow virus infections is that they have shown us the sort of things that *can* happen, and have suggested the sort of research approaches that might be useful. Indeed, the other slow virus infections, such as subacute sclerosing panencephalitis and progressive multifocal leukoencephalitis have given the whole field of MS research a fantastic new impetus. It was not long ago that one could define "virus" as a Latin term used by physicians to mean "your guess is as good as mine." Now we can be a little more precise, and at the same time the possibilities have expanded. If, for instance, I ask the visna experts whether there is a primate representative of visna virus or whether this virus is ridiculously unique to sheep and goats, they have to admit that they do not know. There are low titer visna virus neutralizing factors in the sera of many people, but these factors may be nonspecific inhibitors. Again, could the human oligodendrocyte, the cell especially involved in MS, be uniquely susceptible to a human C type virus? Whenever one grows mouse brain cells in bottles, C type particles seem to emerge. What about the human coronaviruses? They have always been regarded as respiratory viruses, but we really do not know very much about them. We never include them in our antibody studies for MS, and we must remember that many viruses reach unexpected parts of the body, especially in the immature host. After all, mouse hepatitis virus, a virus that causes one of the few primary demyelinating diseases, is a coronavirus.

One other way of looking at the slow and persistent infectious agents is to ask ourselves how they persist in the body and how they evade the normal host resistance factors that are designed to eliminate invading microorganisms. We have, in fact, identified some of the ways in which the immune defenses can be bypassed. But we must remember that many persistent infectious agents cause no lesions or illness. We are persistently infected with adenoviruses, herpes simplex, varicella-zoster, and cytomegalovirus; we carry the Epstein–Barr virus genome, and we probably all have the human C type virus. Nevertheless, with some exceptions, we have escaped any harmful consequences. Like all good parasites, these persisting viruses cause little trouble for the most part.

When a possible infectious agent for MS was discussed, I was reminded very strongly of chronic glomerulonephritis in man. Most of this glomerulonephritis is thought to be caused by immune complexes, and in this particular disease we have superb animal models that have told us how immune complexes cause glomerulonephritis. Although the pathogenesis has been worked out, we still know almost nothing of the (possibly microbial) antigens that are present in the complexes. In MS, however, we know very little of the pathogenesis and even less of the possible virus. Norrby told us of the oligoclonal antibodies in the CSF in MS, but no one knows what antigen provoked them. This problem should be investigated because it may be possible to study the antigen specificities of the oligoclonal antibodies. Such a study might be more promising than a search for viral antigens in the glomerular deposit from a kidney biopsy in glomerulonephritis. We should also look at nucleic acid sequences in brain cells, just as tumor virologists have had to do in tumor cells. One of the difficulties with our modern approach to MS is that we need live cells from the human brain for cocultivation, fusion, and so on. In the old days of virology, the great standby in the isolation of viruses was the availability of deep frozen tissues that could be used for reisolation. If we must grow the cells from a brain specimen, this type of reisolation becomes impossible.

Other difficulties abound. It is possible that the infectious agent gets into the body, initiates the changes in the CNS that lead to MS, and then totally disappears leaving nothing of itself behind. The changes that slowly evolve are no longer dependent on the presence of the virus. We have good precedent for this in Richard Johnson's studies of hamster neonatal infections with mumps and influenza viruses. It is necessary, therefore, to look at infected animals for long periods of time, as we have learned from slow virus research in general.

I have always been astounded at people's prejudiced, or perhaps weighted, attitudes to experimental animals. If I wrote a paper describing the results of my experiments on three mice, I would be laughed at. But if I use a large and expensive animal, small numbers do not seem to matter. Benedict based his entire book, *The Physiology of the Elephant*, on a single circus elephant called something like Clarabella. It is said that in the early days of immunology there was an entire text on immunochemistry that was literally a one-horse textbook. Yet each little mouse is as complete an individual and as complete a host for an infectious disease as a horse, elephant, or chimpanzee. This is a serious problem if we cannot help using large expensive animals, as Gajdusek discovered in his classic pioneering studies with primates, but wherever possible we must use a convenient, small, and inexpensive laboratory animal. Our progress is then more rapid. Research on scrapie leaped ahead when Chandler discovered that mice were susceptible. The mouse is the ideal animal. We know so much about its genetics, its immunology, and so on, that one can go so far as to say that we are frankly foolish if we do not pursue our studies in a mouse, if it is at all possible and not too irrelevant a host.

It has been crippling for research on equine infectious anemia that one must have horses. Experiments, therefore, have to be done with just a few animals. If only some magician–geneticist could have devised a minihorse so that we could keep six of them in a mouse cage, hearing the thunder of little hoofs as we lifted the lid, then I am sure we'd know as much about equine infectious anemia as we do about lymphocytic choriomeningitis.

If MS is an infection, the disease evolves over a long period of time. Millar did a study of 700 MS patients over many years and showed that the average time from when MS was first diagnosed until death was 21.5 years. That is the median time, and it is not the picture of any progressive infectious process that we know about. To understand the highly irregular course of the disease process in MS, we have to think, for instance, of a disease such as tuberculosis where the defense system is waxing and waning over the years. In other words, there is a long drawn out, sometimes life long, battle between infectious agent and host defenses. We might also ask whether in the normal aging process there are changes in the ability of cells in the CNS to regenerate damaged cell membrane, so that a steady, low grade, and initially reversible pathologic process would progress with age. If we are pessimists, we might suggest that it is more complicated, and there are infections or associated immunologic events that also wax and wane and contribute to this very long drawn out type of infection.

At the fundamental level we need to learn a great deal more about neurons and glial cells and their responses to injury and to infection with all varieties of viruses. Even if the virus etiology of MS should prove to be incorrect, it will, nevertheless, have been of immense importance, simply because the virologic interest has generated so much work relevant to MS. We have learned how to grow brain cells, and we can now study them in bottles; we are investigating immune events in the CNS. Until recently MS research was a neglected field, which did not attract the young and interested people. The focusing of modern virology and immunology on to the problem of MS has, in fact, been a transfusion of life and hope.

I must counter, therefore, Porter's sober but very depressing survey of the virologic approach to MS. It is not that we are necessarily going to discover that this or that virus causes MS, but that we have generated a great ground swell of research effort and active interest on the part of young people. It is this interest that will enable us to assault and conquer the MS mountain. We need the general biologic studies on glial and tumor cells. The oligodendrocyte must be our central focus, but unfortunately 90% of this cell in the intact brain is wrapped spirally around the axon, producing myelin. If we study in the bottle only the little cell that was sitting beside the neuron, we will miss out a lot of what, in fact, the oligodendrocyte is in the body. But studies are progressing, and Ponten in Uppsala can now clone glial cells. He studies their replication in little tissue culture gardens on the surface of agar, and he can make studies of the offspring of single cells. There is a great future in the general biologic approach to MS.

Finally, we must keep our options open about the virus being considered, but advance against the MS mountain on all fronts. The infectious hypothesis is the most important one for the moment, and as we study the infection and immunology of the CNS, the pathophysiology of neurons and glial cells, the prospects of success will be high. As good scientists, we have to temper our enthusiasm and hope with self-criticism and skepticism.

Index

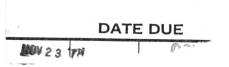